Risk, Reproduction, and Narratives of Experience

Risk, Reproduction, and Narratives of Experience

*Edited by Lauren Fordyce
and Amínata Maraesa*

Foreword by Carole H. Browner
Afterword by Rayna Rapp

Vanderbilt University Press ■ Nashville

© 2012 by Vanderbilt University Press
Nashville, Tennessee 37235
All rights reserved
First printing 2012

This book is printed on acid-free paper
Manufactured in the United States of America

Library of Congress Cataloging-in-Publication Data

Risk, reproduction, and narratives of experience /
edited by Lauren Fordyce and Amínata Maraesa ;
foreword by Carole H. Browner and afterword
by Rayna Rapp.
p. cm.
Includes bibliographical references and index.
ISBN 978-0-8265-1819-4 (cloth edition : alk. paper)
ISBN 978-0-8265-1820-0 (pbk. edition : alk. paper)
1. Childbirth—Cross-cultural studies. 2. Maternal health
services—Cross-cultural studies. 3. Health risk assessment—
Cross-cultural studies.
I. Fordyce, Lauren. II. Maraesa, Amínata.
GN482.1.R57 2012
362.198′2—dc23
2011018130

For my parents, William and Patricia. —*L.F.*

To everyone who has ever taken a risk on me. And to Afinatou, Safouane, and Douniya, who have no choice but to come along for the ride. —*A.M.*

Contents

Foreword

Carole H. Browner

Women have been bearing and caring for children since the dawn of time. And as best we know, pregnancy and the act of giving birth have always been recognized as times of vulnerability, uncertainty, and danger—as much for pregnant women and new mothers as for the larger groups to which they belong. It is for this reason that in contrast with nonhuman primates, who give birth on their own, the evolution of the human species favored assisted reproduction.

Given that disparate interests and values are inextricably linked to the reproduction of every social group, the social relations of human reproduction were potential sites for conflict in the earliest societies: between spouses, co-wives, and generations; between fertile women and the extended families, bands, tribes, villages, neighborhoods, communities, and nation-states to which they belonged.

The chapters in Lauren Fordyce and Amínata Maraesa's fascinating new collection focus mainly on one particular type of reproductive conflict: that between pregnant women and mothers and the nation-states in which they reside. They reveal that in a growing number of countries throughout the world today, women are expected—if not required—to participate in the biomedical health care system through prenatal care regimens administered by Western-trained and biomedically certified providers, to give birth in state-sanctioned hospitals or clinics, and to extend biomedical protocols of care to their children.

These chapters also compellingly reveal that although we anthropologists tend to speak of biomedicine in hegemonic terms, in fact, its penetration is quite variable and often ambivalently met. To some extent this is because throughout the world today, many women do not consider pregnancy an illness and continue to have confidence in their bodies' own ability to bear healthy children without the need for state-sanctioned interventions. Yet, at the same time, growing numbers of women simply do not feel free to turn down the monitoring, measuring, and other interventions that are part of modern prenatal care, or to insist on giving birth in the location of their choosing. *Risk, Reproduction, and Narratives of Experience* sheds new light on a troubling core aspect of medicalization processes, which simultaneously render pregnant women more docile subjects even as they are impelled to actively engage with biomedicalized prenatal care regimes.

The chapters vividly show that many pregnant women and mothers do not necessarily wish to reject biomedical reproductive care out of hand, but to select only those aspects they consider most valuable and avoid the rest. This means that contrary to conventional wisdom, "traditional" and "modern" reproductive care practices are not inherently in opposition, nor on a linear trajectory with one inevitably supplanting the other: we see in several chapters that multiple knowledge systems can—and do—productively coexist.

We also see that a consummate means by which states seek to consolidate power in the reproductive realm is through expansion of the biomedical concept of risk. This critical observation emerges repeatedly in this collection. I was fascinated to learn that the term "risk" came into use centuries ago in the transition to modern society, and that in its original sense, "risk" simply denoted the precise probability of a specific outcome; no value judgment was implied. While today, the notion of risk is associated only with danger, back then, one could be considered "at risk" for becoming fabulously wealthy, for instance, or for rising to a powerful position. Only over time did the term come to be strictly associated with potential negative outcomes that might arise from some uncertain future event.

Moreover, we learn from Fordyce and Maraesa's collection that over time, the concept of risk has also increasingly become politicized, especially when deployed by modern state governments seeking greater control over particular groups. Not surprisingly, pregnant women are key targets. In part, this is because one of the most significant functions of the modern state lies in the creation of cultural identities, which necessarily include ideas as to what constitutes a good mother and, ultimately, a good citizen. This cultural identity–building project justifies the implementation of policies designed to regulate which groups will be encouraged to have children and which will not; what ideal family size and gender composition should be; whether "assisted" reproduction will be allowed, and for whom. Because the regulation of reproduction is central to the modernization agendas of all contemporary states, women who fail to conform to their society's expectations around reproduction, including the kinds of dynamics analyzed in detail in this collection (such as how to manage a pregnancy, where to give birth, and how to care for babies and small children), are seen as impeding their state's modernization efforts.

Reading these chapters led me to further reflect not only on who benefits from framing health research and policy through risk concepts and discourses, but also on what the consequences might be for those whose life experiences, reproductive or otherwise, are framed through risk concepts and discourses—that is, how risk as a specific mathematical probability bleeds into its becoming an absolute or near certainty and, ultimately, an intrinsic attribute of a given class of people, thereby inhering to all the individuals who constitute the particular group. One obvious example concerns the intense debates about childbirth by cesarean section: because some women who had one cesarean birth were subsequently unable to deliver vaginally during successive trials of labor, the mandate "once a cesarean, always a cesarean" was generalized to all pregnant women, even in the face of weak medical evidence.

Readers of *Risk, Reproduction, and Narratives of Experience* may be surprised to learn that in many parts of the global South, hospital births are significantly more dangerous than home births, with higher rates of both maternal and infant mortality. We learn this is the case not only for the obvious reason that women with more complicated pregnancies are more likely to be referred to hospitals. Equally if not more important is the dismal state of primary and secondary care facilities throughout developing and postcolonial nations. The need for beds, supplies, and personnel far outstrip their availability, requiring some women who actually do make it to hospitals to deliver their own babies while waiting their turn. Yet the idea that hospital birth is always best still manages to prevail, while women who resist are labeled noncompliant, selfish, and ignorant.

Today, as I write this Foreword, the dynamics of reproduction have become increasingly subsumed by larger political agendas. Impassioned struggles over women's reproductive rights continue to intensify globally as well as here in the United States. *Risk, Reproduction, and Narratives of Experience* provides a wealth of powerful ammunition to inform those debates and struggles and the ones that inevitably lie ahead.

Acknowledgments

Lauren Fordyce and Amínata Maraesa would like to thank all the contributors to this volume for their hard work and patience in seeing this text from the planning stages through to its completion. We are very grateful to Carole Browner, who generously agreed to write the Foreword to this text, sent us helpful feedback in the editing process, and provided valuable mentorship to young reproductive scholars, including us, over the years. Special thanks to Rayna Rapp, who wrote the Afterword; contributed her editorial expertise to earlier stages of Amínata's, Becca's, and Alyshia's writing; and has been an active supporter of this project since its inception.

We are very thankful and grateful for the amazing experience and support we have had at Vanderbilt University Press. Michael Ames has been helpful and encouraging throughout the process, from seeing first drafts of chapters through imagining the finished product. Ed Huddleston was very patient and helpful through our numerous and specific e-mails about copyediting questions. We would also like to thank Rachel Chapman and an anonymous reviewer, whose incisive comments and feedback were instrumental in shaping this volume into its final form.

Finally, Lauren and Amínata would like to acknowledge that we serendipitously met to turn this project into a fruitful and inspiring partnership—one that will be long lasting and that we anticipate will produce many more collaborative ventures.

Introduction

The Development of Discourses Surrounding Reproductive Risks

Lauren Fordyce
and Aminata Maraesa

With the rise of reproductive technologies, contested struggles over reproductive choice, and the global proliferation and normalization of reproductive freedoms has come an increase in the attention and scrutiny surrounding individual behaviors and group actions associated with poor reproductive outcomes. What was once the domain of chance, fate, or divine will has been repositioned as behavioral "risk," both scientifically calculable and technologically avoidable. Reproductive risks can now be measured, and, through behavior modification and the use of technological intervention, these risks are deemed preventable. The existence of these preventive measures, while often undertaken as matters of policy by national governments, links the notions of risk to individual choice, responsibility, and blame, whereby women, as gatekeepers of a population's health, are the recipients of moral imperatives related to child and family well-being. At other times, entire cultural collectives are situated as at odds with reproductive propriety and social good. This labeling of individuals or their communities as being "at risk" for reproductive danger has triggered a host of intervention programs, public health campaigns, and development initiatives. Subsequently, individual reproductive freedoms, and the bodies through which these freedoms are exhibited, have come under increasing surveillance and ideological control.

But such macro-understandings of risk do not take into account the myriad lived experiences that demonstrate how individual and collective interactions with reproductive risks vary both locally and globally. To this end, this volume explores contemporary understandings of reproductive risks from a cross-cultural and ethnographic perspective. By examining how risk is mobilized in debates about maternal and child health, perinatal decision making, nationalized reproductive policy, and international public health commitments, the following chapters provide insight into the many ways risk is formulated, deployed, experienced, embodied, and contested by cultural actors and their social networks.

Charting New Terrain in the Definition of Risk

Various scholars across disciplines have defined and operationalized risk in a number of ways, including its conceptualization as an absolute: true and real dangers exist in the biological world that can be measured independently of social and cultural processes. The rationalizing discourse of science and expert bureaucracies have laid claim to the transformation of human precariousness into categories of risk that can be neatly measured and quantified (Lupton 1999; Reddy 1996). In this way, calculable scientific knowledge about risk has become the manner through which life's uncertainties can be recognized and avoided—or contained (Castel 1991; Ewald 1991; Hacking 1990; Lupton 1999). But this claim is not without challenge from qualitative analyses that call for a nuanced and flexible understanding of risk that takes into account sociocultural human variation (including the often hidden cultural and qualitative judgment of the scientific observer)—and cultural beliefs in a higher spiritual ordering of existence (Denham, this volume; Dudgeon, this volume).

Indeed, many scholars have argued that social and cultural frameworks complicate the assumption and absolute authority of neutral and objective scientific knowledge about risk (Herr Hawthorne and Oaks 2003; Lupton 1999; Trostle 2005). *Risk, Reproduction, and Narratives of Experience* joins this body of literature in examining the epistemological complications of measuring and defining risk in cross-cultural contexts. Building on the work of Hayes (1992) and Herr Hawthorne and Oaks (2003:3) and their call for a "critical analysis of the way risk is discussed, deployed, and disentangled by multiple actors across varied cultural and social divides," Part I, "Complications in Measuring and Defining Risk," reexamines the ways that risks are defined, measured, and thereby lived by both the biomedical community and local stakeholders.

In Chapter 1, Matthew Dudgeon examines how different meanings of risk attach to pregnancy and its management for three groups of health care providers in the western highlands of Guatemala: local physicians, regional workers for an international NGO working to improve health quality in maternal and infant health services, and K'iche' Maya traditional birth attendants (TBAs). He argues that theories of risk that focus on the state as a source of power and the administration of risk may be inadequate for conceptualizing local meanings of reproductive risks for TBAs. In contrast, many TBAs work within a multilayered discourse of risk within which they rate their clients' pregnancies as well as evaluate each other's worthiness of the title *comadrona* (midwife). Indeed, TBAs perceive their relationship to the supernatural as a mitigating force against the risks associated with pregnancy in rural Guatemala, substantiating their midwifery practices through a divine connection.

In Chapter 2, Alyshia Gálvez explores how birth outcomes among Mexican women living in New York City begin to resemble those of other similarly situated socioeconomic groups, effecting a reduction in the benefits of the "birth weight paradox" as their "cultural advantage" wears off the longer they reside in the United States. Gálvez argues that the rise in unfavorable birth outcomes may be the result of a shift in reproductive understanding and behavior: the women are slowly convinced of the riskiness of their own reproduction and come to behave in ways that actually erode their cultural advantage. Despite these changes, Gálvez points out, Mexican immigrant women continue to assert their understanding of pregnancy as something they were born to successfully accomplish, calling into question some of the prenatal standards of care they encounter in New York while continuing various traditions from their homeland.

Alison Hamilton, in Chapter 3, looks at the medically and subjectively defined risks associated with prenatal methamphetamine use, suggesting that the numerous medically defined risks are distant from women users' subjective concerns during and after pregnancy. Though perceiving few effects of their illicit drug use on the health of their babies, women in Hamilton's study are far from carefree; they daily confront challenging and interacting life circumstances that place them at great risk for ongoing substance dependence or relapse, and thus for exposing their children to the physical and psychological effects of methamphetamine dependence. Hamilton also examines the state's absolutist conceptualization of risks and responsibility during pregnancy, which ignores the social context in which pregnant women with drug addiction embody and enact their struggles.

Toward a Theory of Reproductive Risk and the Politics of the Body

Mary Douglas was perhaps the first to highlight the cultural relativity of judgments about risk (1985, 1992; Douglas and Wildavsky 1982). While acknowledging the existence of "real" dangers out in the world, Douglas argues that the responses to these dangers have been socially constructed, in that any universalizing language of risk is always culturally and socially interpreted: "each form of social life has its own typical risk portfolio" based on the "shared confidence and shared fears" of a particular community (1992:8). The chapters in this volume examine and build upon this argument as it relates to reproductive behaviors and experiences in cross-cultural settings.

Although a collective risk portfolio might be shaped by shared cultural understandings of social roles and practices, many of the women and their families in the following chapters form their ideas about risk through concrete experiences and interactions with governing bodies that seek to position risk and risk management at the gateway to health, development, and modernity. Indeed, risk is a highly politicized and strategic union that often leads to finger pointing and blaming of certain individuals and groups for actions that purportedly cause danger to themselves and the larger public health measures of social well-being (Lupton 1999). Many of the women discussed in this volume find themselves on the receiving end of personal accusations or collective social blame for behaviors slated as causing perinatal complications and maternal, infant, or child death (Cosminsky, this volume; Hamilton, this volume). Their stories provide an important counterpoint for those interested in looking beyond a realist perspective that assumes risk to be an objective fact or absolute truth, ignoring the political, social, and moral influences on risk judgments emphasized in this volume (Douglas 1992; Lupton 1999).

According to sociologists Ulrich Beck (1992[1986]) and Anthony Giddens (1991) the rise of modernity is inextricably linked to the development of discourses of risk and risk avoidance. Beck and Giddens describe modern life as preoccupied with the future and tied to risk scenarios that influence present decision-making processes. Both portray society as evolving into a new stage—"reflexive modernization" (Beck 1992[1986]) or "late modernity" (Giddens 1991)—in which the certainties of science and technology are under question, their self-assuredness scrutinized and itself linked to new forms of risk. While Bujra (2000) has questioned whether the term "modernity"—much less "late modernity" as defined by Giddens (1991:15–16)—can be rightfully applied to developing populations, this volume argues that the global penetration of reproductive technologies has created localized counternarratives of risk and risk reduction that call into question the confidence of scientific discourses. Although developing populations have become accustomed to and even welcome many forms of technological advancement, they also have very articulated concerns about the risks of certain technologies. These concerns remain rooted in personal memories or "a practical sense of community epidemiology" (Rapp 1999:176) steeped in shared beliefs and embodied experiences. Highlighted throughout the volume are the ethical dilemmas posed by the availability and purported superiority of medical machines and medicines that obviate certain risks—while giving rise to others (Gálvez, this volume).

Other analyses of risk within contemporary theory take a Foucauldian perspective that integrates the theory of governmentality in order to investigate the ways in which specific discourses, strategies, practices, and institutions help bring risk into being and then construct it as a phenomenon (Lupton 1999). Foucauldian scholars of risk and responsibility have argued that understanding the changing notions of risk is more complicated than following its shifts from global to local contexts. As Lupton argues, "changes in risk rationalities have occurred which have resulted in risk being conceptualized and dealt with in diverse ways that have strong links to ideas about how individuals should deport themselves in relation to the state" (1999:102). Indeed, tests for "risk potential," "risk profiling," and other diagnostic information can be used at the level of the state or local bureaucracy to justify enforcement of conformity, hierarchical classification, and regulation of access—all of which could infringe upon basic human rights—while espousing a rationalizing discourse of economic benefit and administrative streamlining necessary to social governance (Chua 2003; Gammeltoft 2007; Ma, this volume; Nelkin and Tancredi 1994; Rose 2006).

Reproduction has long remained an important case study within biopolitics, particularly as pregnancy care today includes increasing prescriptions for risk management and risk-related technologies (Franklin 2007; Rapp 1999). Rabinow and Rose note that reproduction provides an important problem space "in which an array of connections appear between the individual and the collective, the technological and the political, the legal and the ethical. This is a biopolitical space par excellence" (2006:208). Much of the risk talk related to pregnancies enforces the notion that a woman is responsible for the health of her fetus; women are taught that ignoring expert advice could result in harm to the fetus or a poor birth outcome (Howes-Mischel, this volume; Lupton 1999, 2000; Oaks 2001; Ruhl 1999; Smith-Oka, this volume).

Yet a growing number of scholars have criticized the Foucauldian perspective on risk as focused too closely on the discourses and strategies of governmentality, with little attention to how these practices are experienced in daily life (Lock and Kaufert 1998; Lupton 1999). Feminist scholars have found Foucault's work lacking focus on the specificity of women's bodies as an important site for new forms of biopower (Sawicki 1991), as well as neglectful of the gendered dynamics of disciplinary techniques of power (McNay 1992). Building on theories of governmentality, and taking into account criticisms of its macroconceptualizations of subjects, this volume examines the ways in which women in particular reflect on and respond to risk in their everyday lives.

Gendering the focus of population health, discourses of risk rationalize the use of reproductive technologies and biomedical care to avoid the seemingly inherent risks associated with certain types of reproductive practices deemed contrary to the health of the social body. Discussions about the intersections of risk and reproduction circulate in the debates surrounding the causes of maternal and child death and are explicitly addressed in public health mandates and government referenda. While these discourses are developed at the level of state officials and disembodied actors, they proliferate and are enacted at the local level of the intimate body. As the bearers and keepers of children, women are by and large the targets of reproductive risk talk.

Notions of risk permeate the core of women's reproductive lives; without addressing the larger social and structural world in which women reproduce, biomedical discourses of risk and risk avoidance lead us to believe that certain individual behaviors and practices can decrease women's reproductive risk. Nichter (2003) has argued that a deployment of risk under the rubric of "harm reduction" produces a sense of agency and self-control over risk scenarios while potentially drawing attention away from the larger structural factors that contribute to risky circumstances to begin with. Yet, increased surveillance of the individual does nothing to address the structural impediments that often impact women's ability to heed purportedly harm-reducing directives, thereby exacerbating preexisting risk conditions or creating new risk factors. Chapters in this volume look at the ways institutionalized risk management strategies are enacted on female bodies and how these embodied actors engage with and redirect discourses of individual risk avoidance care to correspond to their realities.

In their analyses of the interactions of risk, health, and power, and the role of individual responses to the implementation of top-down health care measures and public health mandates, Herr Harthorn and Oaks (2003) call attention to the political nature of risk assessment and how it can be deployed by both an overarching governing apparatus and the many individual and collective social actors who are likewise appropriating definitions of risk for their own measures. Part II, "Biopolitical Narratives of Risk and Responsibility," explores the ways individuals are creatively circumventing the increasing invasiveness of the state over their reproductive and familial lives by creating narratives of counterrisk and risk assessment that contest the absolute authority of the state and its deployment of universalist and universalizing public health measures and mandates. In Chapter 4, Sheila Cosminsky examines the legal restrictions placed on midwives in Guatemala that mandate hospital births as a result of particular maternal "risk factors," arguing that the subtext of the WHO Safe Motherhood policy is that the greatest "risk factor" is the midwife. Cosminsky interrogates three interrelated issues: the use of infant and maternal mortality rates as a criteria for evaluating the midwives and the effectiveness of their training, the concept of "risk"—what is defined as "high risk" and by whom—and the use of "referrals" as an evaluative criteria.

In Chapter 5, Vania Smith-Oka discusses how the concept of being a "modern" woman has been promoted with great enthusiasm by the Mexican state. Receiving biomedical reproductive care is viewed as a necessary step toward achieving this modernity. Women who fall outside the norm of reproduction—through their prenatal, labor, or mothering choices—are perceived to be engaging in highly risky practices, as well as challenging the state's efforts at modernity. Using ethnographic data from two contexts in Mexico—rural and urban—Smith-Oka explores the state's efforts to produce and reproduce good motherhood through women's engagement with biomedical reproductive care. This chapter examines local women's and biomedical practitioners' ideas of reproductive health and investigates the risks and consequences of these women's "disobedience."

Building on this discussion of risks and notions of modernity in Mexico, Rebecca Howes-Mischel explores in Chapter 6 how sociomedical narratives of health encourage women to negotiate their control over and responsibility for prenatal health in specific ways. Grounded in ethnographic research in public health clinics in Oaxaca, Mexico, and in Southern California, her analysis examines how discourses of "reproductive risks" become discourses of citizenship. Rather than discussing biological or genetic risks, doctors encourage women to look to their individual life choices as the sites of risk production and alleviation. Community health teams reinforce these narratives in local instantiations of national health campaigns, advocating a neoliberal sensibility of self-care, or *autocuidado*, as incumbent on modern individuals. Pregnant women and their kin reaffirm this emphasis on individual self-care, articulating a sense of responsibility for risk reduction that parallels the professional narratives that frame the women as irresponsible reproductive subjects.

Concluding this section, Qingyan Ma in Chapter 7 examines the reproductive practices in the southwestern Chinese borderland of Weixi County, Yunnan Province, that have arisen out of the negotiations between state and local discourses of reproductive propriety. As part of a post-Mao national plan to create a "new countryside" and "new family" by modernizing rural health care, the Larger Shangri-la Project indicates the changing strategy of state control over women's reproductive bodies. Exploring how women's reproductive bodies and fertility are imagined and regulated by state policy makers, public health experts, local officials, health providers, and residents, this chapter is primarily concerned with the relationship between the state and its multiethnic constituency, shedding light on nationalist strategies of knowledge production and social control, as well as on local responses to China's ongoing modernizing project.

Struggles over the Embodiment of Reproductive Risk

As reproduction and childbirth transitioned away from the domain of women to enter the world of male obstetricians, their mechanized tools of extraction, and chemically induced avoidance, women have moved from compliance to advocacy to proactive desire to engage with and contest the medicalization of childbirth (Davis-Floyd 1992; Martin 1992[1987]; Oakley 1984)—quite often taking the issue, as Morgen (2002) points out, into their own hands. Women's struggles to reclaim their reproductive bodies are not necessarily coterminous with an opposition to biomedicine. Rather, women often exhibit particular strategies of engagement with available medical practices, using them creatively as well as actively to reflect on individual choice (Cussins 1998; Lock and Kaufert 1998; Riessman 1983) and in consideration of sociocultural constructs (Lopez 2008).

Situating pregnant women as agents in their own pregnancies was a logical outcome of the feminist movement and the critique of biomedicine that aimed to highlight women as active participants in their own reproductive lives (BWHBC 1973; Davis 2007; Ruhl 1999). Yet, the reproductive risk model makes assumptions that are inappropriate in relation to pregnancy; women do not "control" their pregnancies in the way this model suggests (Landsman 2009; Layne 2003; Rapp 1999). Regulatory health agencies project all responsibility for the health and control of "risk factors" on pregnant women, raising the specter of the "irresponsible pregnant woman" who threatens the health and well-being of her "unborn child" (Kaufert and O'Neil 1993; Maraesa, this volume; Ruhl 1999; Smith-Oka, this volume; Tsing 1992; Weir 2006). The moral panic generated by this bestowal of absolute responsibility is reinforced by invoking the purportedly risk-taking "bad mother"—the alcoholic, the crack addict, the chain smoker, the teen mom (and do not forget the single mother and the lesbian); the list is truly endless and quite subjective—obscuring the many factors that influence reproductive behavior (Armstrong 2008; Armstrong and Abel 2000; Balsamo 1996; Hamilton, this volume; Lewin 1993; Murphy and Rosenbaum 1999; Oaks 2001; Roberts 1998; Roth 2000; Ward 1995).

Placing full blame for reproductive outcomes on pregnant women as the sole authorities and agents in the care of themselves and their fetus ignores many of the practical realties of women's lived experiences and certainly leaves no room for force majeure when discussing reproductive malfeasance (Denham, this volume; Fordyce, this volume; Young, this volume). Attention to the on-the-ground negotiation of risk is extremely significant to this volume and to theories about the power hierarchies inherent in reproduction, reflecting a long legacy of feminist scholarship around the politics of reproduction and, in particular, stratified reproduction, whereby some women are empowered to reproduce while others are disempowered (Cohen 1995; Davis-Floyd 1992; Davis-Floyd and Sargent 1997; Ginsburg and Rapp 1991, 1995; Martin 1992[1987]; Rapp 1999).

Finally, Part III of this volume, "Struggles over the Embodiment of Reproductive Risk," takes a closer look at the ways in which local practices and definitions of risk intersect with and challenge biomedical authority. Reminiscent of Jordan's (1993[1978], 1997) early work on reproduction and authoritative knowledge (see also Davis-Floyd and Sargent 1997), the contributors to this section argue for the existence of parallel reproductive knowledge systems among which pregnant women and their caregivers often move seamlessly but not without substantial effort and awareness. Indeed, biomedical knowledge of reproductive health and propriety is powerfully—and politically—constructed as more legitimate and as imbued with expertise, while alternative forms of knowledge are portrayed as backward, ignorant, and "risky."

In Chapter 8, Alyson Young addresses the gaps in understanding between biomedical and cultural conceptions of childhood diarrheal illness among the pastoral Datoga in Tanzania. Young examines the meanings maternal caregivers attribute to ethnomedical knowledge and practices associated with risks for disease transmission, as well as local ways to avoid—and comprehend—infant death. This examination of Datoga constructions of risk and vulnerability makes explicit the "naturalization" of Western biomedicine and helps us better understand the creation, representation, legitimization, and application of knowledge about reproduction and the body.

Aaron Denham describes in Chapter 9 how biomedical knowledge about maternal and early childhood risk factors in the Kassena-Nankana District of Ghana has not supplanted traditional or socially grounded notions of risk; rather, families have incorporated it as an additional way to understand the broader management of reproductive vulnerabilities. Viewed from the intersection of local and biomedical reproductive epistemologies, this chapter presents Nankani understandings of maternal and infant risks and the contemporaneous behavioral taboos and reproductive technologies (local and transnational) used to mitigate them. Denham concludes that local understandings frame motherhood as the grounds for biological dangers, as well as the embodiment of social dissonance, ancestral demands, and spiritual concerns.

In Chapter 10, Lauren Fordyce uses ethnographic data from her research among Haitians living in South Florida to examine the narratives of risk and responsibility that accompany the practice of prenatal diagnosis in biomedical prenatal care in the United States. Underlying the choice to use diagnostic technologies such as ultrasound or amniocentesis is the notion that pregnant women have a responsibility both to understand the genetic "risks" to their unborn child and to use biomedicine to discover these risks. The majority of the Haitian women interviewed saw ultrasound as a valuable part of the pregnancy experience and therefore a necessary expense for their families. Questions about their own experiences with ultrasound exams solicited a show-and-tell of fetal photos, yet providers' comments on the necessity of ultrasound for prenatal diagnosis speak precisely to what makes ultrasound such an interesting study—the ways in which this technology is situated as a both a diagnostic tool and a pleasurable experience.

Closing out this section's discussion of intersections of embodied knowledge and biomedical expertise, in Chapter 11 Amínata Maraesa illustrates how the prenatal examination room at the local hospital in southern Belize is the site of competing knowledge systems where nurse-midwives and pregnant women often negotiate opposing viewpoints concerning prenatal care and maternal and child health. As nurse-midwives work hard to convey and maintain the authority of international biomedical standards and discourses of risk that rely on a fictitiously constructed objectivity to validate its superiority, pregnant women construct their own definitions of risk based on subjective experience and an embodied understanding of their reproductive condition. It is in this oppositional cultural matrix that Maraesa examines some of the heated arguments that erupt as pregnant women disregard the biomedical discourses of risk and make reproductive decisions based on their subjective embodiment of pregnancy and a culturally defined interpretation of sickness and health.

Conclusion

This volume explores the multitude of ways ideas about risk have targeted women, their bodies, and their reproductive behaviors, and how women as cultural actors in cross-cultural settings have constructed their own metanarratives of the coupling of risk and reproduction. As a collective, this work emphasizes that risk can never be reduced to a static list of behavioral imperatives; rather, it is a messy concept that is highly cultural, often traced to communal rather than individualistic understandings. In many cases, ways of thinking about risk in reproduction take into account mutual obligations and expectations among women, families, and society. The counternarratives highlighted in this volume bring to light how women's local moral worlds—in addition to larger factors such as structural barriers, economic access, and the natural environment—contribute to risk assessment and management in reproductive life. Finally, this volume emphasizes that while a regulating discourse of risk might (un)comfortably situate itself on the "unruly" and "porous" female body (Kukla 2005), women are not "docile" (Martin 1992[1987]) recipients of statistical risk categories. Rather, they are pragmatic actors whose interactions with statistical risk assessment and risk-managing protocols often reflect particular strategies aimed at achieving personal goals or conforming to socioculturally appropriate practices.

References

Armstrong, Elizabeth
   2008   Conceiving Risk, Bearing Responsibility: Fetal Alcohol Syndrome and the
           Diagnosis of Moral Disorder. Baltimore: Johns Hopkins University Press.

Armstrong, Elizabeth, and Ernest Abel
  2000   Fetal Alcohol Syndrome: The Origins of a Moral Panic. Alcohol and Alcoholism 35(3):276–82.
Balsamo, Anne
  1996   Technologies of the Gendered Body: Reading Cyborg Women. Durham, NC: Duke University Press.
Beck, Ulrich
  1992[1986] Risk Society: Towards a New Modernity. London: Sage Publications.
Boston Women's Health Book Collective (BWHBC)
  1973   Our Bodies, Ourselves. New York: Simon and Schuster.
Bujra, Janet
  2000   Risk and Trust: Unsafe Sex, Gender and AIDS in Tanzania. *In* Risk Revisited. Pat Caplan, ed. Pp. 59–84. London: Pluto Press.
Castel, Robert
  1991   From Dangerousness to Risk. *In* The Foucault Effect: Studies in Governmentality. Graham Burchell, Colin Gordon, and Peter Miller, eds. Pp. 281–98. Chicago: University of Chicago Press.
Chau, Peter
  2003   Governing Migrants' Sexual Behavior: Work, HIV/AIDS, and Condom Use Campaigns in Southeast Asia. *In* Risk, Culture, and Health Inequality. Barbara Herr Harthorn and Laury Oaks, eds. Pp. 165–84. Westport, CT: Praeger.
Cohen, Shellee
  1995   "Like a Mother to Them": Stratified Reproduction and West Indian Childcare Workers and Employers in New York. *In* Conceiving the New World Order. Faye Ginsburg and Rayna Rapp, eds. Pp. 78–102. Berkeley: University of California Press.
Cussins, Charis
  1998   Ontological Choreography: Agency for Women Patients in an Infertility Clinic. *In* Difference in Medicine: Unraveling Practices, Techniques and Bodies. Marc Berg and Annemarie Mol, eds. Pp. 166–201. Durham, NC: Duke University Press.
Davis, Kathy
  2007   The Making of Our Bodies, Ourselves: How Feminism Travels across Borders. Durham, NC: Duke University Press.
Davis-Floyd, Robbie
  1992   Birth as an American Rite of Passage. Berkeley: University of California Press.
Davis-Floyd, Robbie, and Carolyn Sargent, eds.
  1997   Childbirth and Authoritative Knowledge: Cross-Cultural Perspectives. Berkeley: University of California Press.
Douglas, Mary
  1985   Risk Acceptability According to the Social Sciences. New York: Russell Sage Foundation.
  1992   Risk and Blame: Essays in Cultural Theory. London: Routledge.
Douglas, Mary, and Aaron Wildavsky
  1982   Risk and Culture: An Essay on the Selection of Environmental and Technological Dangers. Berkeley: University of California Press.

Ewald, François
  1991   Insurance and Risk. *In* The Foucault Effect: Studies in Governmentality. Graham Burchell, Colin Gordon, and Peter Miller, eds. Pp. 197–210. Chicago: University of Chicago Press.

Franklin, Sarah
  2007   Dolly Mixtures: The Remaking of Genealogy. Durham, NC: Duke University Press.

Gammeltoft, Tine
  2007   Sonography and Sociality: Obstetrical Ultrasound Imaging in Urban Vietnam. Medical Anthropology Quarterly 21(2):133–53.

Giddens, Anthony
  1991   Modernity and Self-Identity: Self and Society in the Late Modern Age. Cambridge: Polity Press.

Ginsburg, Faye, and Rayna Rapp
  1991   Politics of Reproduction. Annual Review of Anthropology 20:311–43.
  1995   Introduction: Conceiving the New World Order. *In* Conceiving the New World Order. Faye Ginsburg and Rayna Rapp, eds. Pp. 1–18. Berkeley: University of California Press.

Hacking, Ian
  1990   The Taming of Chance. Cambridge: Cambridge University Press.

Hayes, Michael
  1992   On the Epistemology of Risk: Language, Logic and Social Science. Social Science and Medicine 35(1):401–7.

Herr Harthorn, Barbara, and Laury Oaks, eds.
  2003   Risk, Culture, and Health Inequality: Shifting Perceptions of Danger and Blame. Westport, CT: Praeger.

Jordan, Brigitte
  1993[1978] Birth in Four Cultures: A Crosscultural Investigation of Childbirth in Yucatan, Holland, Sweden, and the United States. Prospect Heights, IL: Waveland Press.
  1997   Authoritative Knowledge and Its Construction. *In* Childbirth and Authoritative Knowledge: Cross-Cultural Perspectives. Robbie Davis-Floyd and Carolyn Sargent, eds. Pp. 55–79. Berkeley: University of California Press.

Kaufert, Patricia, and John O'Neil
  1993   Analysis of a Dialogue on Risks in Childbirth: Clinicians, Epidemiologists, and Inuit Women. *In* Knowledge, Power, and Practice. Shirley Lindenbaum and Margaret Lock, eds. Pp. 32–54. Berkeley: University of California Press.

Kukla, Rebecca
  2005   Mass Hysteria: Medicine, Culture, and Mothers' Bodies. Lanham, MD: Rowman and Littlefield.

Landsman, Gail
  2009   Reconstructing Motherhood and Disability in the Age of Perfect Babies. New York: Routledge.

Layne, Linda
  2003   Motherhood Lost: A Feminist Account of Pregnancy Loss in America. New York: Routledge.

Lewin, Ellen
    1993   Lesbian Mothers: Accounts of Gender in American Culture. Ithaca, NY: Cornell
            University Press.
Lock, Margaret, and Patricia Kaufert
    1998   Introduction. *In* Pragmatic Women and Body Politics. Margaret Lock and Patricia
            Kaufert, eds. Pp. 1–27. Cambridge: Cambridge University Press.
Lopez, Iris Ofelia
    2008   Matters of Choice: Puerto Rican Women's Struggle for Reproductive Freedom.
            New Brunswick, NJ: Rutgers University Press.
Lupton, Deborah
    1999   Risk. London: Routledge.
    2000   Risk and the Ontology of Pregnant Embodiment. *In* Risk and Sociocultural
            Theory: New Directions and Perspectives. Deborah Lupton, ed. Pp. 59–85.
            Cambridge: Cambridge University Press.
Martin, Emily
    1992[1987] The Woman in the Body: A Cultural Analysis of Reproduction. Boston:
            Beacon Press.
McNay, Lois
    1992   Foucault and Feminism: Power, Gender and the Self. Boston: Northeastern
            University Press.
Morgen, Sandra
    2002   Into Our Own Hands: The Women's Health Movement in the United States,
            1969–1990. New Brunswick, NJ: Rutgers University Press.
Murphy, Sheigla, and Marsha Rosenbaum
    1999   Pregnant Women on Drugs: Combating Stereotypes and Stigma. New Brunswick,
            NJ: Rutgers University Press.
Nelkin, Dorothy, and Laurence Tancredi
    1994   Dangerous Diagnostics: The Social Power of Biological Information. Chicago:
            University of Chicago Press.
Nichter, Mark
    2003   Harm Reduction: A Core Concern for Medical Anthropology. *In* Risk, Culture,
            and Health Inequality: Shifting Perceptions of Danger and Blame. Barbara Herr
            Harthorn and Laury Oaks, eds. Pp. 15–33. Westport, CT: Praeger.
Oakley, Ann
    1984   The Captured Womb: A History of the Medical Care of Pregnant Women.
            Oxford: Basil Blackwell.
Oaks, Laury
    2001   Smoking and Pregnancy: The Politics of Fetal Protection. New Brunswick, NJ:
            Rutgers University Press.
Rabinow, Paul, and Nikolas Rose
    2006   Biopower Today. Biosocieties 1(2):195–217.
Rapp, Rayna
    1999   Testing Women, Testing the Fetus: The Social Impact of Amniocentesis in
            America. New York: Routledge.
Reddy, Sanjay
    1996   Claims to Expert Knowledge and the Subversion of Democracy: The Triumph of
            Risk over Uncertainty. Economy and Society 25(2):222–54.

Riessman, Catherine
   1983   Women and Medicalization: A New Perspective. Social Policy 14(1):3–18.
Roberts, Dorothy
   1998   Killing the Black Body: Race, Reproduction, and the Meaning of Liberty. New
           York: Vintage House.
Rose, Nikolas
   2006   The Politics of Life Itself: Biomedicine, Power, and Subjectivity in the Twenty-
           First Century. Princeton, NJ: Princeton University Press.
Roth, Rachel
   2000   Making Women Pay: The Hidden Costs of Fetal Rights. Ithaca, NY: Cornell
           University Press.
Ruhl, Lealle
   1999   Liberal Governance and Prenatal Care: Risk and Regulation in Pregnancy.
           Economy and Society 28(1):95–117.
Sawicki, Jana
   1991   Disciplining Foucault: Feminism, Power, and the Body. New York: Routledge.
Trostle, James
   2005   Epidemiology and Culture. Cambridge: Cambridge University Press.
Tsing, Anna
   1992   Women Charged with Perinatal Endangerment. *In* Uncertain Terms: Negotiating
           Gender in American Culture. Faye Ginsburg and Anna Tsing, eds. Pp. 282–89.
           Boston: Beacon Press.
Ward, Martha
   1995   Early Childbearing: What Is the Problem and Who Owns It? *In* Conceiving the
           New World Order: The Global Politics of Reproduction. Faye Ginsburg and
           Rayna Rapp, eds. Pp. 140–58. Berkeley: University of California Press.
Weir, Lorna
   2006   Pregnancy, Risk, and Biopolitics: On the Threshold of the Living Subject.
           London: Routledge Press.

PART I

Complications in Measuring and Defining Risk

CHAPTER 1

Conceiving Risk in K'iche' Maya Reproduction

Matthew R. Dudgeon

In the department of Quetzaltenango in Guatemala's western highlands, different meanings of risk attach to pregnancy and its management for three distinct groups of health care providers: local physicians, regional workers for an international NGO working to improve health quality in maternal and infant health services, and K'iche' Maya traditional birth attendants (TBAs)—midwives, or, in Spanish, *comadronas*.[1] Moreover, theories of risk that focus on the state as a source of power and the administration of risk may be inadequate for conceptualizing local TBAs' meanings of reproductive risks. Many TBAs work with a multilayered discourse of risk within which they rate their clients' pregnancies, as well as evaluate each other's worthiness of the title comadrona. Indeed, midwives in rural Guatemala perceive their relationship to the supernatural as a mitigating force against the risks associated with pregnancy. Midwives who purportedly strike a pact with the devil may find themselves outside the parameters of local definitions of what makes a good midwife.

Background to Experiences of Reproduction in Cantel, Guatemala

For most of the twentieth century, the government of Guatemala interacted with its rural population as a sovereign power. State administration of that population was achieved primarily through force rather than infrastructure or social services, and it has differed according to locally recognized ethic distinctions between indigenous Maya and *ladino* groups of Spanish ancestry. Such regulation of the rural population has helped exclude indigenous groups from state politics, maintained a semi-feudal concentration of land and resources in the hands of a small minority, and supported some of the highest levels of inequality between the richest and poorest in the Latin American region (Suarez-Berenguela 2001). Throughout Guatemala's postcolonial history, national political debate has focused less on the inclusion of indigenous communities and more on the degree to which sovereign versus disciplinary and regulatory power should be exercised by elites in the administration of those communities; strategies have included privatization of land and indigence laws with forced labor directed at indigenous groups (Handy 1984).

While in the nineteenth and twentieth centuries Quetzaltenango's indigenous K'iche' elite class has wielded political power, much of its authority rested on administration of land and community relations of reciprocity, increasingly under-mined as K'iche' elites depended more heavily on the state and its punitive powers. At the same time, a growing K'iche' middle class of merchants and artisans called for health and educational reforms and increasing integration of the Guatemalan state into local administration in the departmental capital (Grandin 2000). The prevalence of sovereign power has produced both fragmentation among indige-nous communities and a limited degree of autonomy within them—an autonomy shattered for many communities as the state shifted from isolated massacres to total war, development poles (army-administered communities), and community policing during Guatemala's civil war in the 1980s. In the aftermath, and in paral-lel with the activities of international organizations such as the United Nations and bilateral and multilateral NGOs, Guatemala has seen increased administration of the biopolitical life of rural Maya, with a particular emphasis on reproduction and reproductive health. Most recently this shift has included the establishment of a Ministry of Reproductive Health and the pursuit of a plan for indigenous health, both implemented under Guatemala's Integrated National Health System (SIAS) and with the stated goals of reducing infant and maternal mortality (Cosminsky, this volume; Maupin 2008, 2009).

While conducting research on reproductive health in a K'iche' Maya com-munity in the municipality of Cantel in Quetzaltenango, I encountered great variation among groups of health care providers in the meanings they attached to infant illness and death.[2] Conducted from December 2001 until May 2003, my ethnographic and epidemiological fieldwork focused on Maya men's experiences of reproduction, as well as men's influences on maternal and infant health. The peri-urban municipality provided an ideal location to investigate reproductive health in a Maya community that had, relatively speaking, good access to the health facilities of the urban center of Quetzaltenango and yet, like many parts of Guatemala, still experienced relatively high rates of infant mortality. With a population of nearly 99 percent indigenous K'iche' Maya, the municipality of Cantel had 729 live births in 2001 and an infant mortality rate of 53.5 per thousand, higher than Guatemala's overall rate, estimated between 39 per thousand in 2000 and 45.8 in 2001 (CIA 2011).

I located my research in one *aldea* (hamlet) of Cantel, a community with a population of approximately 3,500, where I also conducted multisited ethno-graphic fieldwork with several groups of health professionals. These included phy-sicians and epidemiologists working with the Ministry of Health, several local and regional health NGOs, and collective organizations of TBAs. I conducted semi-structured and open-ended interviews and attended planning and training meet-ings, gathering data via observation of physician training in reproductive health, interviews with traditional midwives, and verbal autopsies from families in the community after stillbirths and perinatal and infant deaths. Those data provide in-sight into the differences and similarities in concepts of reproductive risk between groups, as well as implications for the provision of health care by those groups.

Risk among Biomedical Health Care Providers

One dimension of my fieldwork involved characterizing the levels of reproductive health care. I worked with TBAs as well as physicians, nurses, and other biomedical health care providers. In the departmental capital of Quetzaltenango, I attended a conference and training session on maternal and infant health at the departmental office of the Ministry of Health for regional doctors and hospital staff. The conference included lectures and slide presentations that focused on measurements of mortality and morbidity, vaccination campaigns and their outcomes, and epidemiological data on the quality of health care provided by the Ministry of Health.

The concept of risk arose concretely during a presentation by a local physician who had worked for the last several years with maternal and infant health NGOs receiving funding from USAID. His current work with an NGO had shifted focus from the training of TBAs (cf. Cosminsky, this volume) to the assessment of indicators of quality in different health care settings run by the Ministry of Health, such as hospitals and health clinics. Factors measured included the presence and quantities of essential supplies and medicines, number of beds in different wards, and sanitation in and around the facility. In his presentation on quality control, he spoke of the creation of "emergency plans" with couples during their pregnancy. The NGO's focus on education regarding preventive measures for obstetric emergency was targeting the vast majority of the couples in indigenous communities like the K'iche' community in Cantel in which I worked, who planned to deliver in their own homes with TBAs rather than in a hospital. Although some of these same couples would readily go to the hospital if the pregnancy proved complicated, others were resistant. Emergency plans ostensibly allowed couples to have a course of action in place in the event of an obstetric crisis—planning ahead who might drive if delivery occurred at a time when buses were not running, having some money set aside for the transportation, and deciding the roles husband, extended family, in-laws, and TBA would play. Each plan included training in how to recognize signs of danger in the pregnancy and during labor. This effort incorporated some elements of training given to TBAs in Maya communities by earlier NGO projects, along with some focus on education for couples.

The theme of the physician's talk, introduced as part of the justification for emergency plans, was that providers' understanding of the risks of pregnancy had to change. Rather than the "old" way of thinking about pregnancy—that some subset of pregnancies had complications that had to be managed, such as obstetric emergencies that required physician intervention—the speaker's project advocated the perspective that "every pregnancy is at risk." Pregnancy was to be thought of as an inherently unstable period during which the health of both mother and fetus was at risk. Rather than wait for an obstetric emergency, or rely on prenatal care to sort women into categories of complications, pregnancies by their very nature should be thought of as risky.

This view brought immediate murmurs of dissent from the crowd of physicians and mutterings throughout the rest of the talk. Discussion afterward was brief but heated and revolved around the statements of several physicians in the audience that pregnancy is a normal, healthy biological process, a part of life, and that to call pregnancy inherently risky flew in the face of basic reproductive physiology. The presenter was conciliatory, saying that much of the risk of pregnancy depended on context—limited resources, rural, poorly educated, and indigenous. But he did defend his position that pregnancy and delivery are complex physiological processes, that some part of that process might go wrong with any pregnancy, and that every pregnancy is at risk.

I was initially surprised by the other physicians' vehement reaction to the premise that all pregnancies are risky. At face value, it seemed a rather subtle shift, and a realistic one in a setting of limited resources and historically poor indicators of maternal and infant mortality. My first assumption was that physicians would embrace any expansion of the field of health care (making every pregnancy, rather than just a few high-risk pregnancies, the domain of doctors) rather than reject it outright. In speaking with some of the physicians in the audience after the talk, I did hear this perspective voiced—but about the presenter and the NGO, not about themselves. As one physician put it: "This idea of all pregnancy being risky, it's nonsense. Look around. Look in the hospital and in people's homes. The vast majority of pregnancies turn out fine. Saying that every pregnancy is risky is just a way for projects to expand, to self-justify, and to get more funding. We need to spend money on the pregnancies that are actually in trouble, rather than projects with fancy talk about risk."

The presenter had his own insight into the crowd's reaction: "I've seen this reaction before, when I give this talk. They have an older idea of risk, one that's based on their training as doctors, that risk is about pathology, about being sick. They see risk as out there somewhere, a germ or an accident, rather than a part of the process of pregnancy and childbirth."

Between these two views I see a fundamental shift in the way risk connects the individual pregnant woman to the population served by biomedicine. For the physicians, risk is more discrete, with pathology an outside threat. For the NGO worker, however, it is more pervasive, a field to be navigated rather than a threat encountered. Moreover, physicians are removed from the universe of blame unless they fail in their intervention in a pathological pregnancy. But from the perspective of the NGO worker, blame extends in all directions, making lack of prenatal care a risk factor for poor pregnancy outcome. This second perspective resonates strongly with Agamben's (1998) state of exception, in which a condition of constant emergency allows the powers that be to suspend rights and exert total control—a mechanism to import the older sovereign rules into modern structures of power.

Implicit in the discussion—and much more explicit in my ongoing work with physicians and hospital workers—is the idea that the reproduction of some groups is riskier than that of others. The reproduction of indigenous Maya occurs in a dense cloud of risk, not unlike the fog that hangs over the chilly cornfields of their highland mountain communities, where distance, inaccessibility, poverty, illiteracy, and culture obscure access to biomedical facilities and blur perceptions of dangerous reproductive practices. Hospital staff I had previously interviewed in two neighboring departments (Dudgeon 2000) felt a major contributor to Guatemala's high infant and maternal mortality was the late arrival of complicated deliveries to the hospital such as those that included prolonged or obstructed labor, hemorrhaging, and asphyxia. Arriving at a health facility far into the course of the complication, many of these cases were "too late" to be managed by biomedicine. This lateness was framed as needless and exacerbated by informational and cultural barriers, including the TBA/midwife, who perhaps did not recognize the complication in time or who, along with the patient and her family, did not want to go to the hospital until the final moment (see Cosminsky this volume for an extended discussion of TBA training in Guatemala). This differential field of risk echoes Ginsburg and Rapp's (1995) use of the concept of stratified reproduction (cf. Colen 1995), by which the reproduction of members of some groups is encouraged and facilitated, while that of others is limited and hindered.

These attitudes contrast with the attitudes toward risk held by some K'iche' TBAs in the communities of Cantel. Each hamlet of that community is served by a handful of TBAs, locally known as comadronas and as *iyom* or *ilonel* (in K'iche'). Some of these TBAs practice only in the hamlet in which they live, while others may have clients spread over several communities in the municipality. Some work only with a few patients, such as members of their extended family, while others have many more clients and support themselves through their work as midwives. Some of the women are in their seventies and have been practicing for decades with little formal training, while others are in their twenties and have received government or NGO training courses but have little real-world experience. Many of them have delivered numerous infants both before and after receiving government or NGO training. While some are relatively isolated in their practice, most participate in a loosely organized guild, which focuses on facilitating training by outside groups and on soliciting material contributions. The most active TBAs and those with the highest client load tend to be in their fifties and sixties, delivering from a dozen or fewer to more than one hundred infants a year.

As informal and poorly integrated members of the biomedical obstetric care community, any interaction with other health care providers has meant for many midwives a risk to both their personal integrity and their professional credibility. Obstetric emergencies that resulted in trips to the hospital were failures for these TBAs, rather than the smooth shift in levels of care envisioned by NGOs and hospital staff (cf. Berry 2006). The antagonism and derision they met in hospitals was often humiliating, but more damaging for many was the insult to their reputations as professionals and, less commonly, the potential animosity and retribution they might face from families that had a difficult delivery or a poor delivery outcome. False alarms—trips made that are later deemed unnecessary—can be equally damaging.

The importance of professional credibility depended in large part on the zero-sum dynamics of midwifery practice in a small community, in which professional rivalries and jealousies created a fairly continuous background hum of blame and insinuation with and about other midwives. Such discourse in large part operates to maintain a hierarchy of reputation of good and bad midwives in an area in which no one midwife can attend all deliveries, but many work to function as health care providers at as high a capacity as possible. Such friction between midwives is balanced by the solidarity they maintain as a group in order to prevent other midwives from infringing on their territory and to compete as a group for positive attention from outside organizations such as the Ministry of Health and NGOs. Comadronas that work together to form groups are more likely to receive support (like funding, training, and equipment) and less likely to encounter problems when they do go to hospitals or interact with physicians, because they may develop ties with hospital staff and physicians and may, therefore, be perceived as cooperative, albeit ancillary, pieces of a larger technobureaucratic health care system (see Davis-Floyd 1996). Locally, however, comadronas negotiate the complex, risky moral landscape of relationships among the group of midwives themselves.

Traditional Birth Attendants in Guatemala

Ample evidence suggests that midwives delivered women and their neonates among indigenous Maya in Mesoamerica before contact with the Old World, and TBAs continue to attend a high percentage of births in rural Guatemala. The Guatemalan government began issuing permits to these midwives based on examinations in 1935, and Guatemala's Ministry of Health has engaged in the training of midwives since 1955. In 1969, the Maternal Child Health Division of the Ministry of Health was created, with concomitant growth of TBA training; by the mid-1970s, approximately six thousand of an estimated sixteen thousand practicing midwives had received training.

The training of TBAs has fallen from favor among international policy makers. WHO examined the training of TBAs beginning in the 1970s, promoting their integration into formal health care to extend coverage of maternal and child health services (Verderese and Turnbull 1975) into the mid-1980s. By the 1990s, however, stakeholders such as WHO had begun to shift funding away from TBA training because of its unclear impact (Replogle 2007). In *World Health Report 2005*, WHO said of TBA training that "the strategy is increasingly seen as a failure," with provision of professional skilled care the most effective intervention (WHO 2005:70).

The impact of TBA training has been difficult to assess in Guatemala and elsewhere because of the ecological nature of the intervention and the quasi-experimental assessment of outcomes before and after the intervention in or between locations where multiple other variables are left uncontrolled (and uncontrollable). Outcomes that have been assessed include improved referral by TBAs, increases in women's antenatal and emergency obstetric care, and improved maternal and neonatal mortality and morbidity. Multicountry meta-analyses of the impact of TBA training found that such training in Guatemala may have led to nonsignificant improvement in TBA knowledge and significant, if small, positive association with TBA referral and maternal use of services (Sibley, Sipe, and Koblinsky 2004) and reduction in perinatal mortality and birth asphyxia mortality (Sibley and Sipe 2004). These results were limited, however, by the quality of TBA training evaluation. Focusing on four randomized control trials, the authors found that one study reported significant reductions in stillbirths, perinatal death rate, and neonatal death rate (Sibley et al. 2007).

In 1995, only 35 percent of women in Guatemala delivered with a doctor or nurse, while 55 percent delivered with a TBA, and 10 percent delivered with a family member or alone ([Anon] 1997). In 1990, the Institute of Nutrition of Central America and Panama (INCAP) began the Maternal and Neonatal Health Project, which focused on the predominantly indigenous highland population of Quetzaltenango of approximately 150,000. This project was funded by USAID and MotherCare Project (Proyecto Cuidado Materno) of John Snow Inc. A major component of that intervention was the training of TBAs from March to May 1991 to detect, manage, and refer obstetric and neonatal emergencies and complications. Training in the region continued through the 1990s. In 1999, USAID did not renew MotherCare's funding and instead funded the Johns Hopkins affiliate, JHPIEGO. Many of the same in-country staff continued to work with the new JHPIEGO projects, with some continuity of TBA training. In analyzing the effects of the MotherCare intervention, O'Rourke (1995) found an overall increase in TBA referral after the intervention. Another study found, however, that from 1990 to 1993, the intervention might have increased referral of postpartum complications but did not seem to have had any effect on referral of obstetric and neonatal complications generally (Bailey, Szászdi, and Glover 2002).

Social science research on TBAs in Guatemala has contrasted comadronas who have received some formal training with those who attend births with knowledge and practices based on their experiences of their own pregnancies or attending the deliveries of others (see Berry 2006; Cosminsky 1982; Glei, Goldman, and Rodríguez 2003; Goldman and Glei 2003; Greenberg 1982; Maupin 2008). The distinction to some extent was based on TBAs' self-identification, but boundaries between the two categories are not rigidly fixed and have blurred over time. Many comadronas in communities like Cantel began attending births without formal training. However, during their careers as midwives, most of these women have received some formal training from either the Ministry of Health or organizations like the Institute of Nutrition of Central America and Panama (INCAP), Mother-Care, or JHPIEGO. Comadronas are generally categorized not as valuable and legitimate health care providers in their own right but as unskilled providers and auxiliary health care workers that best serve the needs of their patients in the referral of emergent complications and in the management of uncomplicated pregnancies up to the point at which biomedical health care has adequately expanded to provide those services. That being said, many Guatemalan physicians, nurses, and other allied health care providers work closely with comadronas and respect them as individual providers, even if they may not highly value their structural position as TBAs. As Hinojosa (2004) observed among Kaqchikel Maya in Guatemala, formal health care providers often value midwives primarily as a means to the ends of biomedicine rather than as legitimate health care providers. In other words, formal health care workers may pursue the administration of reproductive life *through* the comadrona rather than *by* the comadrona.

Supernatural Pacts

The distinction between trained and untrained TBAs is a contested political issue among comadronas themselves in Cantel, because registration carries with it some authority, recognition, and qualification for benefits like medical supplies. Some comadronas even distinguish between real and fake midwives, but not according to training—rather, according to destiny.

A familiar narrative throughout Latin America is the pact with the devil, in which some member of the community is said to have struck a Faustian bargain for money, sex, and power, explaining their rapid, easy, or sizeable acquisition of material goods. In his classic treatise on the subject, Taussig discusses devil pacts at sugar plantations of the Cauca Valley in western Colombia and tin mines in Oruro, Bolivia, to argue that as labor becomes commodified for rural peasant groups in the shift from household to capitalist economy, peasants lose control of the means of production, and commodities, rather than labor, appear to be the source of value and profit. Rather than suggesting envy of or repressed desire for these material goods, devil pact narratives represent moral condemnation of the clash between use-value and exchange-value, in which social relationships among things hide, replace, and supersede those among people. "Instead of reducing the devil-beliefs to the desire for material gain, anxiety, 'limited good,' and so on, why not see them in their own right with all their vividness and detail as the response of people to what they see as an evil and destructive way of ordering economic life?" (Taussig 1980:17).

In a subsequent interpretation of devil pact narratives from northern Costa Rica, Edelman emphasizes not a universal transition to agrarian capitalism and wage labor, but instead to local forms of exploitation, with a focus on the gendered and reproductive dimensions of those relations of power, such as male sexual dominance. For example, Edelman highlights an important element also contained in Taussig's analysis: the barren, transient nature of the profits of the devil pact: "Those making contracts are believed to die prematurely and in pain, land purchased with ill-gotten gains will become depleted, livestock will not thrive" (1994:59), which suggests an incompatibility of the evil fruits of devil pacts with the previous local cycles of production and reproduction. Edelman specifically notes that women do not enter into devil pacts, which may represent community fears that women's pregnancies and births may no longer be sustainable on the basis of a precapitalist economy. Women, I would argue, are not allowed to enter into narratives of deals with the devil because of the perceived threat to their reproductive capacity, such as infertility, and the frightening reproductive possibilities following such a pact. In the Costa Rican context, Edelman argues that devil-pact stories grew up around one wealthy landowner in particular and not others in part because of his sexual promiscuity, again pointing to the sex/gendered nature of devil pacts. A more general formulation is that new social and economic relations are interpreted and represented as supernatural: "The basic argument is that in rural Latin America devil-pact stories constitute a significant, nearly ubiquitous cultural matrix through which to view relations of power and exploitation and through which to express a variety of socially conditioned anxieties and psychic conflicts" (60).

Dealings with the supernatural in Latin America are not limited to the diabolical. Paul's work in San Pedro La Laguna on Lake Atitlán in the department of Sololá in the 1960s and 1970s describes the recruitment of comadronas and their roles in the community (Paul 1975, 1978; Paul and Paul 1975). Women in San Pedro, as in other communities, had dreams in which they were called by supernatural beings to become midwives and underwent illness and suffering before entering the midwife role. Paul interprets these dreams and illnesses as elements in the transformation of identity from an ordinary woman to an extraordinary midwife, resolving the identity crisis through rites of transition and psychic dramas and allowing women to overcome their husbands' resistance to their new roles. While Paul's analysis alludes to forces of modernization, both in terms of comadronas who use modern contraceptives like the birth control pill and the IUD and in the economic benefits that accrue to comadronas, she suggests that supernatural election of comadronas in large part conflicts with these modernizing trends.

More recent ethnographic work shows continuity with Paul's descriptions. In discussing beliefs and rituals among comadronas in the Kaqchikel community of San Lucas Tolimán, also on Lake Atitlán, Walsh (2006) explores three thematic domains: sacred calling, sacred knowledge, and sacred ritual. I encountered similar themes in my work in Cantel, where many, although not all, women in the *aldea* who worked as comadronas reported very similar dreams and visions in which they received direct instructions or some sign that they were destined to attend births. Kaqchikel women described having dreams or visions in which they received communication from a divine force, such as God or a saint, instructing them to become a midwife or to symbolize that they had a sacred calling. Walsh notes that all the women with whom she worked initially rejected that calling. At some later point, sometimes years after the initial call, they described falling ill and regaining their health only once they had begun their work as a comadrona.

Angel Pacts in Cantel

Doña Magdalena is a thin, soft-spoken woman who was not sure of her exact age but believed herself to be around sixty-one or sixty-two.[3] She describes herself as *muy humilde* (very humble), and indeed she made little eye contact during our discussions. Her slow answers suggested limited fluency in Spanish. Nonetheless, her answers were full and expressive, and she kept meticulous written records of her patients over time. Magdalena learned in a dream she was destined to become a comadrona.

> I had a dream. It was before there was a session for training for comadronas—sixteen years ago, maybe more. I was lifted up into the sky and there were angels. There were three girls and one man, and they were tall and had

blue eyes, and their skin was white, white, white, like yours—they looked like gringos like you. They smiled at me and gave me a little white cloth, the kind you use to clean the face of the child when it is born. Then I had another dream and I saw this same white cloth again.

She said that her husband was also having dreams at that time. He did not want his wife to work as a midwife, because it meant that she would be learning new concepts. However, he had dreams in which a doctor dressed in white came to him and said not to punish his wife but instead to allow her to work as a comadrona. In the dream, the doctor assured him that this was Magdalena's destiny and that, even though she would be learning, this was what she was supposed to do, as it would help others.

Another midwife, Doña Sebastiana, is a plump woman even by local standards, in her late forties, with a round, smiling face, tiny bright eyes, and perpetually rosy cheeks. Her husband, an even more impressively rotund man with a bushy graying beard, worked as a self-described *hombre de negocios* (businessman) as a dealer in *corte* (a textile) that he sold in Quetzaltenango. He also held a position in the municipal government. The two of them have thirteen children together, the youngest a four-year-old who would appear periodically with his siblings during our interview. When I interviewed her, Sebastiana said that she had been a midwife for eight years. She said that she started as a comadrona because a physician from INCAP had come to give a training session. All the women who attended the training session were already comadronas except for her and her friend. Before that she had never attended a birth but felt as if she could become a midwife because she had already had several pregnancies. The training lasted only five days, at the culmination of which she felt ill prepared to attend any deliveries. When she asked the physician for more training, he suggested that she observe births at the hospital. So, for the next seven months, she went several days a week to observe how deliveries took place at the regional hospital in Quetzaltenango.

Doña Romelia was fifty years old when I interviewed her. She too had been working as a comadrona for about eight years. A heavy-set, energetic woman whose hair, unlike that of many women in the community her age, had gone completely gray, she was the mother of four surviving children: a daughter who brought us a cup of hot *atole* (a corn-based beverage) during the interview and three sons. She would have had six children, but her first child died after a month and her third after eight days. She did not know exactly why they had died, but she thought that the first had had a cough, and both were small and weak when they were born and did not want to take milk. Her husband is a fifty-one-year-old field laborer who owns his own *milpa* (cornfield) but also works on occasion weaving or baking bread. Although Romelia feels that she was destined to become a comadrona, she did not feel that way because of dreams or visions. Instead, her mother had been a comadrona, and Romelia had seen how she practiced throughout her lifetime, as well as during the deliveries of Romelia's own children. One day her mother was not at home when someone came to fetch her for a delivery, so Romelia took her place. She said that first delivery was not at all difficult, and so she started working as a comadrona, with training at the hospital in Quetzaltenango on the weekends for eight months, sometimes for twelve or even twenty-four hours at a time. Romelia's mother lived with her but died while she was training. With less help at home, Romelia's husband wanted her to stop the training. Nonetheless, Romelia persisted.

Women may not recognize their dreams immediately as indicating a vocation, or they may choose not to take up the obligation of midwifery. Many women emphasize their reluctance to work as a comadrona for fear of their husband's disapproval, community gossip, and the work outside the home. However, women who avoid their destiny invariably encounter problems like bad luck or failing health. Such was the case for Doña Francisca, who, at fifty-two, towers over many of the other women in the community. Despite her size, Francisca is a quiet woman who enjoys talking about the months she spent in the United States visiting a son and working as a housekeeper. While there, and upon her return to Guatemala, she thought she would not continue as a midwife: "For several years I decided that I no longer wanted to be a comadrona. However, I became sick. My back hurt, and I had no energy. I did not know what was wrong, but a *kamal b'e* (traditional healer) told me that it was my destiny to be a comadrona, and if I avoided it I would always suffer. It is a burden, to work this way, but I have to do it."

These narratives of sacred calling—what I term "angel pact" narratives—parallel those of devil pacts but with some important structural oppositional qualities beyond the dichotomy of good and evil. These are women rather than men. Men in the community may also discuss themselves as involved in a sacred calling, in particular men who work as Mayan priests (*sacerdotes Maya* or *kamal b'e*). But in both Taussig's (1980) and Edelman's (1994) discussions, women did not participate in devil pacts, and for Edelman the aspect of reproduction and fertility associated with women was of particular importance to the social practice of assigning devil pacts. The comadronas in my study profess to have received the sacred calling and entered into service themselves, rather than ascribing the narrative to someone else. These women were all reluctant to follow a sacred calling that was thrust upon them. Rather than eager to seek out a deal, they saw their pact as a burden to be avoided rather than a boon, and as an offer that was unavoidable. In contrast, it is the consequences of the bargain, not the deal itself, that become the unavoidable destiny of the bargainer in a devil pact.

The comadronas work for the benefit of others rather than themselves through a positive, divine force, while in the devil pact the gains accrue directly to the individual bargainer. Although the maker of the devil pact may choose to share some of his wealth, the overall effect of the presence of the diabolical in the community is a negative one. Finally, while both sets of narratives include a departure from baseline, the negative and positive effects of the agreement occur at very different times in the narrative. In the devil pact, the positive benefits are immediate, but the long-term consequences are stagnation, ruination, and ultimately damnation. For comadronas, it is the initial rejection of the offer that has demonstrable negative consequences in terms of health and well-being, while the benefits accrued for accepting the sacred calling may be somewhat equivocal. Many of the midwives I interviewed were straightforward about enjoying their work and spoke with pride about their proficiency as comadronas. Some worked to translate that into other areas of women's health and advocacy, both within the group of comadronas and in the community. But many women also professed that their activities were an ongoing burden from which they would seek reprieve if it did not mean forfeiting their health.

However, similar to devil-pact narratives, these angel-pact narratives do aid in the interpretation of changing social relations along several dimensions, as they work to resolve and justify some contradictions in the work of comadronas. When women become comadronas, they enter into a vocation that carries both responsibilities and respect. They become responsible for attending births and delivering infants, a painful and difficult process with unique risks and potentially horrible outcomes. That vocation, if it is their true calling, confers on them the right to walk freely in the streets at any time of night or day, an autonomy denied most women. They are also allowed to enter into a community of other women, many of whom become strong friends and allies through their work as comadronas. Finally, women who work as comadronas, now more than in the past, enter into relations with their patients in which they are paid for their services. Most midwives acknowledge that, in the past, comadronas might receive some reciprocity, such as a meal or some local produce for their services. Now, most have a payment scale according to which they either charge a fixed fee for antenatal visits, delivery, and postpartum massages and steam baths, or charge per visit, with a larger fee for delivery. Some women go so far as to say that the receipt of money, or large sums of money, for work as a comadrona is *awa's* (K'iche') or *pecado* (Spanish), that is, a sin.

The angel-pact narratives help justify this different position comadronas hold in the community with respect to other women, while they continue to operate as women in what has been in Cantel a very woman-centered sphere of knowledge and practice. Angel-pact narratives allow women to negotiate the risks inherent in the local, shifting moral economy surrounding their work as women, as well as the changing risks of operating as medical providers in a field increasingly penetrated by governmental and nongovernmental administrators of maternal and infant health. Comadronas mobilize these narratives to complement and to resist government and NGO programs for training comadronas, pointing to an authority beyond those programs that legitimates their own practice—with respect both to less authentic comadronas who have been trained but were not called, and to the biomedical model of pregnancy and delivery, which would question their abilities to deliver infants safely and without complication or to recognize complications should they occur.

Interestingly, there are elements of the devil pact in comadrona discussions of their practice and their reflections on the practice of other comadronas in Cantel who use oxytocin. Oxytocin is a hormone naturally produced during labor that strengthens uterine contractions, and a synthetic analog of oxytocin can be administered to facilitate birth. Injections of oxytocin are widely used by many comadronas with whom I worked to induce or speed labor and delivery, often at the request of the laboring woman and her family, despite cautions against this practice in TBA training sessions because of the difficulties in dosing. While no comadrona will admit to using oxytocin herself, many I interviewed were more than willing to indict other comadronas. What follows is a conversation I had with one comadrona that was repeated in its general outline with many others.

> Matthew Dudgeon: Do you ever use injections during delivery?
> Comadrona X: No, I never use injections [of oxytocin].
> Matthew: Do you know anyone who does?
> Comadrona X: Oh, many do [lists some names]. . . . You know who uses it a lot? [Name]. She has so many patients that she is running back and forth between deliveries, so she will give the injection to one patient to hurry [the delivery] up, then she goes to the other delivery.

Most comadronas I interviewed gave similar answers to questions about the use of injections to hasten deliveries, and some preferred not to answer the question at all. Accusations of the use of oxytocin are associated with the distinctions made between real and study-only comadronas. Those destined to deliver babies need not use oxytocin, while those who have merely studied use the drug because of their lack of natural ability and sacred calling. Indeed, some midwives' use of biomedical technology may raise questions as to their authenticity—provoking claims that they have entered into a kind of devilish pact with a medical system that shuns the ways of the traditional comadrona and her belief in the supernatural forces that keep risk at bay.

Men and Destiny

My complementary research on men's influences on the household production of reproductive health afforded me the opportunity to talk with men, women, and comadronas about the different roles they perceived men played during pregnancy and delivery and in child care. While few of my closest male informants had direct experience with obstetric emergencies, some had heard of instances in which women had been taken to the hospital during childbirth, and many had strong opinions about the proper course of action in such an emergency. Among couples that received prenatal care from comadronas, the vast majority of both men and women expressed views on the subject of complications during delivery ranging from absolutely no travel to a hospital under any circumstances to having an emergency transport plan in place. I want to focus here on some of the dynamics of the decision-making process in obstetric emergencies, with attention to men's roles.

A number of recent quantitative studies in western Guatemala have discussed the importance of considering multiple actors, including men, in analyses of decisions surrounding delivery complications. Fonseca-Becker et al. (2004) found that men are the primary decision makers about the use of biomedical care in obstetric emergencies, with mothers-in-law and comadronas also exerting influence. Carter (2002) found that women reported their husbands to be the principal decision maker in emergencies that required immediate use of funds. Becker,

Fonseca-Becker, and Schenck-Yglesias (2006) reported that most women were included in a variety of decisions, among them, household purchases, child illness, medicine purchases, and obstetric emergency, but fully 38 percent of couples were concordant in reporting that the wife was not involved in the final decision in obstetric emergencies. Moreover, these women tended to underestimate rather than overestimate their role in decisions relative to their husbands' reports. Collectively, these studies point to the privileged position many men occupy in households in western highland Guatemala.

My own qualitative interview data with men, women, and comadronas provide context for these survey data. When asked about decision making in the household relative to emergent situations such as an obstetric emergency, many men state that others in the household might be involved in the decision to go to a doctor or hospital, including a comadrona, a female relative (sometimes that same comadrona) such as his mother or the mother of his wife, or a male relative such as his father or the father of his wife. Men's comments suggest that relatives are more likely to be involved if the couple lives with those relatives, especially if the couple is younger or if this is the woman's first pregnancy. As in the quantitative studies, men's responses to questions about decisions to go to a hospital or physician varied from including their wives or deferring to them completely to maintaining that they would make the decision themselves in such an event. Many men said that, because she was the health care provider attending the delivery, the comadrona would necessarily be involved in the decision, if not herself the decision maker.

An important distinction I found in men's comments about obstetric emergencies and reproductive decision making in general (e.g., contraception use, pregnancy timing, family size, etc.) was that, while many men said that women should be included in decisions, and that they in fact did include them in reproductive decisions, ultimate authority in making and executing those decisions lay with the husband. Many men felt that their wives' opinions were valuable and that discussing such matters as reproductive decision making *entre las chamarras* (literally "between the covers," or in bed with one's partner) could improve a relationship and build trust and intimacy. However, the final authority rested with the man; were the couple to disagree about a decision, his would necessarily be the last word in the matter.

Returning to the specific example of emergency obstetric decisions, comadronas agree that men exert authority in such situations, and several cited examples in which they had to argue, plead, or in some cases bargain with husbands to prompt transport to a biomedical provider (see Cosminsky, this volume). Doña Elena, a youthful-at-fiftyish comadrona as well as local contraceptive provider, told of how she had, in the face of refusals from a husband, written up on the spot a "legal document" she asked him to sign absolving her of responsibility, at which point he acquiesced. Men's authority could be swayed or subverted, but it was a reality comadronas acknowledged.

At the same time, men acknowledge the authority—and the authoritative knowledge (Davis-Floyd and Sargent 1997)—of the comadrona within the domain of pregnancy and childbirth. Many men do not equivocate in expressing that pregnancy and childbirth are *cosas de las mujeres* (women's things) and, while they may be present in the house during a delivery, the details are best left to the professional—the comadrona. Men occupy, therefore, a tenuous position in which they have both given over and maintain authority simultaneously, and that tenuous position becomes less tenable in an obstetric emergency in which they may be quickly required to make decisions about a process they have remained apart from, in accordance with longstanding mores regarding women's privacy during childbirth (Cosminsky 1982; Paul 1974; Ruz 2000).

The cultural logic of the angel pact—the call to service—operates in such moments both to legitimate the decision making of the comadrona and to contradict the imperative of biomedical intervention. Midwives who have received a spiritual call can take a more authoritative position than those who have not in the households in which they deliver—their knowledge and practice based on a mutually understood foundation of divine inspiration and intervention. Yet midwives who have been called should, therefore, be less likely to encounter complications and more capable of surmounting them when they do, obviating the need for biomedicine. While men were less explicit on this point, my impression was that the authority of called comadronas with established records of successful deliveries continues to leverage their influence on men's decisions in obstetric emergencies, while comadronas who have training but do not subscribe to a calling may be more likely to be challenged by men (or other family members) in the event of an obstetric emergency. Under such circumstances a called comadrona may be brought in to manage the emergency, which may resolve under her supervision or may progress to emergency transport but with further delay. The importance of the angel-pact narrative and its disruption of typical gendered patterns of decision making, however, goes to the heart of the attending deliveries in the context of masculine authority.

Conclusion: Risk and Reproduction in Guatemala

Variations in the meaning of risk among different groups of health providers point to the distinct vested interests of those stakeholders. Health care professionals, physicians, NGO workers, and TBAs operate as mediators of the risky state of pregnancy and childbirth. Yet each of these groups operationalizes risk differently. As has been pointed out by physician informants, NGOs may appear to expand definitions of risk to justify their projects, vacillating among different poles of risk (midwife training, quality control, emergency plans) and perpetuating a state of emergency, albeit local and focal. Physicians and hospital workers, as purveyors of biomedicine, focus instead on the heroic mastery of risk when it arises as pathology rather than on its constant presence as part of normal pregnancy. However, hospitals may also recognize the limits of their resources and abilities. Knowing that they cannot possibly handle the patient load, they in fact depend heavily on the labor of TBAs to manage the vast majority of uncomplicated deliveries.

Moreover, health care providers occupy different locations in the field of obstetric risk. In particular, TBAs, unlike their physician and NGO counterparts, maintain highly risky positions because of their occupations. In the angel-pact narratives, comadronas manage the risks that their practices pose *to themselves*: the risk of poor outcome within the community, as well as the risks they encounter as marginalized health care providers.

For hospital and NGO workers who are caught between biomedicine and traditional birth practices, risk serves as a merographic bridge (Davis-Floyd and Sargent 1997); medicalized risk factors differ from lay discourse insofar as they encompass and extend beyond what TBAs are trained to recognize and rectify. For physicians, risk captures the moment of transition of the division of labor from comadronas to hospitals, and indicates when a delivery should pass from the one to the other. The uneven distribution of danger between bodies—calculated, assessed, and managed through quality assurance—brings with it the forensic threats of accountability and compensation. For many Guatemalan physicians, this means excluding pregnant Maya women and their midwives until a moment of crisis is reached. From the more global perspective of the NGO worker, that state of exception extends to the entirety of pregnancy and birth, including the provision of health care.

Ultimately, Maya women and the comadronas who attend them remain objects of administration and repositories of blame. The risks they run in their own communities are often minimized, unattended, or obscured by the management of the statistical risks of reproduction. Angel-pact narratives emerge, I argue, as TBAs resist the biomedicalization of their field and negotiate competition among themselves in an occupation that is, as a cultural ideal, without personal reward. The shadow of oxytocin parallels devil pacts as an extranatural explanation for ill-gotten rewards and exploitation of natural abilities. Rather than lying outside the forces of modernization, however, angel-pact narratives, like their devil-pact counterparts, show the connections between traditional roles like that of the midwife and the powers of the Guatemalan state and capitalism. Finally, because the role of the comadrona requires ongoing negotiation of one's position in a field of competing midwives, many comadronas' identity and authenticity are constantly redreamed or threatened by illness rather than accomplished once and for all.

Acknowledgments

I would like to thank the physicians of the Ministry of Health in Quetzaltenango who worked with me during my fieldwork, as well as the physicians of JHPIEGO who helped make my fieldwork possible. I would especially like to thank the families of Cantel, in particular the comadronas, who opened their homes to share their stories over a hot cup of *atole*.

Notes

1. I use the terms "traditional birth attendant," "midwife," and "*comadrona*" somewhat interchangeably here, referring to (predominantly) women without extended, formal biomedical training who attend births. I distinguish these women's levels of training when relevant.
2. Funding for fieldwork in Cantel was provided by the National Science Foundation and Fulbright-Hays/Department of Education.
3. All names are fictitious.

References

[Anon]
   1997   Guatemala 1995: Results from the Demographic and Health Survey. Studies in Family Planning 28(2):151–55.
Agamben, Giorgio
   1998   Homo Sacer: Sovereign Power and Bare Life. Stanford, CA: Stanford University Press.
Bailey, Patricia, José Szászdi, and Lucinda Glover
   2002   Obstetric Complications: Does Training Traditional Birth Attendants Make a Difference? Revista Panamericana de Salud Pública 11(1):15–23.
Becker, Stan, Fannie Fonseca-Becker, and Catherine Schenck-Yglesias
   2006   Husbands' and Wives' Reports of Women's Decision-Making Power in Western Guatemala and Their Effects on Preventive Health Behaviors. Social Science and Medicine 62(9):2313–26.
Berry, Nicole
   2006   Kaqchikel Midwives, Home Births, and Emergency Obstetric Referrals in Guatemala: Contextualizing the Choice to Stay at Home. Social Science and Medicine 62(8):1958–69.
Carter, Marion
   2002   Husbands and Maternal Health Matters in Rural Guatemala: Wives' Reports on Spouses' Involvement in Pregnancy and Birth. Social Science and Medicine 55(3):437–50.
Central Intelligence Agency (CIA)
   2011   The World Factbook. www.cia.gov/library/publications/the-world-factbook/index.html, accessed February 16, 2011.
Colen, Shellee
   1995   "Like a Mother to Them": Stratified Reproduction and West Indian Childcare Workers and Employers in New York. *In* Conceiving the New World Order: The Global Politics of Reproduction. Faye Ginsburg and Rayna Rapp, eds. Pp. 78–102. Berkeley: University of California Press.
Cosminsky, Sheila
   1982   Childbirth and Change: A Guatemalan Study. *In* Ethnography of Fertility and Birth. Pp. 205–29. London: Academic Press.
Davis-Floyd, Robbie
   1996   The Technocratic Body and the Organic Body: Hegemony and Heresy in Women's Birth Choices. *In* Gender and Health: An International Perspective.

Carolyn Sargent and Caroline Brettel, eds. Pp. 123–66. Upper Saddle River, NJ: Prentice Hall.

Davis-Floyd, Robbie, and Carolyn Sargent
  1997   Introduction: The Anthropology of Birth. *In* Childbirth and Authoritative Knowledge: Cross-Cultural Perspectives. Robbie Davis-Floyd and Carolyn Sargent, eds. Pp. 1–51. Berkeley: University of California Press.

Dudgeon, Matthew
  2000   Slippery Subjects: Reproductive Health in International Health Discourse and Highland Guatemala. Annual Meeting of the Society of Medical Anthropology, San Francisco. November 15–19.

Edelman, Marc
  1994   Landlords and the Devil: Class, Ethnic, and Gender Dimensions of Central American Peasant Narratives. Cultural Anthropology 9(1):58–93.

Fonseca-Becker, F., O. Cordon, C. Schenck-Yglesias, L. Hurtado,
R. Valladares, and R. Ainslie
  2004   Case Study Report: Impact Evaluation, Community Mobilization and Behavior Change, Maternal and Neonatal Health Component, Ministry of Health and Public Assistance of Guatemala. Baltimore: Johns Hopkins University, Bloomberg School of Public Health, Center for Communication Programs. www.jhuccp .org/sites/all/files/Case%20Study-Impact%20Evaluation,%20Community%20 Mobilization%20and%20BC%20MNH.pdf, accessed June 11, 2011.

Ginsburg, Faye, and Rayna Rapp
  1995   Introduction: Conceiving the New World Order. *In* Conceiving the New World Order: The Global Politics of Reproduction. Faye Ginsburg and Rayna Rapp, eds. Pp. 1–17. Berkeley: University of California Press.

Glei, Dana, Noreen Goldman, and Germán Rodríguez
  2003   Utilization of Care during Pregnancy in Rural Guatemala: Does Obstetrical Need Matter? Social Science and Medicine 57(12):2447–63.

Goldman, Noreen, and Dana Glei
  2003   Evaluation of Midwifery Care: Results from a Survey in Rural Guatemala. Social Science and Medicine 56(4):685–700.

Grandin, Greg
  2000   The Blood of Guatemala: A History of Race and Nation. Durham, NC: Duke University Press.

Greenberg, Linda
  1982   Midwife Training Programs in Highland Guatemala. Social Science and Medicine 16(18):1599–1609.

Handy, Jim
  1984   Gift of the Devil: A History of Guatemala. Boston: South End Press.

Hinojosa, Servando
  2004   Authorizing Tradition: Vectors of Contention in Highland Maya Midwifery. Social Science and Medicine 59(3):637–51.

Maupin, Jonathan
  2008   Remaking the Guatemalan Midwife: Health Care Reform and Midwifery Training Programs in Highland Guatemala. Medical Anthropology 27(4):353–82.
  2009   "Fruit of the Accords": Healthcare Reform and Civil Participation in Highland Guatemala. Social Science and Medicine 68(8):1456–63.

Ministry of Health and Public Assistance, Proyecto de Salud Materna y Neonatal,
Center for Communication, and JHPIEGO.
  2004   Impact Evaluation: Community Mobilization and Behavior Change, Maternal
          and Neonatal Health Component, Ministry of Health and Public Assistance. Case
          Study. Johns Hopkins University, Bloomberg School of Public Health, Center for
          Communication Programs.
O'Rourke, Kathleen
  1995   The Effect of Hospital Staff Training on Management of Obstetrical Patients
          Referred by Traditional Birth Attendants. International Journal of Gynecology
          and Obstetrics 48 Suppl.:S95–S102.
Paul, Lois
  1974   The Mastery of Work and the Mystery of Sex in a Guatemalan Village. *In*
          Women, Culture, and Society. Michelle Zimbalist Rosaldo and Louise Lamphere,
          eds. Pp. 281–99. Stanford, CA: Stanford University Press.
  1975   Recruitment to a Ritual Role: The Midwife in a Maya Community. Ethos
          3(3):449–67.
  1978   Careers of Midwives in a Mayan Community. *In* Women in Ritual and Symbolic
          Roles. Judith Hoch-Smith and Anita Spring, eds. Pp. 129–50. New York:
          Plenum.
Paul, Lois, and Benjamin David Paul
  1975   The Maya Midwife as Sacred Specialist: A Guatemalan Case. *In* American
          Ethnologist. 2(4):707–26.
Replogle, Jill
  2007   Training Traditional Birth Attendants in Guatemala. Lancet 369(9557):177–78.
Ruz, Mario Humberto
  2000   The Seeds of Man: Ethnological Notes on Male Sexuality and Fecundity among
          the Maya. *In* Fertility and the Male Life-Cycle in the Era of Fertility Decline.
          Caroline Bledsoe, Jane Guyer, and Susana Lerner, eds. Pp. 93–118. New York:
          Oxford University Press.
Sibley, Lynn, and Theresa Ann Sipe
  2004   What Can a Meta-Analysis Tell Us about Traditional Birth Attendant Training
          and Pregnancy Outcomes? Midwifery 20(1):51–60.
Sibley, Lynn, Theresa Ann Sipe, Carolyn Brown, Melissa Diallo, Kathryn McNatt,
and Nancy Habarta
  2007   Traditional Birth Attendant Training for Improving Health Behaviours and
          Pregnancy Outcomes. Cochrane Database of Systematic Reviews (3):CD005460.
Sibley, Lynn, Theresa Ann Sipe, and Marge Koblinsky
  2004   Does Traditional Birth Attendant Training Improve Referral of Women with
          Obstetric Complications: A Review of the Evidence. Social Science and Medicine
          59(8):1757–68.
Suarez-Berenguela, Ruben
  2001   Health System Inequalities and Inequities in Latin America and the Caribbean:
          Findings and Policy Implications. *In* Investment in Health: Social and Economic
          Returns. Pp. 119–42. Washington, DC: Pan American Health Organization.
Taussig, Michael
  1980   The Devil and Commodity Fetishism in South America. Chapel Hill: University
          of North Carolina Press.

Verderese, Maria de Lourdes, and Lily Turnbull
   1975   The Traditional Birth Attendant in Maternal and Child Health and Family
          Planning. Geneva: World Health Organization.
Walsh, Linda
   2006   Beliefs and Rituals in Traditional Birth Attendant Practice in Guatemala. Journal
          of Transcultural Nursing 17(2):148–54.
WHO
   2005   World Health Report 2005—Make Every Mother and Child Count. Geneva:
          World Health Organization.

CHAPTER 2

Failing to See the Danger

Conceptions of Pregnancy and Care Practices among Mexican Immigrant Women in New York City

Alyshia Gálvez

Rosa migrated from Puebla's state capital three years before becoming pregnant and seeking prenatal care at Manhattan Hospital.[1] I asked her if she planned to have anesthesia during labor and delivery. While her husband massaged her back, she told me she did not.

> Alyshia: ¿Y anestesia por qué no quiere?
> Rosa: No sé, me gustaría sentir a mi bebé. Pienso que para eso se arriesga
> uno a tener bebes. Si no, ¿qué . . . qué chiste?

> [Alyshia: And why don't you want anesthesia?
> Rosa: I don't know, I'd like to feel my baby. I think that is the reason
> that one risks having babies. If not, what is the point?]

In New York City, babies born to native Mexican women have lower rates of low birth weight and infant mortality than do many other groups, in spite of a greater incidence of the risk factors associated with these problems—a phenomenon known as the "birth weight paradox." However, as such women continue to live in the United States, this cultural advantage wears off, and birth outcomes begin to resemble those of other similarly situated socioeconomic groups. Based on an ethnographic study involving just over one hundred women in a public prenatal clinic at Manhattan Hospital as well as sites outside of institutionalized medicine in New York City, and in Oaxaca and Puebla States, Mexico, I argue here that Mexican immigrant women often share a view of pregnancy as something they are well equipped to accomplish successfully, without any special intervention.[2] Even while they enthusiastically seek what they view as a modern, technologically advanced model of prenatal care (see Howes-Mischel, this volume; cf. Smith-Oka, this volume), they demonstrate some immunity to the view commonly held by providers: that pregnancy and childbirth are inherently risky and to be successful require the management of skilled medical personnel and assessment and mediation of risk factors. The rise in unfavorable birth outcomes with longer residence in or nativity in the United States may be not a biological problem but an epistemological one, in which women are slowly convinced of the riskiness of their own reproduction and come to behave in ways that erode their cultural advantage.

In the interchange at the start of this chapter, Rosa reveals a view common to the participants in this study. Most women interviewed expressed disinclination toward pain medication during labor, as well as a generally negative view of the use of medications, some fetal diagnostic tests, and routine interventions during pregnancy and delivery. Although providers praise Mexican patients for their purported stoicism and docility during pregnancy and labor, I found that many women I interviewed had pronounced contrary views about some of the protocols of prenatal care and labor and delivery that are routine in contemporary biomedical settings. While many of the women in the study eagerly embraced the prenatal care they received, viewing it as more modern, humane, and advanced than the care they might have been able to access in Mexico, they did not unquestioningly consume prenatal care but actively rejected some central components of it. The patterns evident in the aspects of care that women critiqued and rejected reveal certain commonly held ideas about pregnancy and an agentive approach to health care consumption.

As I describe some of the contentions over risk between the biomedical model of care provided in Manhattan's clinic and the norms and expectations of many Mexican immigrant women, it will become apparent that even while Mexican immigrant women are enthusiastic about accessing what they view as a modern and technologically well-equipped hospital, entrance into this mode of care does not erase their deeply rooted understandings of pregnancy and childbirth as something they were born to successfully accomplish. On the contrary, their epistemologies of pregnancy indicate that they negotiate the care they receive in the hospital under certain suppositions about their own abilities to have a healthy pregnancy and successful labor and delivery. These suppositions may be protective and may partly explain the birth weight paradox. Nonetheless, they complicate the relationship between prenatal care providers who follow a medicalized perinatal script and Mexican immigrant women who have their own ideas about what constitutes a healthy diet, views on chemical pain relief and the consumption of medicines during pregnancy and childbirth, and opinions on cesarean section and other increasingly routine interventions during delivery.

Methods

This chapter is based on a multisited ethnographic research study that employed several qualitative methods, including participant-observation, surveys, and life history interviews, as well as quantitative analysis of individual medical records, public vital statistics, and census data. In New York City, participants were found at a major public hospital's prenatal clinic in Manhattan and at a community service organization in Queens, as well as through the snowball method. In Mexico, research occurred in both rural and urban settings in Oaxaca and Puebla states. Research was conducted over two years, from 2006 to 2008, with one- to four-month intensive periods in each location, and informal interviews over a longer period.

In all, approximately one hundred Mexican immigrant women participated in New York City. All but one of the women were immigrants born in Mexico. The exception was a nineteen-year-old woman interviewed during her second pregnancy who was born in New York to Mexican immigrant parents. On average, women in the study had migrated four and a half years before our first interview. They had lived in the United States for from three months to twenty-one years. A few women migrated as children (the 1.5 generation). Research among Mexicans in New York City offers a snapshot of a recent immigrant community in which first-generation immigrants are still an overwhelming majority.

In addition to pregnant women and mothers, I interviewed more than a dozen health care professionals or accompanied them in their clinical practice, including midwives, obstetricians, nutritionists, social workers, nurses, and physician's assistants in the public hospital in New York, as well as a general practitioner, two midwives, and a botanist in the Río Blanco neighborhood of Oaxaca City; Ixtlán de Juárez, Oaxaca; and San Antonio Texcala and Zapotitlán Salinas, Puebla. All but one of the participating practitioners were women. These interviews and participant-observations were aimed at identifying some of the opinions and perceptions of health care providers toward the patients in their care. While the emphasis in this study is on pregnant women's practices and experiences, I viewed it also as important for the providers to have an opportunity to share their views. In Mexico, I interviewed a few practitioners with the aim of learning about the political economy of prenatal care and childbirth in immigrant sending communities. Further, I asked them to give providers' perspectives on practices particular to the region that are associated with prenatal care and childbirth, including the use of herbs and thermal baths.

Background

The purported cultural advantage of Mexican immigrant women in pregnancy and childbirth is the puzzle identified by epidemiologists as the "birth weight paradox" (Buekens et al. 2000; also Hayes-Bautista 2002; Forbes and Frisbie 1991; Guendelman and Abrams 1995; Hessol and Fuentes-Afflick 2000; Landale et al. 2000; Liu and Laraque 2006; Morenoff 2000:12; Palloni and Arias 2004; Palloni and Morenoff 2001). This is a subset of the "immigrant paradox" by which first-generation immigrants have more favorable health indicators than their U.S.-born counterparts in spite of a high prevalence of risk factors (Abraído-Lanza et al. 1999; Alegría et al. 2007; Forbes and Frisbie 1991; Landale et al. 1999; Rumbaut and Weeks 1996; Shai and Rosenwaike 1987; Sorlie 1993; and Taningco 2007). The immigrant paradox is comprised of subsets including the "Hispanic" or "Latino paradox," that is, Latino immigrants demonstrate an advantage over U.S.-born Latinos and other groups on a number of health indicators.

According to research studies on the birth weight paradox, mothers born in Mexico tend in the United States to have lower rates of pregnancy complications, such as low birth weight, premature births, intrauterine growth retardation, and infant mortality, than might be predicted by their "disadvantageous risk profiles" (Buekens et al. 2000; Cramer 1987; Forbes and Frisbie 1991; Hessol and Fuentes-Afflick 2000; Landale, Oropesa, and Gorman 2000; Liu and Laraque 2006; Morenoff 2000:12; Palloni and Morenoff 2001). This rupture in the formula that "wealth equals health" is considered paradoxical, first, because it conflicts with expectations that poorer women with greater incidence of risk factors will have more complicated pregnancies and childbirths, and, second, because this protection declines over time and across generations, that is, greater assimilation results in worse outcomes (Guendelman and Abrams 1995; Hayes-Bautista 2002).

The risk factors associated with low birth weight and infant death cited in studies of the birth weight paradox include socioeconomic and behavioral correlates such as low income, low levels of education, late or no prenatal care, teen mother or advanced maternal age, unmarried mother, and lack of access to health insurance. While more strictly medical causes such as maternal infection or other health problems, placental problems, and birth defects are associated with low birth weight and infant death, they are not considered elements of the birth weight paradox. In turn, the protective factors that have been hypothesized to contribute to the favorable birth outcomes of Latina immigrant women include cultural factors like diet, social support, religious faith, and positive attitudes regarding pregnancy (Fernández and Newby 2010; Fuentes-Afflick, Hessol, and Perez-Stable 1999; Guendelman and Abrams 1995; Harley 2004; Hessol and Fuentes-Afflick 2000; Scribner and Dwyer 1989; Sherraden and Barrera 1996). How cultural and behavioral correlates translate into biological outcomes in the perinatal period is a mystery larger than the puzzle surrounding the birth weight paradox (Conley, Strully, and Bennet 2003). Even more puzzling are the ways in which risk calculation can amount to risk attribution and event-risk accretion. Although this chapter does not resolve this puzzle, it provides clues that inserting risk into families' understandings of reproduction can heighten reproductive risk, even while activating protocols designed to minimize risk.

Risk

How might risk calculation contribute, paradoxically, to greater risk in the perinatal context? Operating under etiologies of pregnancy that do not conceive of pregnancy as an inherently dangerous endeavor, many Mexican immigrant women ignore or reject providers' classification of their pregnancies as risky, and with good reason: their birth outcomes are enviably favorable compared to those of many other groups. Nonetheless, in public prenatal care settings like Manhattan Hospital, they are subject to care protocols that may inject their pregnancy experiences with concepts of risk that can ultimately be detrimental to the norms of self-care with which they migrated.

The ever more elaborate calculation of risk is one of the great accomplishments of contemporary epidemiology. Rather than making assumptions about health-fulness, behavior, habits, and genetics based on specious racialized categories and overly simplified health indicators, or subjecting all patients to a one-size-fits-all, prohibitively expensive, highly interventionist model of care, public health care providers' risk calculations allow a greater degree of customization based on specific indicators that an individual is likely to experience a given complication, disease, or other problem. Nonetheless, the very nature of public health and epidemiology requires the grouping and categorization of individuals, presumably for the greater good, in terms of treatment, allocation of resources, and disease prevention. Such grouping necessarily elides individual variation, and the logic of any categorization can be questionable. Even setting aside the systems for categorizing social groups, the calculation of risk in itself is not as transparent or objective as it might seem. Mary Douglas articulated an influential anthropological critique of risk as cul-turally embedded and socially constructed (1985, 1992; Douglas and Wildavsky 1982). And Rapp, in her work on prenatal diagnostic testing, found a tremendous amount of variability in the ways that prenatal patients interpreted the calculations of risk made for them—such as the mathematical probabilities that a child may be born with a disability indicated in prenatal testing (2000; for further critiques of risk, see Bridges 2011:198; Glick Schiller 1992; Layne 1996:648n56; Martin 1994; Rabinow 1992; Susser 1973).

Mexican immigrant women may harbor different attitudes about risk than those of their care providers in public prenatal clinics. Sesia (1996) noted that risk was a largely unknown concept for the Oaxacan midwives with whom she conducted research. Mexican immigrant women living in New York City and con-suming public prenatal care do not have the luxury of ignoring epidemiological formulations of risk, but they may operate under different assumptions than those of their providers. Nelkin posits that risk is a "surrogate issue, a proxy for many other concerns," that is, "the way people interpret risks and benefits may be influ-enced less by the details of scientific evidence than by social, political and ethical concerns, and especially by questions of participation and control" (2003:viii).

Indeed, in spite of being bombarded with constant information regarding the ways that their pregnancies were or were not anticipated to be risky in the pre-natal clinic—the tracking of care into distinct high- and low-risk protocols, the frequency and mandatory nature of interactions with health educators, nurses, nu-tritionists, and social workers—Mexican immigrant patients subscribed to their own notions about the relative riskiness or lack thereof of their pregnancies. The vast majority of women reported that their mothers and grandmothers (and some-times their sisters and the women themselves) delivered babies without complica-tions in settings far more technologically primitive. While they described life in New York City as posing challenges to their efforts to care for their pregnancies as they knew how to do, it also brought benefits, especially increased buying power and access to hospital-based prenatal care and delivery. Increased buying power is primarily linked in interviews with the ability to overcome the food insecurity with which many women described growing up and living in Mexico. Women who said they felt the need to quiet their cravings because of economic constraints during pregnancies in Mexico described indulging them in New York, with these cravings often interpreted as the baby, or the body, asking for a needed nutrient.

Importantly, Frank and Hummer (2002) have found that migration is correlated with favorable birth outcomes even for those who do not migrate: infants born in households in Mexico with members who have migrated are less likely to be born low birth weight than infants in nonmigrant households. Results from this study indicate that recent migrants may enjoy favorable pregnancy outcomes in part because they do what they learned to do to care for their pregnancies from their mothers and grandmothers, enabled by the additional resources afforded by their own and their partners' better-remunerated work in the United States. In this way, they describe their pregnancies in the United States as being favored by greater economic means and access to biomedical prenatal care, without altering their notions of pregnancy as an endeavor they are equipped to successfully accomplish.

Some women therefore view the risk of complications as lessened by their migration. Women who have been told they might consider additional prenatal diagnostic testing to determine the probability of occurrence for chromosomal irregularities, for example, may refuse such tests on the grounds that "no one in my family has had a baby with problems," and that, if anything, receiving technologically advanced medical care meant they were at less risk than were their female relatives in Mexico (cf. Browner, Preloran, and Cox 1999).

Women in my study placed a far greater emphasis on care practices for the laboring and postpartum mother and child than on gestation. Care practices associated with pregnancy were remarkably simple, with the advice most women describe receiving reducible to a few simple mandates: eat well, walk a lot, and do not carry heavy things. Women in this study did not explicitly remark on pregnancy as being less susceptible to intervention than childbirth and the postpartum period; however, if following Ivry, the practices and attitudes associated with gestation are examined, we may locate among the population included in this study certain "etiologies of fetal [and maternal] health and illness" (2010:233). While pregnancy is not an illness, nor is it inherently dangerous under normal circumstances, it is thought that certain complications may arise during gestation and labor that require supervision by specialists.

In discussing theories about pregnancy and childbirth among women living in rural Mexico and migrants from there, we might even choose to discard Ivry's (2010) claim that "etiologies" refers, by definition, to origins of an illness or disease. Maternal health and illness have not necessarily been considered together in rural Mexican contexts historically, although with greater diffusion of biomedical models of obstetric care, risk is certainly more commonly discussed today (Howes-Mischel, this volume). When women describe caring for themselves and obtaining care from others during pregnancy, then, they do not necessarily do so within a context of implicit risk. These benign views of pregnancy accompany women to the United States but are almost immediately countered upon arrival to public prenatal care settings with implications that pregnancy, especially pregnancies of women with so many risk factors, is inherently dangerous (Smith-Oka, this volume).

Pregnancy and Prenatal Care in General

Columba migrated only seven months before I met her at Manhattan Hospital. She was twenty weeks into her fourth pregnancy. She left her elder three children in Ocuapa, Guerrero, in the care of her mother after asking her partner to help her migrate because of economic necessity, as the remittances he was sending were not sufficient for their children's needs. Twenty-four years old and one of the youngest of thirteen siblings, she was the only member of her natal family to migrate. She worked sewing in a textile factory. As soon as the baby was born, she hoped to return to Mexico.

Before she migrated to the United States, Columba explained, her first three children were delivered by her mother at home. I asked her how her mother knew how to deliver babies, and she said that her grandmother had been a *partera* (empirical midwife), and also her mother had herself given birth to thirteen children. When I asked if her mother knew how to cut the umbilical cord and take care of the newborn and the postpartum woman, Columba said yes, of course she did.

Columba explained that when she realized she was pregnant in New York, a friend had brought her to Manhattan Hospital. I asked Columba what opinion she held of the prenatal care she was receiving at Manhattan. She told me that she felt it was too much: "Pues en México no nos están checando a cada rato y acá nos están checando siempre. . . . No pues a mí, no me gusta que me estén revisando a cada rato. Me molesto como no estoy acostumbrada" [Well, in Mexico, they aren't checking us all the time, and here they're always checking us. . . . And, well, I don't like that they're always examining me. It bothers me because I am not used to it]. Columba indexes here a point of great variation in prenatal care: the "appropriate" number and frequency of prenatal visits in mainstream care varies dramatically around the world (Davis-Floyd et al. 2009; Ivry 2010; Strong 2000). She had resolved not to go to all of her appointments. She told me that she felt the pregnancy was normal and that she felt the same as with her earlier pregnancies. She did not see the need for constant examinations when her embodied experience was of a normal, uncomplicated pregnancy.

Mexican immigrant women in this study frequently described pregnancy as a normal, expected part of life that they are well equipped to successfully accomplish. Flora told me that she had no worries associated with her pregnancy; she simply wished to eat well, avoid frustration and anger, and take care of herself (cf. Ramírez 2001:1). In the view of these women, a pregnant woman requires no special care. While labor, delivery, and the postpartum period require specific interventions largely centered on enabling the body to rapidly recuperate and return to normal—avoiding *aire* (drafts or cold), promoting the return of the uterus to its normal shape and size, and restoring the abdomen and bone structure—pregnancy itself is not viewed as inherently risky.[3]

When I asked women what they thought they should do to ensure a healthy pregnancy, they frequently named a short list of common recommendations. They reported consistency in the advice given them by their mothers, grandmothers, and mothers-in-law, and also by medical prenatal care providers. In addition to a common recommendation that they regulate their emotions to avoid *coraje* (anger) and remain *tranquila* (calm), they needed to eat well, walk, avoid heavy work, and get sufficient rest.[4]

Brenda echoed many of the women when she told me what constituted a healthy diet:

> A nosotros nos gusta lo natural. En mi caso, mis hijos pesaron nueve libras. . . . Yo siento que todas las mexicanas comemos lo normal lo que es de siempre. Nosotros comemos comidas como nopales. En mi caso, a veces me hago un licuado de avena. A muchas mexicanas no les gusta la leche pero sí comen lo que son tortillas, sopas, frijoles, carnes. O sea yo siento que ellas no son de tener una dieta, o sea, nosotros comemos lo normal.

> [We like everything that is natural. In my case, my sons weighed nine pounds. . . . I feel that we Mexican women eat what is normal, what we always eat. We eat foods like *nopales* (cactus paddles), and in my case, I sometimes make myself an oatmeal shake. Many Mexican women don't like milk, but what they eat are tortillas, soups, beans, meats. I feel that most women are not going to have a diet; what I mean is, we eat what is normal.]

Food plays an important role in discussions of pregnancy self-care among Mexican immigrant women, even though they say that one should simply eat what is "normal." Women told me they experienced *antojos* (cravings), in which they eagerly indulged, for fruit (often with lime and chili powder), oatmeal, and *licuados* (smoothies). They told me they sought to avoid pork, spicy foods, and fried foods. The most common foods women told me they consumed during pregnancy are *licuados de fruta o leche* (fruit or milk smoothies), yogurt, fruit, oatmeal, beans, eggs, milk, chicken broth or soup, stews, tortillas, and *atole* (a drink made of corn flour).

Janette told me that she started to eat "normally" during pregnancy, although she had not cared for herself before, eating only one meal a day. When she became pregnant, she said, she had to think about her baby and could no longer be selfish. While Janette said she was able to do what she thought she should to care for her pregnancy by eating meals throughout the day, other women said that some aspects of life in New York inhibit families' abilities to do what they think they should. They named fast-paced lifestyles, demanding work schedules, and kitchens shared with unrelated housemates as some of the factors constraining their ability to eat as they thought they should.

Apart from foods, many women in the study mentioned walking to be an important part of pregnancy care. Virtually all said that *caminar mucho* (walking a lot) is an important way to care for oneself and avoid risk during pregnancy. While no one mentioned engaging in formal exercise regimens or more rigorous forms of exercise such as biking, swimming, or running, and they did not say such exercise was something they thought they should do or refrain from doing during pregnancy, almost all discussed walking as an important healthful activity. Walking during pregnancy was described as a means to get the baby into a proper head-down position for delivery, to prevent excessive weight gain, to maintain strength needed for delivery, and to keep the baby from being *flojo* (lazy).

Walking during labor was said to speed dilation of the cervix and aid delivery. Some women said they even walked to the hospital during labor to deliver their babies. One woman told me she walked to Elmhurst Hospital, about two miles from her home in Jackson Heights, Queens, during early labor, with her partner and toddler. Lila, a *bañera* (specialist in herbal steam baths to aid a woman's postpartum recovery), said that she knew to walk during labor because her mother had suggested this to her and her sisters. Here she describes a dialogue with her mother during labor:

> Porque mi mamá nos decía que cuando tuviéramos los dolores que no nos acostáramos, "¡Caminen, caminen, caminen!" Y es cierto es bien bueno eso. Llegábamos y caminábamos. "Acuéstate si quieres," me dijo. "No, yo quiero caminar," y caminaba. Y ya cuando tenía los dolores, "Ya ahora sí, me voy a aliviar." "¿Y cómo sabes?" "Ya me voy a aliviar."[5]

> [Because my mother told us when we had labor pains that we should not lie down, "Walk, walk, walk!" And it's true, that's really good. We got there and we walked. "Lie down if you want," she said. "No, I want to walk." And I walked. And when the pains came, I said, "Now, yes, the baby is coming." "And how do you know?" "The baby is coming."]

Perhaps her mother felt sympathy for her daughter's pain when she told her: "Lie down if you want." But Lila knew that she should continue to walk, so she told her mother that she *wanted* to walk. Walking probably hastened Lila's labor such that when Lila's mother asked Lila how she knew she was ready to give birth, Lila replied that she just knew. Lila here describes the process by which she came to know for herself what had previously been a mandate delivered by her mother. Her acquisition of embodied knowledge of what to do in pregnancy and labor was similar to that she described in her practice as a *bañera*, an expertise earned through training combined with intuition.

Several women mentioned in interviews that if one does not walk enough or is otherwise too *floja*, her baby may be lazy when born. The adjective *flojo* was used to describe babies who had poor suckling reflexes and who seemed "too sleepy" to nurse or were otherwise viewed as frail or weak. It was also thought that the risk of laziness could extend to adolescence and adulthood—a woman who was lazy during pregnancy could have a lazy baby who would become a lazy adult, unwilling to do the work that life requires.

Many women described feeling lazy during pregnancy, especially in the first trimester, but said they sought to conquer these sensations through activity and walking. Elba told me that if a pregnant woman "se lo pasa durmiendo el día, es más doloroso el parto, porque se le pega el bebé" [spends all of her time sleeping, labor is more painful because the baby gets stuck to her]. To give in to feelings of sleepiness or tiredness was described as a failure to care for oneself and one's fetus. Even though many women ceased working early in pregnancy to care for their pregnancies, get rest, and avoid heavy labor, they described being as worried about excess rest as they were about too little rest.

Refraining from carrying heavy loads and from heavy exertion was another mandate women in the study frequently mentioned (cf. Masley 2007:110). This mandate was often corroborated in advice from providers in prenatal clinics. There seemed to be little controversy about its wisdom, although many women had a hard time following it, given the demands of their daily lives. One woman said she felt that a miscarriage she had experienced the year after her first child was born was caused by lifting heavy things. Floridia told me that her cesarean scar opened following the birth of her first child because she had to get back to doing household work too soon.

Many women expressed concern that they had no choice but to do hard work and lift heavy objects in spite of this mandate, a fact that caused them distress. Many said they lived in walk-up apartments, as many as six flights up. One woman said that she avoided carrying heavy objects by asking someone from the supermarket to carry her groceries up the four flights of stairs to the door of her apartment. Once there, she said, her four-year-old son helped her by dragging the bags across the floor to the kitchen. María, who lives in a fifth-floor walk-up, told me she had no choice but to carry her baby's stroller up the stairs, as her building was not secure enough for her to leave the stroller in the lobby. Other women described having to carry strollers with sleeping children up and down subway stairs or to their apartments. Some said that during their pregnancies, their partners carried dirty clothing to the self-service laundry, carried groceries, and took their older children to school or the park so they could rest. But Emilia said: "Si no hago los quehaceres, ¿quién los hará?" [If I don't do the chores, who will do them?].

While some women were able to alleviate some of the burden of carrying heavy things and doing chores with help from their partner and other family members, for many women, life in New York City involved some unavoidable exertions. In Mexico, many said, there were more members of their family available to share labor burdens and relieve a pregnant woman from rigorous tasks. One woman told me that her mother and mother-in-law argued about who got to take care of her after the birth of her first child. Living in Queens, however: "No va a haber quien me ayude. Le traté de contar a mi prima, pero no acepta que es como una enfermedad que hay que cuidar" (There is no one who will help me. I tried to convince my cousin, but she doesn't accept that it is like an illness that one should care for). However, in Mexico, some women said such burdens were worse, with demands from mothers-in-law to do domestic chores, and the routine labor required by a rural or semi-rural life with animals, homes, gardens, and children to tend.

Some women consider not only hard physical labor risky, but all work. Even though Mexican families widely view one's working while pregnant as dangerous for the fetus, only one woman I spoke with was told by her medical provider to discontinue working outside the home during pregnancy. She had experienced break-through bleeding toward the end of her first trimester and was told that if she did not stop working and stay on partial bed rest, her pregnancy was at risk. In spite of their providers' silence about working during pregnancy, many women said that their partners and families encouraged them to stop working upon learning they were pregnant, and in some cases demanded that they stop. That providers either have no opinion about working during pregnancy or encourage women to keep working until late in their pregnancy is routinely ignored by pregnant women and their families. Further, a man who insists his pregnant partner stop working is generally viewed as benevolent, taking proper care of his partner.[6] Many women work in spite of their husbands' commands and amid claims that their actions are selfish and put their child at risk. Yet far from resisting patriarchal demands, women choose to work outside the home to avoid loneliness and boredom or for the necessary extra income.

Chemical Pain Relief and Medication during Pregnancy and Childbirth

Brenda told me her greatest worry in her first pregnancy was that she had perhaps inadvertently brought harm to her fetus by consuming cold medication when she thought she had the flu. When the medicine did not relieve her symptoms, she said, a member of her family told her: "You don't have the flu. You're pregnant."[7] She said she counted back the days to her last menstrual period and knew that it could be true. When she realized she had taken the cold medication at a month of gestation, she immediately made an appointment with the prenatal clinic at Coney Island Hospital.

In retrospect, Brenda and her husband told me, there were home remedies they use to treat common illnesses that they believe would not have incurred the types of risk they were afraid of when Brenda consumed the cold medication. They said that if someone has a cold, they should be given a mixture of honey, grated radish, onion, and garlic that works "like an antibiotic" to relieve a cough. They said they give their elder son tea made of cinnamon and onion for flu symptoms as well, although they said cinnamon tea during pregnancy can be dangerous. For diarrhea, Brenda recommended a tea made of corn silk. She referred to these practices as being traditional Mexican customs of provincial origin, "son tradiciones Mexicanas de provincia." Even though she and her husband were well versed in and avid practitioners of various home remedies, they dismissed others, such as avoiding lemon during pregnancy, as *creencias* (beliefs) and *supersticiones* (superstitions).

While fewer women said they avoided medication during pregnancy than the number who believed in the other prescriptions for having a healthy pregnancy mentioned earlier, it was a common theme in interviews (cf. Root and Browner 2001:210). Brenda told me that the greater exposure to chemicals in food and the air in the United States made it more difficult for families to avoid using medications. She told me that she had never heard of anyone suffering from allergies or asthma in Mexico, but that here she sensed these were a common problem.

Claudia received a great deal of advice from her mother and mother-in-law while pregnant. Her mother-in-law commanded her son to take good care of Claudia. Claudia's mother told her to drink hot water with lemon to boost her immunity and to use cool washcloths on her forehead if she had headaches. When she came down with a cold while pregnant and living in Brooklyn, she missed the herbal drops her mother bought for her from a naturopath. In fact, Claudia's main differences with her husband's family centered on the use of natural foods and products. In her natal home, she was accustomed to consuming meals based on vegetables and herbs, while in her mother-in-law's house, meat played a starring role in each meal. In spite of what she described as commitment to "todo lo natural" [everything natural], Claudia felt that a hospital birth was superior to a midwife-attended home birth. Claudia and her siblings were born in a clinic, and she felt that having a baby in a hospital or clinic was the only safe and hygienic place to deliver. When I asked her why giving birth in a clinic or hospital is better than having a child at home, she told me: "Pues están más preparados y tienes más experiencia, y está más desarrollado. Y estaba convencida de que iba a salir todo bien" [Well, they are more prepared and more experienced, and it's more developed. I was convinced that everything was going to turn out well].

The antitechnology natural childbirth movement that gained headway in the United States in the early 1970s (see, e.g., Arms 1975) was not a movement that any Mexican immigrant woman in this study professed an interest in or an allegiance to. Nonetheless, many women in the study were assertive about their desire for what they called a "normal" or "natural" childbirth.[8] Brenda told me: "A nosotros nos gusta lo natural" [We like that which is natural]. When women asked me about my own childbirth experiences, one of their first questions was frequently, "¿Los tuviste normal?" [You had them normally?]. I learned that by "normal," they meant a vaginal delivery as opposed to a cesarean section. When I asked women in interviews if they planned to have epidural anesthesia during labor, what some women called *la raquidia*, the way they phrased their response was typically: "No, prefiero tenerlo natural" [No, I prefer to have it naturally].[9] Jessy told me that she preferred not to have anesthesia on the grounds that "antes no les ponían" [it was not done in the past]. She said she preferred to use her strength and have her baby "normally." She had an epidural with her first delivery but declined it with her second: "Me dijeron que con el segundo no era necesario" [I was told I did not need it with the second]. But with the third, her labor was induced, and she was again given epidural anesthesia. She also told me that her biggest fear as she approached her fourth delivery was of the pain. Some women, including Claudia, told me that they would accept an epidural if the pain became too much for them to handle.

Napolitano (2002) found in her research that women living in the metropolitan area of Guadalajara, Mexico, were more likely than their rural-dwelling mothers and grandmothers to accept pain relief during labor. Rural women saw "a positive connection between female endurance and the experience of coping in a labor. For them, opting for a painless delivery undermines the central rite of womanhood." Napolitano refers to the difference in opinion between older and younger and rural and urban women as "an intragenerational dialogical field where there is a tension of modernity between a self-choosing subject versus a reification of suffering and motherhood as a claim for agency" (2002:166). This difference seemed present in my study as well. For example, while some women who migrated at an early age, before having children, described wishing to try labor without anesthesia, they were less likely to express opposition to epidural anesthesia than were more recently arrived immigrants and those who had experienced births in Mexico. Women who had borne children in Mexico, irrespective of the length of time they had lived in the United States, were the most likely to express confidence in their ability to deliver their babies without chemical pain relief. Among the women in this study for whom I have data regarding their use of pain relief during labor, slightly more than 50 percent had an epidural during their most recent delivery, significantly lower than the 58.5 percent nationwide for Hispanic mothers and 68 percent for all mothers (Martin and Menacker 2007:6). However, far more than 50 percent told me in interviews that they wished to avoid an epidural, and even more were opposed to the idea of cesarean section except in an emergency. Although rates of epidural administration tell us nothing about desires to avoid or consume chemical pain relief, Mexican women who wished to avoid an epidural may have been more successful in doing so than women from some other groups.[10]

Extramedical Interventions

Conducting research in New York City, I did not encounter or hear of a practicing midwife from Mexico, but I did find other practicing and nonpracticing specialists, including *bañeras* (herbal bath specialists), *yerberas* (herbalists), a particularly renowned *huesero* (specialist who adjusts bones and does *sobadas* [deep-tissue massages]), and *brujos* (roughly translated as "witch doctors," but often used as a general term for any of these other specialists). In addition to care they received in the public prenatal care system, some Mexican women also solicited care from these specialists, who bring knowledge with which the women are familiar from their hometowns. Often, care specialists are from the same hometowns as their clients and operate on the basis of their reputation in Mexico. Women recounted seeking care from these specialists during pregnancy and after delivery for generalized aches and pains, sciatica, discomfort, incontinence, indigestion, skin problems, uterine cramps, and bleeding. They generally described this care as supplemental to their prenatal care, although sometimes they described it as offering assistance that they could not obtain in a public clinic or hospital.

María's first baby was in a breech position at twenty weeks of pregnancy, and the high-risk practitioners at a Manhattan public hospital told her that she would need a cesarean section. Distressed and determined to have a vaginal delivery, she sought the help of the huesero. Over several visits, he manually turned her fetus. She told me it was painful but ultimately successful. She did not inform her prenatal care providers that she had sought outside assistance to turn her baby, and she ultimately delivered vaginally. This technique, external cephalic version, is commonly known by midwives but rarely learned by obstetrical students in the United States today (see Cosminsky, this volume). It was mentioned by women in interviews as one of many strategies midwives in Mexico use to avoid delivery complications. The same huesero gave María massages to ease sciatica and other pregnancy-related pains. Some months after giving birth, she solicited the huesero's help in relieving severe back pain that immobilized her.

Cesarean Section and Other Routine Medical Interventions during Delivery

Floridia told me she delivered her first child with a cesarean section at Metropolitan Hospital in Manhattan. In spite of a previous cesarean delivery, Floridia continued to believe that vaginal birth was more natural and better, the "normal" way to deliver babies. Further, even though she was getting ready to have a second hospital birth, she was of the opinion that her mother's experiences birthing at home were preferable, enabling a woman to avoid exposing herself to strangers. She retained hope she might still have what she considered a normal birth, even though she was told she was likely to need a second cesarean because of the earlier cesarean and absent any explanation she could recall for her first cesarean beyond a failure to dilate.

Karen also sought to deliver vaginally in spite of a cesarean with her first child at Sunnyside Hospital in Queens. Then she returned to Mexico, where she had her second child. Her third was born at St. Vincent's Hospital in Manhattan, and I met her during prenatal care for her fourth at Manhattan. She explained that in Mexico she was told that all her births would need to be by cesarean section because the incision had not healed well. Indeed, all three were delivered by that means. However, with her fourth she still wanted to attempt to have her baby "normally," what providers refer to as VBAC (vaginal birth after cesarean). The providers at Manhattan told her that if she attempted a vaginal birth, it would be at her own risk; they would not be held responsible. She told me: "Yo sé que puedo tenerlo normal" [I know I can have it normally]. Here, Karen disregards the risk that VBAC delivery has been assumed to carry and asserts as more reliable her embodied understanding of her ability to deliver her fetus safely, despite previous cesarean sections.[11]

Rosario also sought to avoid a cesarean with her second delivery. Her first child was born by cesarean section in a private clinic in Toluca, Estado de México, after she was told that she was not dilating and her baby was not descending into the birth canal. With her second pregnancy, nine years later, her medical providers at Manhattan told her that she would likely need a second cesarean if they did not know more about the reasons for the first one. Rosario experienced symptoms of miscarriage and preterm labor between the fourth and eighth months of her pregnancy and was being seen by an obstetrician because her pregnancy was classified as high risk. She asked her mother to withdraw her medical record from the clinic where her first baby had been born and send it to her in New York. Her mother made two trips to the clinic but was unsuccessful in getting the record and was finally told that the record was in storage or destroyed because nine years had passed. Unable to provide the kind of data her doctors at Manhattan Hospital said they needed to analyze her first cesarean, Rosario was likely to have another.

Rosa, quoted at the start of this chapter, also told me she wished to avoid a cesarean, as well as epidural anesthesia. She said she did not want marks on her body, and she wished to feel her baby being born. Brenda was able to avoid a cesarean, although her incredulous doctor asked how she had delivered her first two children vaginally when each weighed more than nine pounds.

In all these instances, women insisted that a vaginal birth was the only normal means of childbirth and held to their view that a cesarean, far from the routine procedure it is increasingly becoming in the United States (Grady 2010; Menacker and Hamilton 2010), is an intervention to be reserved only for extreme situations of necessity. Nonetheless, they are given indications by medical providers that having a large baby without cesarean is remarkable, that having a previous cesarean implies the necessity of future cesarean deliveries, and that any lacuna of data in their medical record can be grounds for a cesarean. In this way, their assumptions about childbirth being normal and natural except in extreme circumstances are challenged by clues that cesarean section and other interventions are increasingly default procedures.

Concluding Thoughts

Rubi told me that she thought the childbirth practices common to her hometown, San Felipe Xochiltepec, Puebla, were better than those typical in New York City, although she expressed this opinion with a caveat. She said that in her town of origin, anesthesia was not an option. Although she framed this as a shortcoming, she said that anesthesia was not particularly necessary there. While one gave birth at home with only *una señora que atiende en las casas* (a woman who comes to the house), the midwife took charge from early in the pregnancy to *acomodar* (properly situate) the fetus to minimize pain during childbirth. Rubi felt that if one had a real complication in labor and delivery, New York was a safer place, given greater access to medical intervention; however, she implied that this was not necessary in a normal pregnancy. She said that the number of appointments to which she was subjected in New York was excessive and bothersome but made clear that if someone were to have a complicated pregnancy, they were better off in New York than in Mexico.

Soliciting the care of a huesero and, importantly, not mentioning that care to biomedical care providers are indications that some Mexican immigrant women hold views of traditional medicine as valuable and efficacious. It would be valuable for additional research to be conducted on what is likely a very small number of Mexican women who obtain all their pregnancy care and also deliver their babies outside hospital settings in New York. While I did not encounter any women who did this, several women told me of stories they had heard of women who had "delivered their own babies" at home, usually because they had not left for the hospital in time—but possibly on purpose. Other women mentioned considering this possibility but feared that it would complicate issuance of the infant's birth certificate. Although this study was not constructed to access such a population, it does reveal that biomedical and traditional approaches to pregnancy care co-exist for many women interviewed. In some cases, women and their families actively sought out the care of specialists, requested the shipment of herbs from their hometowns, and constructed makeshift *temazcales* (steam baths) in their apartment bathtubs. In other cases, women did not actively seek out alternative care but operated under assumptions regarding their pregnancies and their abilities to deliver their babies without pain medication, cesarean sections, and other medicalized risk-based interventions that ran contrary to the technoscientific approach to their care they received in the prenatal clinic or labor and delivery department (cf. Martin 1992[1987]).

Many of the immigrant mothers I interviewed described changing their practices or choosing not to reveal their behavior to their providers because of the opinions and preferences they anticipated these providers would offer. Further, providers' concern about risks and reliance on intervention-rich protocols of care may increase the risks of Mexican immigrant women's pregnancies because of women's heightened apprehension about self-care in a context of excessive biomedical care. If pregnancy itself is increasingly viewed as inherently risky as women are incorporated into biomedical prenatal care regimens, it is logical that they are ever more likely to view expert intervention as necessary for its successful completion. In these ways, a disjuncture is evident between providers' assumptions about medicalized perinatal risk reduction and the views of recent immigrant patients from Mexico about their pregnancies and labors. On one hand, this disjuncture produces friction that may contribute to the wearing down of culturally based care practices. On the other hand, these tensions may also serve to strengthen cultural practices as a mode of active resistance to the subjectifying aspects of medicalized risk reduction prevalent in the public health care system.

Acknowledgments

I am grateful to the editors of this volume, Amínata Maraesa and Lauren Fordyce, for their vision and energies in putting this volume together and seeing it to its realization. Thanks also to Rayna Rapp and Carole Browner for their sound advice on the chapter, and to all at Vanderbilt University Press for their work on the book. I am thankful also to the funders that enabled the research on which this chapter is based: New York University, the Professional Staff Congress–City University of New York, and Lehman College.

Notes

1. All names of individuals used in this chapter are pseudonyms, as is Manhattan Hospital.
2. Parts of this chapter are excerpted from my forthcoming book *Patient Citizens, Immigrant Mothers: Mexican Women, Public Prenatal Care, and the Birth Weight Paradox.* Copyright © 2011 by Alyshia Gálvez. Reprinted by permission of Rutgers University Press.
3. Avoidance of cold, *frío* or *aire*, is important in the postpartum woman's physical sur-

roundings: avoiding a draft or in food that is ingested. Food can be considered "cold" or "hot," characteristics derived from its reputed effect on the body, not its temperature or piquance (see Howes-Mischel, this volume, for additional information regarding humoral medical beliefs among Mexican women).

4. Elba told me that she tended to be quick to anger, but that during pregnancy she tried to remain calm, as people had told her that her baby would cry a lot if she spent a lot of time angry during pregnancy (see Laderman 1983 for an in-depth discussion of associated illness).

5. *Aliviarse* (to alleviate oneself) is the verb most participants in this study used for "to give birth." The most standard Spanish translation for giving birth is *dar a luz* (to give or bring to light). *Aliviarse* may be commonly used only in Mexico.

6. This may be different than when a male partner discourages or prohibits a female partner from working at all, which Harvey et al. find more likely an exertion of male authority than benevolence (2002:288).

7. Interestingly, many women in the study recounted being told by housemates that they were pregnant, because of the color of their face, dark circles under their eyes, sleepiness, fatigue, and other clues.

8. These are the terms they used, which are both identical cognates in Spanish and English.

9. *Raquídia* comes from the Spanish term *anestesia neuraxial raquidia*, which actually refers to a spinal (or subarachnoid) blockade, as opposed to epidural blockade anesthesia, the difference lying in the location of the injection of anesthetic. With epidural anesthesia, the medication is injected into the epidural space in cranial and caudal directions, while with a subarachnoid block the anesthetic acts directly on the spinal column itself (Anaesthesia UK 2005).

10. Bridges (2011) suggests that women of color, perceived as stoic and having a high pain threshold, may be *denied* pain relief more often than are white women, under the assumption that they do not experience pain in the same way.

11. Karen's insistence is in keeping with recent developments in biomedical care. In July 2010, the American College of Obstetricians and Gynecologists relaxed its policy on VBAC delivery, stating it "is a safe and appropriate choice for most women who have had a prior cesarean delivery, including for some women who have had two previous cesareans" (Steinweg 2010; see also Martin 1992[1987]).

References

Abraído-Lanza, Ana, Bruce Dohrenwend, Daisy Ng-Mak, and J. Blake-Turner
    1999   The Latino Mortality Paradox: A Test of the "Salmon Bias" and Healthy Migrant Hypotheses. American Journal of Public Health 89(10):1543–48.

Alegría, Margarita, William Sribney, Meghan Woo, Maria Torres, and Peter Guarnaccia
    2007   Looking beyond Nativity: The Relation of Age of Immigration, Length of Residence, and Birth Cohorts to the Risk of Onset of Psychiatric Disorders for Latinos. Research on Human Development 4(1):19–47.

Anaesthesia UK
    2005   Conduct of Epidural and Subarachnoid Blockade. www.frca.co.uk/article .aspx?articleid=100445, accessed March 21, 2011.

Arms, Suzanne
  1975   Immaculate Deception: A New Look at Women and Childbirth in America. Boston: Houghton Mifflin.
Bridges, Khiara.
  2011   Reproducing Race: An Ethnography of Pregnancy As a Site of Racialization. Berkeley: University of California Press.
Browner, Carole, H. Mabel Preloran, and Simon Cox
  1999   Ethnicity, Bioethics, and Prenatal Diagnosis: The Amniocentesis Decisions of Mexican-Origin Women and Their Partners. American Journal of Public Health 89(11):1658–66.
Buekens, P., F. Notzon, M. Kotelchuck, and A. Wilcox
  2000   Why Do Mexican Americans Give Birth to Few Low-Birth-Weight Infants? American Journal of Epidemiology 152:347–51.
Conley, Dalton, Kate Strully, and Neil Bennet
  2003   Starting Gate: Birth Weight and Life Chances. Berkeley: University of California Press.
Cook, B., M. Alegría, Y. Lin, and J. Guo
  2009   Pathways and Correlates Connecting Latinos' Mental Health with Exposure to the United States. American Journal of Public Health 99(12):2247–54.
Cramer, James
  1987   Social Factors and Infant Mortality: Identifying High-Risk Groups and Proximate Causes. Demography 24(3):299–322.
Davis-Floyd, Robbie, Lesley Barclay, Betty-Anne Daviss, and Jan Tritten, eds.
  2009   Birth Models That Work. Berkeley: University of California Press.
Douglas, Mary
  1985   Risk Acceptability According to the Social Sciences. New York: Routledge.
  1992   Risk and Blame: Essays in Cultural Theory. London and New York: Routledge.
Douglas, Mary, and Aaron Wildavsky
  1982   Risk and Culture: An Essay on the Selection of Environmental and Technological Dangers. Berkeley: University of California Press.
Fernández, Leticia, and Alison Newby
  2010   Family Support and Pregnancy Behavior among Women in Two Mexican Border Cities. Frontera Norte 22(43):7–34.
Forbes, Douglas, and Parker Frisbie
  1991   Spanish Surname and Anglo Infant Mortality: Differentials over a Half-Century. Demography 28(4):639–60.
Frank, Reanne, and Robert Hummer
  2002   The Other Side of the Paradox: The Risk of Low Birth Weight among Infants of Migrant and Nonmigrant Households within Mexico. International Migration Review 36(3):746–65.
Fuentes-Afflick, E., N. Hessol, and E. Perez-Stable
  1999   Testing the Epidemiologic Paradox of Low Birth Weight in Latinos. Archives of Pediatrics and Adolescent Medicine 153:147–53.
Glick Schiller, Nina
  1992   What's Wrong with This Picture? The Hegemonic Construction of Culture in AIDS Research in the United States. Medical Anthropology 6(3):237–54.

Grady, Denise
  2010   Cesarean Births Are at a High in U.S. New York Times, March 23.
Guendelman, Sylvia, and Barbara Abrams
  1995   Dietary Intake among Mexican-American Women: Generational Differences and
         a Comparison with White Non-Hispanic Women. American Journal of Public
         Health 85(1):20–25.
Harley, Kim
  2004   Examining an Epidemiological Paradox: The Role of Acculturation, Nutrition
         and Social Support in the Birth Outcomes of Women of Mexican Descent. Ph.D.
         dissertation, University of California at Berkeley.
Harvey, Marie, Linda Beckman, Carole Browner, and Christy Sherman
  2002   Relationship Power, Decision Making, and Sexual Relations: An Exploratory
         Study with Couples of Mexican Origin. Journal of Sex Research 39(4):284–91.
Hayes-Bautista, David
  2002   The Latino Health Agenda for the Twenty-First Century. In Latinos: Remaking
         America. Marcelo Suárez-Orozco and Mariela Páez, eds. Pp. 215–35. Berkeley:
         University of California Press.
Hessol, N., and E. Fuentes-Afflick
  2000   The Perinatal Advantage of Mexican-Origin Latina Women. Annals of
         Epidemiology 10:516–23.
Ivry, Tsipy
  2010   Embodying Culture: Pregnancy in Japan and Israel. New Brunswick, NJ: Rutgers
         University Press.
Laderman, Carol
  1983   Wives and Midwives: Childbirth and Nutrition in Rural Malaysia. Berkeley:
         University of California Press.
Landale, N., R. S. Oropesa, and B. Gorman
  1999   Immigration and Infant Health: Birth Outcomes of Immigrant and Native-Born
         Women. In Children of Immigrants: Health, Adjustment, and Public Assistance.
         D. J. Hernandez, ed. Pp. 244–85. Washington, DC: National Academy Press.
  2000   Migration and Infant Death: Assimilation or Selective Migration among Puerto
         Ricans. American Sociological Review 65(6):888–909.
Layne, Linda
  1996   "How's the Baby Doing?" Struggling with Narratives of Progress in a Neonatal
         Intensive Care Unit. Medical Anthropology Quarterly 10(4):624–56.
Liu, Kai-Li, and Fabienne Laraque
  2006   Higher Mortality Rate among Infants of US-Born Mothers Compared to Foreign-
         Born Mothers in New York City. Journal of Immigrant and Minority Health
         8(3):281–89.
Martin, Emily
  1992[1987]   The Woman in the Body. Boston: Beacon Press.
  1994   Flexible Bodies: The Role of Immunity in American Culture from the Days of
         Polio to the Age of AIDS. Boston: Beacon Press.
Martin, Joyce, and Fay Menacker
  2007   Expanded Health Data from the New Birth Certificate, 2004. National Vital
         Statistics Reports 55(12):1–23.

Masley, Kate
  2007   Living the "Latina Paradox": An Ethnography of Pregnant and Postpartum
         Mexican Immigrants in Northeast Ohio. Ph.D. dissertation, Case Western
         Reserve University.
Menacker, Fay, and Brady Hamilton
  2010   Recent Trends in Cesarean Delivery in the United States. National Center for
         Health Statistics Brief 35. Centers for Disease Control and Prevention. March.
Morenoff, Jeffrey
  2000   Unraveling Paradoxes of Public Health: Neighborhood Environments and Racial/
         Ethnic Differences in Birth Outcomes. Ph.D. dissertation, University of Chicago.
Napolitano, Valentina
  2002   Migration, Mujercitas, and Medicine Men: Living in Urban Mexico. Berkeley:
         University of California Press.
Nelkin, Dorothy
  2003   Foreword: The Social Meaning of Risk. *In* Risk, Culture, and Health Inequality:
         Shifting Perceptions of Danger and Blame. Barbara Harthorn and Laury Oaks,
         eds. Pp. vii–xiv. New York: Praeger.
New York City Department of Health and Mental Hygiene
  2008   Summary of Vital Statistics 2000–2007. www.nyc.gov/html/doh/html/vs/
         vs.shtml, accessed November 11, 2009.
Palloni, Alberto, and Elizabeth Arias
  2004   Paradox Lost: Explaining the Hispanic Adult Mortality Advantage. Demography
         41(3):385–415.
Palloni, Alberto, and Jeffrey Morenoff
  2001   Interpreting the Paradoxical in the Hispanic Paradox: Demographic and
         Epidemiologic Approaches. Annals of the New York Academy of Sciences
         954:140–74.
Rabinow, Paul
  1992   Artificiality and Enlightenment: From Sociobiology to Biosociality. *In*
         Incorporations. Jonathan Crary and Sanford Kwinter, eds. Pp. 234–52. New
         York: Zone Books.
Ramírez Carillo, Cristina
  2001   Evolución del Cuidado Materno Infantil. *In* Revista de Enfermería 9(1):1–4.
Rapp, Rayna
  1999   Testing Women, Testing the Fetus: The Social Impact of Amniocentesis in
         America. New York: Routledge.
Root, Robin, and Carole Browner
  2001   Practices of the Pregnant Self: Compliance with and Resistance to Prenatal
         Norms. Culture, Medicine and Psychiatry 25:195–223.
Rumbaut, R., and J. Weeks
  1996   Unraveling a Public Health Enigma: Why Do Immigrants Experience Superior
         Perinatal Health Outcomes? Research in the Sociology of Health Care
         13(B):337–91.
Scribner, Richard, and J. Dwyer
  1989   Acculturation and Low Birthweight among Latinos in the Hispanic HANES.
         American Journal of Public Health 79(9):1263–67.

Sesia, Paola
  1996   "Women Come Here on Their Own When They Need To": Prenatal Care,
          Authoritative Knowledge and Maternal Health in Oaxaca. Medical Anthropology
          Quarterly 10(2):121–14.

Shai, D., and I. Rosenwaike
  1987   Mortality among Hispanics in Metropolitan Chicago: An Examination Based on
          Vital Statistics Data. Journal of Chronic Disease 40:445–51.

Sherraden, Margaret, and Rossana Barrera
  1996   Maternal Support and Cultural Influences among Mexican Immigrant Mothers.
          Families in Society 77(5):298–313.

Sorlie, Paul, Eric Backlund, Norman Johnson, and Eugene Rogot
  1993   Mortality by Hispanic Status in the United States. Journal of the American
          Medical Association 270:2464–68.

Steinweg, Carrie
  2010   American College of Obstetricians and Gynecologists Relaxes VBAC Guidelines.
          Chicago Examiner. www.examiner.com/family-in-chicago/american-college-of-
          obstetricians-and-gynecologists-relaxes-vbac-guidelines, accessed July 24, 2010.

Strong, Thomas
  2000   Expecting Trouble: What Expectant Parents Should Know about Prenatal Care in
          America. New York: New York University Press.

Susser, Merwyn
  1973   Causal Thinking in the Social Sciences: Concepts and Strategies of Epidemiology.
          New York: Oxford University Press.

Taningco, María Teresa
  2007   Revisiting the Latino Health Paradox. Policy Brief. Los Angeles: Tomás Rivera
          Policy Institute, University of Southern California. August.

CHAPTER 3

The Vital Conjuncture of Methamphetamine-Involved Pregnancy
Objective Risks and Subjective Realities

Alison B. Hamilton

Vital Conjuncture #1

Claudia, a twenty-eight-year-old, went into the hospital during labor and called her "connect" (drug dealer) to bring her some methamphetamine (meth) because the doctors were "not doing anything" to stop her contractions.[1] She snorted some meth and then prayed not to "test dirty," that is, positive for drug use. Claudia recalls: "I felt so ashamed. I wanted to kill myself, but I just prayed to God and thanked God for my mom and my dad and the nurses that were telling me, 'It's okay, you're gonna get help. You're not a bad person,' but shoot, I was being self-ish and not thinking that I coulda harmed my daughter." Claudia could not tell her mother that she had used throughout her pregnancy: "I can't tell that to my mom. She asked me just recently, 'Did you use when you were pregnant with [your daughter]? Is that why she, you know, tested dirty?' I said, 'No, I didn't use.' I was lying. How am I gonna admit to it, you know? I'm a bad parent. Using always made me a bad parent, because I was there, but not there."

Claudia also didn't tell anyone that she had been raped during that pregnancy. She described a particularly hard time with staying clean during the pregnancy; the longest she stopped using was three days. In the week before she had her daughter, she said she had to have meth "every single day," explaining: "I had to have it. I had to. I couldn't stop. I could not stop." That experience convinced Claudia that she could not stop using on her own, and she stayed in treatment after having her daughter, who remained in her custody unlike her two other children who had been "taken away."

Vital Conjuncture #2

Thirty-one-year-old Rachel said she did not know why she used during five of her six pregnancies, especially because meth did not have the same effect on her when she was pregnant. She felt that meth went straight to the fetus:

I don't think it would affect me. I think it would just go straight to my child, because I don't remember feeling the same [high] being pregnant as I did when I wasn't pregnant. I would, like, just take a couple of hits just so my body wouldn't hurt anymore, but I don't ever remember feeling the same. . . . I don't know why I did it when I was pregnant. I don't know why. I think it's 'cause I did gain so much weight and I was like, I don't wanna be in this predicament anymore. I don't wanna feel this way anymore.

Rachel had lost custody of three of her children in Arizona, where her experience was that authorities "automatically remove the child" if the mother or child tests positive.[2] California, she said, is different because "they're able to work with you and get you into some type of treatment." Rachel said that during the earlier pregnancies, she was not concerned with custody: "I was so high that I just didn't care about anything, anything or anyone, or who I hurt to get what I wanted. And that's sad, 'cause I didn't care about my children. I didn't care . . . and that's hard to say when I have two now that I just would die without."

Vital Conjunctures

In her book about motherhood in southern Cameroon, Johnson-Hanks develops the idea of "vital conjunctures," defined as "structures of possibility that emerge around specific periods of potential transformation in the lives of one or more participants." These periods of potential transformation might be thought of as transitions, but Johnson-Hanks stresses that these periods are more than transitions because they are "vital," that is, "more than the usual is in play," and "certain potential futures are galvanized and others made improbable" (2006:3). Conception, pregnancy, and birth serve as prototypical vital conjunctures, which usually involve uncertainty and "potential for radical transformation" (22). Johnson-Hanks is careful to make the point that vital conjunctures are not distinct points during which choices are made but are rather "periods in which a social actor suddenly . . . sees the easy taken-for-granted clarity of the stream of future events as false." Vital conjunctures close or resolve when the future becomes less uncertain, regardless of whether the future is as it was conceived of before the conjuncture. Social actors in vital conjunctures see "socially constructed guideposts" (23), and numerous responses to these guideposts are possible. This concept of vital conjunctures provides an intriguing way to contemplate the highly tenuous situations in which women methamphetamine users find themselves during pregnancy, during labor and delivery, and after childbirth.

In this chapter, I explore both the medically and subjectively defined risks associated with prenatal meth use. I suggest that the numerous medically defined risks are typically distal from women's subjective concerns during and after pregnancy. Though perceiving few effects of their meth use on the health of their babies, women in my study are far from carefree; on a daily basis they confront multiple highly challenging and interacting life circumstances that place them at great risk for ongoing substance dependence or relapse, along with exposure of their children to the physical and psychological effects of meth dependence.

The Context: Women Methamphetamine Users in Los Angeles County

The narratives presented here emerged during four years of research with thirty women in Los Angeles County who were in residential treatment for chronic methamphetamine abuse.[3] The original purpose of the research was to explore the relationship between methamphetamine use and sexuality among these women, but through person-centered life history interviews, many other issues emerged, one of the primary ones being motherhood—being mothered (or not) as young girls, being mothers, bearing children as young women, or all of these. In the context of their own childbearing, women described multiple risky behaviors including but not limited to meth use during their pregnancies. The vital conjuncture of pregnancy for some women represented a time of fear—not always fear for the medical condition of their unborn children but also fear of "testing dirty," of being abandoned by their partners during pregnancy, of feeling too much pain and discomfort associated with the pregnancy, and of not being able to get high on meth because they were pregnant.

Participants in the research started using methamphetamine at an average age of fifteen years old. Ten women were using meth by the age of thirteen. Most were introduced to meth by family or friends, with over one-third of the women having parents who were addicted to drugs, alcohol, or both. Two-thirds of the participants described histories of violence and abuse, with 43 percent describing childhood sexual abuse. The average age at which women had their first child was twenty. All but one of the thirty women had children, and most had more than one child, with eight of the women having four or more children. Over half of the participants were Latina, approximately a third were European American, two women were Native American, and two women were ethnically mixed: Latina/European American and Asian/Latina. At the time of the first in-depth interview, the average age of the participants was twenty-eight and a half years. Over half had not completed high school, and all but one were receiving public assistance.

Of the twenty-nine women who had children, twenty-two (76 percent) discussed continuing to use meth while pregnant. Women who used during pregnancy described not being able to stop using, stopping but starting again later in the pregnancy, using in some but not all pregnancies, having risky sex during pregnancy (e.g., unprotected sex, sex with strangers, sex while high), using more than their usual amount of meth during pregnancy, and seeing minimal effects of their meth use on their children. Often surrounding these themes were relationship dynamics such as using during pregnancy to maintain a relationship with a boyfriend or to cope with changing relationship dynamics related to using (or not using) meth.

Another layer of tenuousness during the vital conjuncture of these women's pregnancies was legal in nature. The risk of "testing dirty" at delivery functioned as a "socially constructed guidepost" (Johnson-Hanks 2006:23) that had greater or lesser influence on a woman's course of meth use during pregnancy, depending on how deeply committed she was to using at the time. For some, the risk of testing dirty (and losing custody, facing incarceration, or facing mandated treatment) was enough of a deterrent for them to stop using days or weeks before delivery. For others, often depending on past delivery and custody experiences, testing dirty was a more minor consideration, especially if the state in which the woman was delivering did not mandate removal of newborns who tested positive.

Prenatal Substance Use, Risk, and Stigma

To those who are not familiar with substance dependence, women's concerns about their personal risks regarding relationships and criminal justice involvement may seem distal to the socially defined crux of the problem of drug use during pregnancy: harm to the fetus. As Lester, Andreozzi, and Appiah have pointed out: "Once the fetus became the central protagonist there was a significant shift in social perception. The concept of harming the fetus by using drugs during pregnancy resulted in sanctions by both the criminal justice system and the child protective system" (2004:n.p.). Is that not what women would be most concerned about? Is the risk of fetal harm not enough of a deterrent to cause women to stop using? Are women who continue to use drugs during pregnancy ignorant of this possibility? These questions are not new, yet they are not questions that have been answered to the extent that women are no longer stigmatized for such behavior.

Murphy and Rosenbaum (1999) asked these questions over a decade ago, presenting compelling stories of 120 women who used drugs during pregnancy. They set out to tell the women's stories, to combat stereotypes, and to emphasize the social and economic contexts of drug use during pregnancy. Their sample of meth users was a small proportion of the overall sample, as meth use was not at its peak during their research.[4] However, they noted trends in meth users' experiences: women were uncertain about the risks of meth use on themselves and their babies, and, accordingly, their views "wavered" regarding the extent to which meth could be harmful to their reproductive lives.

Popular ideas of risk and policies related to risk among pregnant women who use drugs seem almost inevitably to revolve around risk to the fetus, going back to the notion of the "crack baby" in the early 1990s (see Frank et al. 2001). This notion has not completely vanished despite much research indicating that other factors such as the lack of good prenatal care, use of alcohol and tobacco, and poverty are highly powerful predictors of poor fetal development and health outcomes of drug- and alcohol-exposed children (see, e.g., Fisher et al. 2011; Latino-Martel et al. 2010; Stone et al. 2010; Zdravkovic et al. 2005). Even as of 2011, some states such as Alabama prosecute women for "chemical endangerment of a child" (U.S. Legal n.d.) when they, their babies, or both test positive for meth or other illicit drugs at childbirth (but not for alcohol or nicotine, which are firmly causally linked to numerous deleterious fetal and child health outcomes); and several states have statutes that mandate reporting of prenatal substance use to Child Protective Services (U.S. Department of Health and Human Services 2009). Women's fears of criminal justice involvement are not so unfounded.

The Medical Discourse on the Impact of Prenatal Meth Use

Meth is a central nervous system stimulant that is typically smoked, snorted, injected, or taken orally; routes of administration vary by geographic region in the United States, with some regions having higher proportions of injectors and others having few injectors and higher proportions of smokers. Meth is a Schedule II stimulant that results almost instantaneously in increased energy and alertness, decreased appetite, and a positive mood state (Gonzales, Mooney, and Rawson 2010).[5] The effects of meth (or its half-life) last from eight to twelve hours, which is a much longer high than a stimulant such as cocaine provides. Meth is relatively inexpensive and easy to manufacture from commonly available products such as pseudoephedrine, hydrochloric acid, and red phosphorus also found in over-the-counter medications or in readily available kitchen materials. The long and powerful high combined with relatively inexpensive availability make meth highly attractive: meth is one of the few drugs that appeals equally to both men and women. In fact, women tend to become more dependent on meth and are more committed to it than men are, being less likely than men to turn to other drugs in the absence of meth (Dluzen and Liu 2008). Meth use in women often co-occurs with depression, other substance use (especially alcohol, marijuana, and nicotine), a history of trauma and abuse (Cohen et al. 2007), and violence. In a study of over a thousand meth users in outpatient substance abuse treatment, 80 percent of women reported abuse or violence from a partner (Cohen et al. 2003). Problems with aggression and perpetration of violence are also common among women meth users (Hamilton and Goeders 2010; Zweben et al. 2004).

In terms of the impact of prenatal meth use on infants and children, scientific biomedical knowledge is largely driven by the Infant Development, Environment, and Lifestyle (IDEAL) study, a longitudinal multisite study focusing on prevalence of prenatal meth exposure among a sample of 1,632 women who had recently given birth (Arria et al. 2006); the sample included both users and nonusers of alcohol, tobacco, meth, and other drugs.[6] Five percent of the participants were meth users. This study evolved in response to the rise in meth use in certain regions of the United States during the late 1990s and has provided a wealth of information about women who use meth during pregnancy. In their study of meth users in particular, the IDEAL group found that women who used meth during pregnancy had lower maternal perceptions on quality of life, greater likelihood of substance use among those close to them, increased risk for criminal justice involvement, and increased likelihood of developing a substance abuse disorder (Derauf et al. 2007).

They also found that approximately one-third (29 percent) of women maintained high frequency of use throughout pregnancy, 9 percent increased frequency of use, one-fourth (26 percent) maintained low/moderate use, and one-third (36 percent) decreased their use. The latter group had more prenatal visits than the other three groups but was most likely to use alcohol during pregnancy (Della Grotta et al. 2010).

Meth-exposed infants in the IDEAL study were 3.5 times more likely to be small for gestational age than the unexposed group (Smith et al. 2006). Meth exposure was also associated with decreased arousal, increased physiological stress, and poor quality of movement (Paz et al. 2009; Smith et al. 2008). Effects of exposure varied by amount of meth used and timing of use by trimester. These results were consistent with those found in the New Zealand IDEAL study (Lagasse et al. 2011). A three-year follow-up study of the IDEAL mother-infant pairs found meth-exposed infants did not have worse long-term cognitive outcomes compared to nonexposed infants, and only modest negative motor effects were found at one year of age, which were mostly resolved by three years of age (Smith et al. 2011).

Prenatal meth exposure outcomes have been examined in other studies as well. In a chart-review study comparing 276 meth users to 34,055 patients in the general obstetric population, preterm delivery, low Apgar scores, cesarean delivery, and neonatal mortality were all significantly associated with meth use (Good et al. 2010). To investigate the impact of meth on the developing brains of children, diffusion tensor imaging (DTI) was used with both exposed and unexposed three- to four-year-olds (Cloak et al. 2009). DTI revealed a lower diffusion of white matter in the exposed children, suggesting that brain damage—though potentially reversible—is possible with prenatal exposure.

In sum, for women who use meth, especially during pregnancy, risk is pervasive and highly complex for both women and their babies. At a phenomenologic level, much of this risk remains elusive; the multiple outcomes possible in the horizons of drug-involved pregnancies and mothers' lives are relative to one another and to the personal histories that inform women's trajectories. Women in this study did not have specific knowledge of the data just described, but they did have varying levels of concern about the impact of their meth use on their babies. This concern typically interacted with numerous other concerns, including relationship issues.

Risk as an Experience-Distant Construct

Despite objectively identifiable and numerous risks of drug use during pregnancy, in the research study described here, not one woman used the term "risk" to describe her experiences—not even her sexual experiences. One might think that "risk" as a trope would be circulating in publicly funded treatment programs. Women in these programs are definitely being taught about the many types of risk that likely permeate their lives: sexual risk, risk for recurring violence, risk during pregnancy, physical health risk related to drug use, risk of relapse, risk of custody loss, et cetera. Many of the women were pregnant at the time or had been pregnant while in treatment (ostensibly a prime opportunity for education and intervention); some of them had been mandated under California's Proposition 36 to treatment instead of incarceration for drug-related charges. Two-thirds of participants were on probation or parole or both, so they were familiar with criminal justice risk. In addition, women were having multiple pregnancy experiences, and most of them had experienced the loss of at least some of their children to other family members or to the foster care system because of their meth use. Risks, and consequences of taking risks, permeated their lives. Yet, "risk" as an explicit concept was nowhere to be found in their narratives.

Pregnancy, Meth Use, and Motherhood:
Women's Subjective Experiences

How else might these women frame their use during pregnancy, their feelings during pregnancy, their attitudes toward their addiction, and their behaviors and experiences after giving birth? Some important commonalities emerged around pregnancy, meth use, and motherhood. First, the majority of the pregnancies the women described were unintended and were often not desired. Studies have shown that among young women, meth use increases the odds of becoming pregnant almost threefold (Zapata et al. 2008). Women had multiple abortions and miscarriages, along with live births. Pregnancy was a given—a taken-for-granted reality—in the context of drug use, which often involved sex-drug exchanges and, typically, no contraception. Second, as has been described for decades, substance dependence, at its peak (which can last for years), subsumes all else; the drug of choice becomes the only focus, and life happens around the drug. The following narrative illustrates both these points: "From seventeen to twenty is when I was just running around, you know, just doing whatever and getting high. And then I got pregnant when I was nineteen. I had him when I was twenty, and then every two years for the next eight years, I had a kid. And by that time my mom had the kids full-time, you know? And I was just running around doing whatever and getting high."

Finally, losing custody of children was widely acknowledged and accepted as part and parcel of addiction. "My children were the casualty of my addiction," one woman said. In many cases, women did not see their babies grow up, and many did not know where their children were. Loss of children was often described in a very matter-of-fact manner, for example: "With my second [child], I didn't really use—just a little bit. With my third one, I used a little bit more. By the time I had my fourth one, the guy that I was with moved, so I had met someone else, and I got pregnant from him. I used every day of my pregnancy with that one." When asked if the newborn tested positive for meth, she responded neutrally: "Yeah, yeah, and the state [of California] took him."

Although losing custody was a "structural expectation" (Johnson-Hanks 2006:24) within the vital conjuncture of women's meth-involved pregnancies, it was not always taken lightly. For most women, the loss of their children either kept them in their addiction or sent them even deeper into intensified use and increasingly risky circumstances. In my interview with thirty-nine-year-old Laura, the connection between her drug use and her identity as a mother emerged somewhat circuitously. Laura had meth available to her at all times: "I had drugs whenever I wanted—the way I wanted, you know what I mean? As much as I wanted. I'd say that I never had to pay for it anymore, either. You know what I mean? . . . I didn't have to pay for it, but I'd have sex with [my connect]." I asked her if he was the only one with whom she exchanged sex for meth, and she responded: "Yeah, the majority of the time, yeah. I was getting raped so much that it was like he was the only one I really wanted to be with. And to be honest, he made me feel beautiful. He didn't make me feel like a prostitute. He didn't."

Thinking of this partner reminded Laura that he gave her money for Mother's Day: "He told me I was, you know, I'm a good mother, even though the state [of California] was doing what they're doing, you know what I mean?" She became tearful in her transition to talking about losing her children to the Department of Child and Family Services: "I really didn't fall apart until after they took my kids. That's when I couldn't maintain a home no more. I couldn't. I was going crazy, you know what I mean? The only thing that ever meant anything to me was stripped from me—my motherhood. And then I got a record of being negligent, abusive, and all this other stuff. And it was like—it was just heart-wrenching for me."

Crying, Laura then said that losing her children drove her deeper into her addiction:

> And it's weird how when they strip you of your kids, you would think a woman would be able to stop. But it doesn't stop you. It drives you deeper and more towards the drug. 'Cause I know, I tried with all my might to stay clean. . . . And that last year, when I got raped those three times and whatnot, I had two hundred and sixty-four clean days. Only a hundred [days] outta the year being loaded, but it was the worst year of my life. It was hell for me.

This vital conjuncture in Laura's life involved loss of her identity as a mother, despair about the future, being labeled abusive (which has legal ramifications for potential reunification with her children in the future), being driven toward more meth use, and being vulnerable to sexual assault. Laura acknowledged the societal expectation that women would stop using drugs if they were at risk of losing their children but emphasized that this expectation is untenable in the face of heightened stress, violence, and hopelessness.

Intensified Craving and Use during Pregnancy

As evident in previous narratives, some women experienced an intensified craving for meth during pregnancy. For example, thirty-one-year-old Rachel said: "I started using again at seven months [pregnant], I think 'cause like I just like craved it, I craved it so bad. I just wanted to just have something, something in me, besides all this water and salt gain. . . . I just smoked it for like the last two months." Twenty-eight-year-old Monica explained her craving and use as follows:

> The longest I tried to stay sober when I was pregnant was like three [days]. Okay, I'm staying clean. No, I'm going to do it again. Stop two days, do it again. Stop two days, do it again. And that's the way I was the whole time. But the last week, the last week before I had her, I was doing it every day, every day, every day. I would, maybe one day, you know, I would not go do it, you know, if the stuff is still in my system, you know? But every single day I had to have it. I had to. I couldn't stop. I could not stop.

Similarly, twenty-three-year-old Susan explained: "I couldn't stop. I tried, but I couldn't. So I used through my whole pregnancy. He was due on the eighteenth, and I stopped on the eleventh and had him on the fourteenth. It really got worse when he was getting bigger and he started moving and, you know, me being high, I wouldn't eat for days at a time. I knew I was starving my baby, but I just couldn't stop."

Susan highlighted the important point that appetite is suppressed by meth use, which presumably would have an impact on the nutritional status of the fetus. To the best of my knowledge, this issue of prenatal nutrition status related to meth use has not been explored. Moreover, increased craving and use of meth during pregnancy has been underexplored. As noted earlier, one-third of the IDEAL sample either maintained a high level of meth use or intensified their use during pregnancy, and effects of prenatal exposure varied by dose and timing of meth administration. Women in my study were often quite specific about when they used the most and why. Intensified use during the last trimester seems particularly risky, according to the scientific literature. Yet the reasons for intensified use during this period are not well understood. Recent research suggests that adverse childhood experiences are associated with risky behaviors (such as substance abuse) during pregnancy, with women who had more than three adverse experiences being two and a half times more likely to engage in risky behaviors during pregnancy (Chung et al. 2010). Future research should investigate this association more thoroughly, especially among women meth users who have significant histories of trauma and abuse.

The Subjective Discourse on the Risks of Prenatal Meth Use

Women's current experiences with mothering included expressions of what was found to be another phenomenologic commonality related to the risks associated with their meth use: uncertainty about the health of their children because they had used meth during and after pregnancy. This uncertainty was often intertwined with relationship concerns and fear of or actual abandonment during pregnancy. Twenty-four-year-old Rosa described these changing dynamics and the impact they had on her: "I started seeing [my boyfriend] using in front of me and then I started seeing him bringing his friends around and then he'd leave, you know? And I'm just like, 'Don't leave me by myself—I'm pregnant, you know? At least, if you're gonna get high, get high in the bathroom and then come back out and kick it with me, hang out with me.'"

But Rosa's boyfriend did not stick around, so Rosa got lonely and started using again by injecting: "Well, I'd scrape it outta the pipe, put a little bit of water, and stick it in the syringe and shoot myself up while I was pregnant. And I'd, I would cry after—the whole time, for like the ten hours I was high, I'd lay there and cry and cry. What am I doing to myself?" Rosa said that she started to feel "paranoid" as the baby got bigger. She worried when she felt him move "real real fast": "Like when I'd be coming down [from being high], I'd run to my doctor and ask him, 'Is he okay? I haven't felt the baby move and I think my baby's dead.' You know, just being fuckin' so paranoid from using. And I was trying to stop. I was trying to stop the whole time and I just—I couldn't stop."

Similarly, thirty-two-year-old Valerie described her drug habit during pregnancy: "During all three of my pregnancies, I used, and I just couldn't stop. Even being pregnant, even feeling my baby move, I still, you know, did dope." Regarding complications, she responded: "No, all of my kids, all my kids are perfectly fine. But yet, you know, my son's only three, you know, and we don't know whether he is levelheaded, you know? But—so I'm sure [the drugs] affected him some way, somehow, you know?" I asked thirty-three-year-old Ana whether she had any problems from using while pregnant: "No, no. I was one of the lucky ones. My kids came out fine. There's no disability with them. I have easy pregnancies." She paused and then added softly: "Well, I had easy pregnancies 'cause I was loaded and I didn't feel the pain."

Ana's depiction of herself as "one of the lucky ones" suggests that she had familiarity with women who were "unlucky," but no one in this study described severe or even pronounced effects of their meth use on the health of their children. In other words, women, for the most part, did not see any visual evidence of the risks of their or their friends' children having been born either with meth in their systems or to women who used meth during pregnancy. Twenty-two-year-old Sherry said that she used heavily during her pregnancy. She and her baby tested positive at delivery, but her son is "fine." She explains: "He doesn't have any mental problems or nothing. He's extremely, extremely smart." This is reminiscent of what Murphy and Rosenbaum (1999) noted about the women meth users in their study: they had either uncertainty about the impact of meth use on their babies, or they did not perceive there to be a pronounced impact. Thirty-nine-year-old Rosie said she had noticed that her children "have no patience or tolerance for crowds, you know? So, yeah, that's probably all that I've ever noticed in them." I asked her if they have any learning disabilities and she responded: "No, unh-uh, no. My one son's actually really smart. I don't even know where he gets that from, but he is very smart, you know?" And her daughter, though exposed to the secondhand smoke of her mother's meth use from age two to four, "seems to be doing good. . . . She doesn't have nothing wrong."

Although there was a consistent, minimizing perception of the risks and consequences of prenatal meth exposure on infants, some women did describe the consequences of their meth-using lifestyles on their children—usually their older children. A mother of five children, Laura, expressed this as follows: "My children are a direct result of me—you know what I mean? My three older kids are. My seventeen-year-old now actually has a year and a half sober. But my other two still battle with it, you know? And it's because it's what I taught them, you know? Johnny, which is my fourteen-year-old—he, he hasn't done any drugs yet, you know? But me and his dad both are drug addicts, you know?"

Laura's fourteen-year-old son had tested positive for meth at birth, as had her six-year-old. Laura's use of the word "yet" suggests that she at least considers it plausible that her son will eventually try drugs.

Women Who Quit Using during Pregnancy

In contrast to women who experienced continued or intensified craving and use during pregnancy, a minority of women (six of the twenty-nine, or 21 percent) stopped using during pregnancy by quitting cold turkey—not through any particular treatment or prenatal care. Twenty-eight-year-old Stacy stopped using during her pregnancies because of her experience being born to an alcoholic mother:

> My mom drank when she was pregnant with me, you know, and it's hard for me to concentrate sometimes. It's like, I wonder if that had anything to do with it. I'm pretty sure it has, you know, has a lot to do with it. And she's all like, "Oh, you guys came out fine. I used to drink with you guys, and I used to pop pills, whites and reds and all those." And she goes, "Nothing happened to you guys." And I go, "Oh, you think nothing happened to us," but I noticed in school, I couldn't concentrate. And I couldn't focus and think right. I said, "Yeah, it might not show, but I could feel it."

Stacy's narrative raises the issue of the intergenerational nature of substance abuse (Messina et al. 2008) and the persistence of the perception that prenatal exposure to substances causes only minimal harm. Stacy also represents the "receiving end" of prenatal exposure: she herself perceived the effects of her mother's substance abuse during pregnancy, and she consciously chose to protect her own babies from these risks.

I asked twenty-eight-year-old Monica if it was hard to stop using when she realized she was pregnant. She replied: "At first, it was hard and then, and then it was easy, 'cause when I would be pregnant, you know, [my boyfriend] would stop with me, you know? But then like the last month [of the pregnancy], you know, he would start again." Monica's situation was unusual in that her partner stopped using with her. In contrast, most women who stopped using did so despite a partner's continued use. This often resulted in conflicts, especially around sex, as described by thirty-year-old Christina:

> I was clean when I was pregnant for my son. I just wasn't interested [in my partner], 'cause I know he wanted to have sex all the time, and I was hurting down there, you know? . . . [He wanted] that hard sex that you have when you're high, and I was like, "I don't know." After not having drugs and alcohol, it was kind of like a depression kicked in, and that's what had a lot to do with our breaking up.

Implicit in Christina's narrative is her use of meth to stave off depression (which she described in more detail in the interview). After Christina gave birth to her son, she went back to using meth because her depression was overwhelming, and she thought she would be able to reunite with her partner if she started using again. They reunited briefly, then broke up again, and then Christina got pregnant from a new partner.

Quitting during pregnancy did not always result in positive outcomes. Sherry explained: "I was clean during my whole pregnancy, and then when we went to have the baby, I lost the baby. It was a stillborn. With both of my [other] kids, I had used—that's why I caught both my [custody] cases." Sherry relapsed on the day of her son's funeral:

> I had got high that one day because, I mean, that was the drug that made me feel nothing. I felt no happiness, I felt no sadness, I felt nothing. I was going through such excruciating pain. I didn't wanna feel it. I didn't wanna feel anything that was going on, and I relapsed and it didn't take anything away. It took nothing away. All the pain was there. The realization was there, everything. Two days later, I didn't get high, and I came in here [to this treatment facility].

Sherry was expressing the frustration with her realization that meth finally did not work for her—it did not take away her pain as she had expected it to.

Although some women were able to quit using meth during their pregnancies, all but one started using again after delivery, as did Christina: "After I would have the baby, right away, you know, I wouldn't even breastfeed, you know, I was just right away back, you know, doing speed, doing meth." Similarly, forty-five-year-old Laura went back to smoking meth after her daughter was born: "I didn't breastfeed, you know, so I could go right back to my dope." These narratives reflect a cognitive decision to reject breastfeeding in order to keep using. Not all women made this particular decision. Twenty-eight-year-old Stephanie explained: "After I had the baby, I still continued using, and I breastfed her while I was using. I breastfed her for a year and a half, 'til my mom took her from me." I asked Stephanie if her daughter developed "normally," and she responded: "Yeah, yeah, she grew okay. She's smart; she's very smart. She knows how to write her name already. She's very smart, you know. She does a lot of things like, like normal four-year-olds."

A high rate of postpartum relapse has been consistently reported in the scientific literature, particularly related to alcohol abuse (Bailey et al. 2008; Crome and Kumar 2007; Spears, Stein, and Koniak-Griffin 2010) but also to cocaine abuse

(Blackwell et al. 1998). Some evidence suggests that relapse may be related to postpartum depression (Ross and Dennis 2009). Postpartum relapse among meth users represents another area that warrants further investigation.

Vital Conjuncture #3

Twenty-four-year-old Rosa, introduced earlier, began injecting meth with her boyfriend:

> When me and my boyfriend got high, I was like so shaking trying to hit [inject] myself the first time that I got high in front of him, and he saw that. I'm like, "You do it for me 'cause I can't do it right now, 'cause you're right here." He saw my arms—how fucked up they were, and he's just like, "What are you doing to yourself?" He's like, "I'm gonna start doing it for you until your arms heal," and so he did it for me. . . . I shoulda never, ever done that with him that day. And then, you know, from then on we were using.

Rosa expressed the intense craving for and commitment to meth that has been reported in the scientific literature: "I wanted it. I wanted more and more—as much as I can get. . . . I started loving it so much that I wanted to fight him if he didn't give me a shot, and that's how bad it got. Like real bad." She realized she was pregnant after "throwing up for a week straight" and went to a clinic:

> One day I was coming down [withdrawing] so hard and I walked over to this clinic right around the corner, the tweaker corner—I walked into this clinic with three of my bags, my stuff that I carried with me all the time, and I told the lady, I'm like, "Look, I'm a drug user, I'm homeless, and I need to find out if I'm pregnant or not." And sure enough [the test] came back that I was pregnant.[7]

Rosa told her boyfriend that the pregnancy test was positive and asked him: "What are we gonna do? I can't have a baby using." When her boyfriend said that he did not believe in abortion, "I'm like, 'Look at the way we live—we live in a fucking garage, sharing somebody else's garage. We don't even have a bathroom. When you go to the bathroom, we peed behind the house and just like, what are we doing to ourselves? You know? What are we gonna do with a baby? You know, how are we gonna support a baby?'"

She spent a month thinking about what to do and decided to have an abortion. She went to the clinic with her boyfriend, and when they arrived, he said he had forgotten his wallet. "I don't know what came over me, but that's what saved my life. At that moment I decided to have my daughter. I told him, 'Just as long as you don't leave me by myself. I don't wanna be by myself. I don't wanna be one of those single moms having to take care of a kid.'"

Her boyfriend promised he would not leave her, and they kept the baby and kept using, but they "slowed down a lot." As her pregnancy progressed, she became increasingly frustrated that her boyfriend kept using but would let her smoke only occasionally. She started to sneak needles from a diabetic friend in order to inject herself. I asked Rosa if they did anything at the clinic to help her:

> No. I told them I was using it. Every single test I gave them was dirty. Never once did they try to help me. And I told 'em, "I'm homeless. I have nowhere to live. I need to find somewhere to go. I don't wanna go back to my boyfriend's house 'cause that's all I do is use and I cannot pull myself away from it." I even told my friend, "Take me with you, take me with you, you know. I don't wanna be here no more. I'm pregnant. I don't wanna get high." And she was pregnant, too. The first time I went over [to her place], me and her got high over there with her boyfriend. We were getting high and getting high. I was already [looking pregnant] at this time. And the whole time I never went up to my mom's house. I stayed away from my mom's house, 'cause I didn't want her to see how fucked up I was.

Implicated in Rosa's experience are the multitude of risks and uncertainties that she confronted during her pregnancy. It is clear that she wanted to stop using, she wanted to be in a different or better place where she could stop using, she did not want to expose herself to her family, and she received no attention for her ongoing meth use from the clinic where she went for prenatal care.

Horizons of Risk and Uncertain Futures

Despite the growing body of evidence about the risks of prenatal meth use, women meth users in my study did not highlight concerns about the health of their fetuses, newborns, or children. Though there was mention of possible effects of their meth use, the term "risk" was never used. Instead, the health of their children was one of the more minor of many risks that women meth users described in their experiences of pregnancy. These risks included, but were not limited to, sexual and physical violence, intensified craving, being arrested/incarcerated, testing "dirty" at delivery, losing their children, losing their partners, having to admit their meth use to family and friends, and being depressed and uncomfortable. All these risks contributed to a great deal of uncertainty about the future after they delivered (if they delivered) their babies. Furthermore, many of these risks contributed to postpregnancy relapse. Clearly, the context of reproductive risk for these women entails much more than the objective determinations of fetal harm. As Whiteford and Vitucci (1997) suggested more than a decade ago, medical and psychological anthropologists can play an important role in studying and untangling the complex reproductive experiences of women with substance abuse problems. Furthermore, public health and psychosocial interventions, along with prenatal care itself, could place more primacy on pregnant women's life histories, cultural and familial contexts, and perceptions of care (Jessup et al. 2003; Whiteford and Szelag 2000).

In 2004, Lester, Andreozzi, and Appiah suggested that it was "time for policy to catch up with research" with regard to substance use during pregnancy. They examined the state-by-state variations in policies, with some states mandating punishment and others advocating treatment. In their policy recommendations in the areas of education, law, assessment, finances, training, treatment, and research, they emphasized that the mother, as well as the fetus, needs to be considered humanely, within social and personal contexts of safety and compassion. As they point out, and as demonstrated throughout this chapter, the issue of prenatal drug use "sits squarely at the intersection of behavioral teratology, jurisprudence, mental health, medicine, child protection, chemical dependency, civil rights, and women's issues perhaps in a way that no other controversy has" (Lester, Andreozzi, and Appiah 2004:n.p.). In policy and practice, this controversy continues to place objective medical risk over women's subjectively defined risks, leaving women to cope with their own risks in their own ways.

Acknowledgments

This research was supported by the National Institute on Drug Abuse (Grant No. DA017647; Principal Investigator: Alison B. Hamilton). The author thanks Southern California Alcohol and Drug Programs, the women who participated in the study, and the anonymous reviewers and book editors who provided constructive feedback on the manuscript.

Notes

1. Pseudonyms have been used throughout this chapter.
2. As of 2009, Arizona had specific reporting requirements in the event of a positive toxicology screen in a newborn infant (i.e., under thirty days of age), but the state did not have mandatory or automatic removal of infants with positive screens (U.S. Department of Health and Human Services 2009).
3. Funded by NIH/NIDA K01DA017647 (A. Hamilton, Principal Investigator).
4. In the United States, meth is currently the primary substance compelling treatment during pregnancy (Terplan et al. 2009).
5. Under the federal Controlled Substances Act, Schedule II substances can be prescribed under highly restrictive guidelines and have the potential for abuse leading to severe psychological or physical dependence.
6. The sites are Des Moines, Iowa; Honolulu; Los Angeles; and Tulsa, Oklahoma.
7. "Tweakers" are meth users, especially injecting meth users.

References

Arria, Amelia, Chris Derauf, Linda Lagasse, Penny Grant, Rizwan Shah, Lynne Smith, William Haning, Marilyn Huestis, Arthur Strauss, Sheri Della Grotta, Jing Liu, and Barry Lester
    2006   Methamphetamine and Other Substance Use during Pregnancy: Preliminary Estimates from the Infant Development, Environment, and Lifestyle (IDEAL) Study. Maternal and Child Health Journal 10(3):293–302.

Bailey, Jennifer, Karl Hill, David Hawkins, Richard Catalano, and Robert Abbott
    2008   Men's and Women's Patterns of Substance Use around Pregnancy. Birth 35(1):50–59.

Blackwell, Patricia, Kathryn Kirkhart, Dorren Schmitt, and Michael Kaiser
    1998   Cocaine/polydrug-affected Dyads: Implications for Infant Cognitive Development and Mother-Infant Interaction during the First Six Postnatal Months. Journal of Applied Developmental Psychology 19(2):235–48.

Chung, Esther, Laila Nurmohamed, Leny Mathew, Irma Elo, James Coyne, and Jennifer Culhane
    2010   Risky Health Behaviors among Mothers-to-Be: The Impact of Adverse Childhood Experiences. Academic Pediatrics 10(4):245–51.

Cloak, Christine, Thomas Ernst, Larissa Fujii, Brooke Hedemark, and Linda Chang
    2009   Lower Diffusion in White Matter of Children with Prenatal Methamphetamine Exposure. Neurology 72(24):2068–75.

Cohen, Judith, Alice Dickow, Kathryn Horner, Joan Zweben, Joseph Balabis, Denna Vandersloot, Christine Reiber, and Methamphetamine Treatment Project Corporate Authors
    2003   Abuse and Violence History of Men and Women in Treatment for Methamphetamine Dependence. American Journal on Addictions 12(5):377–85.

Cohen, Judith, R. Greenberg, J. Uri, M. Halpin, and Joan Zweben
    2007   Women with Methamphetamine Dependence: Research on Etiology and Treatment. Journal of Psychoactive Drugs Suppl. 4:347–51.

Crome, Ilana, and Manoj Kumar
    2007   Epidemiology of Drug and Alcohol Use in Young Women. Seminars in Fetal and Neonatal Medicine 12:98–105.

Della Grotta, Sheri, Linda LaGasse, Amelia Arria, Chris Derauf, Penny Grant, Lynne Smith, Rizwan Shah, Marilyn Huestis, Jing Liu, and Barry Lester
    2010   Patterns of Methamphetamine Use during Pregnancy: Results from the Infant Development, Environment, and Lifestyle (IDEAL) Study. Maternal and Child Health Journal 14(4):519–27.

Derauf, Chris, Linda LaGasse, Lynne Smith, Penny Grant, Rizwan Shah, Amelia Arria, Marilyn Huestis, William Haning, Arthur Strauss, Sheri Della Grotta, Jing Liu, and Barry Lester
    2007   Demographic and Psychosocial Characteristics of Mothers Using Methamphetamine during Pregnancy: Preliminary Results of the Infant Development, Environment, and Lifestyle Study (IDEAL). American Journal of Drug and Alcohol Abuse 33(2):281–89.

Dluzen, Dean, and Bin Liu
    2008   Gender Differences in Methamphetamine Use and Responses: A Review. Gender and Medicine 5(1):24–35.
Fisher, Jane, Meena Cabral de Mello, Takashi Izutsu, and Tuan Tran
    2011   The Ha Noi Expert Statement: Recognition of Maternal Mental Health in Resource-Constrained Settings Is Essential for Achieving the Millennium Development Goals. International Journal of Mental Health Systems 5(1):2.
Frank, Deborah, Marilyn Augustyn, Wanda Grant Knight, Tripler Pell, and Barry Zuckerman
    2001   Growth, Development, and Behavior in Early Childhood following Prenatal Cocaine Exposure: A Systematic Review. Journal of the American Medical Association 285(12):1613–25.
Gonzales, Rachel, Larissa Mooney, and Richard Rawson
    2010   The Methamphetamine Problem in the United States. Annual Reviews of Public Health 21(31):385–98.
Good, Meadow, Ido Solt, Joann Acuna, Siegfried Rotmensch, and Matthew Kim
    2010   Methamphetamine Use during Pregnancy: Maternal and Neonatal Implications. Obstetrics and Gynecology 116(2Pt.1):330–34.
Hamilton, Alison, and Nicholas Goeders
    2010   Violence Perpetrated by Women Who Use Methamphetamine. Journal of Substance Use 15(5):313–29.
Jessup, Martha, Janice Humphreys, Claire Brindis, and Kathryn Lee
    2003   Extrinsic Barriers to Substance Abuse Treatment among Pregnant Drug Dependent Women. Journal of Drug Issues 33(2):295–304.
Johnson-Hanks, Jennifer
    2006   Uncertain Honor: Modern Motherhood in an African Crisis. Chicago: University of Chicago Press.
Lagasse, Linda, Trecia Wouldes, Elana Newman, Lynne Smith, Rizwan Shah, Chris Derauf, Marilyn Huestis, Amelia Arria, Sheri Della Grotta, Tara Wilcox, and Barry Lester
    2011   Prenatal Methamphetamine Exposure and Neonatal Neurobehavioral Outcome in the USA and New Zealand. Neurotoxicology and Teratology 33(1):166–75.
Latino-Martel, Paule, Doris S. Chan, Nathalie Druesne-Pecollo, Emilie Barrandon, Serge Hercberg, and Teresa Norat
    2010   Maternal Alcohol Consumption during Pregnancy and Risk of Childhood Leukemia: Systematic Review and Meta-analysis. Cancer Epidemiology, Biomarkers and Prevention 19(5):1238–60.
Lester, Barry, Lynne Andreozzi, and Lindsey Appiah
    2004   Substance Use during Pregnancy: Time for Policy to Catch Up with Research. Harm Reduction Journal 1:5. doi:10.1186/1477–7517–1–5.
Messina, Nena, Patricia Marinelli-Casey, Maureen Hillhouse, Richard Rawson, Jeremy Hunter, and Alfonso Ang
    2008   Childhood Adverse Events and Methamphetamine Use among Men and Women. Journal of Psychoactive Drugs Suppl. 5:399–409.
Murphy, Sheigla, and Marsha Rosenbaum
    1999   Pregnant Women on Drugs: Combating Stereotypes and Stigma. New Brunswick, NJ: Rutgers University Press.
Paz, Monica, Lynne Smith, Linda LaGasse, Chris Derauf, Penny Grant, Rizwan Shah,

Amelia Arria, Marilyn Huestis, William Haning, Arthur Strauss, Sheri Della Grotta, Jing
Liu, and Barry Lester
   2009   Maternal Depression and Neurobehavior in Newborns Prenatally Exposed to
           Methamphetamine. Neurotoxicology and Teratology 31(3):177–82.
Ross, Lori, and Cindy-Lee Dennis
   2009   The Prevalence of Postpartum Depression among Women with Substance Use,
           an Abuse History, or Chronic Illness: A Systematic Review. Journal of Women's
           Health 18(4):475–86.
Smith, Lynne, Linda LaGasse, Chris Derauf, Penny Grant, Rizwan Shah, Amelia Arria,
Marilyn Huestis, William Haning, Arthur Strauss, Sheri Della Grotta, Jing Liu,
and Barry Lester
   2006   The Infant Development, Environment, and Lifestyle Study: Effects of Prenatal
           Methamphetamine Exposure, Polydrug Exposure, and Poverty on Intrauterine
           Growth. Pediatrics 118(3):1149–56.
Smith, Lynne, Linda Lagasse, Chris Derauf, Penny Grant, Rizwan Shah, Amelia Arria,
Marilyn Huestis, William Haning, Arthur Strauss, Sheri Della Grotta, Melissa Fallone, Jing
Liu, and Barry Lester
   2008   Prenatal Methamphetamine Use and Neonatal Neurobehavioral Outcome.
           Neurotoxicology and Teratology 30(1):20–28.
Smith, Lynne, Linda Lagasse, Chris Derauf, Elana Newman, Rizwan Shah, William
Haning, Amelia Arria, Marilyn Huestis, Arthur Strauss, Sheri Della Grotta, Lynne
Dansereau, Hai Lin, and Barry Lester
   2011   Motor and Cognitive Outcomes through Three Years of Age in Children Exposed
           to Prenatal Methamphetamine. Neurotoxicology and Teratology 33(1):176–84.
Spears, Gwendolyn, Judith Stein, and Deborah Koniak-Griffin
   2010   Latent Growth Trajectories of Substance Use among Pregnant and Parenting
           Adolescents. Psychology of Addictive Behaviors 24(2):322–32.
Stone, Kristen, Linda LaGasse, Barry Lester, Seetha Shankaran, Henrietta Bada, Charles
Bauer, and Jane Hammond
   2010   Sleep Problems in Children with Prenatal Substance Exposure: The Maternal
           Lifestyle Study. Archives of Pediatric and Adolescent Medicine 164(5):452–56.
Terplan, Mishka, Erica Smith, Michael Kozloski, and Harold Pollack
   2009   Methamphetamine Use among Pregnant Women. Obstetrics and Gynecology
           113(6):1285–91.
U.S. Department of Health and Human Services
   2009   Parental Drug Use as Child Abuse: Summary of State Laws. Washington, DC:
           Child Welfare Information Gateway. www.childwelfare.gov/systemwide/laws_
           policies/statutes/drugexposed.pdf, accessed March 21, 2011.
U.S. Legal
   N.d.   Chemical Endangerment of Child Law and Legal Definition. definitions
           .uslegal.com/c/chemical-endangerment-of-child/, accessed March 21, 2011.
Whiteford, Linda, and Barbara Szelag
   2000   Access and Utility as Reflections of Cultural Constructions of Pregnancy. Primary
           Care Update for Obstetricians/Gynecologists 7(3):98–104.
Whiteford, Linda, and Judi Vitucci
   1997   Pregnancy and Addiction: Translating Research into Practice. Social Science and
           Medicine 44(9):1371–80.

Wright, Terry, and E. Tam
  2010   Disparate Rates of Persistent Smoking and Drug Use during Pregnancy of
          Women of Hawaiian Ancestry. Ethnicity and Disease 20:S1–S8.
Zapata, Lauren, Susan Hillis, Polly Marchbanks, Kathryn Curtis, and Richard Lowry
  2008   Methamphetamine Use Is Independently Associated with Recent Risky Sexual
          Behaviors and Adolescent Pregnancy. Journal of School Health 78(12):641–48.
Zdravkovic, Tamara, Olga Genbacev, Michael McMaster, and Susan Fisher
  2005   The Adverse Effects of Maternal Smoking on the Human Placenta: A Review.
          26(Suppl.A):S81–S86.
Zweben, Joan, Judith Cohen, Darrell Christian, Gantt Galloway, Michelle Salinardi, David
Parent, Martin Iguchi, and Methamphetamine Treatment Project Corporate Authors
  2004   Psychiatric Symptoms in Methamphetamine Users. American Journal on
          Addictions 13(2):181–90.

PART II

Biopolitical Narratives of Risk and Responsibility

CHAPTER 4

Birth and Blame
Guatemalan Midwives and Reproductive Risk

Sheila Cosminsky

The beautiful and scenic vistas of Guatemala, the Land of Eternal Spring, mask the realities of a country with one of the highest infant mortality rates and maternal mortality ratios in Central America and the Western hemisphere. With a current infant mortality rate of 26.9/1,000 live births (CIA 2010) and maternal mortality at 153/100,000 live births (Franco de Mendez 2003; PAHO 2007; Repogle 2007), Guatemala's national reproductive statistics obscure intracountry discrepancy and the far greater mortality rates of rural and indigenous populations vis-à-vis their urban and nonindigenous counterparts. In parts of the rural highlands, the maternal mortality ratio is as high as 446/100,000 live births (Bailey, Szaszdi, and Glover 2002). And it is here, among the poorer or indigenous Maya populations, that births occur at home using traditional midwives, and where the choice of birth attendant often becomes conflated with risky reproductive activity.

The Peace Accords of 1996 included the goals of reducing infant and maternal mortality, and the Guatemala government implemented the Sistema Integral de Atención en Salud (SIAS), a health reform program influenced by neoliberal processes and global reproductive health programs formulated by WHO, USAID, and other international organizations (Maupin 2008). In 2007, the government began a new training program for traditional midwives, or traditional birth attendants (TBAs) as they are called by the government and medical personnel, who according to Alejandro Silva of the Guatemalan Health Ministry's National Reproductive Health Program would purportedly be more "culturally sensitive than previous approaches. Over 11,800 TBAs would receive three days of training, during which they learn to identify warning signs, refer problem cases, and develop family and community emergency plans" (Repogle 2007). The main difference in these programs from those that have been offered in Guatemala since the 1950s (see Dudgeon, this volume, for a discussion of some of these programs) seems to be the addition of family and community emergency plans. That is, the family would be encouraged to put aside money and arrange for transportation should complications arise that necessitated a hospital transfer. How realistic this plan is and how it is being carried out has not yet been evaluated.

In September 2008, President Alváro Colom of Guatemala announced an initiative to train fifteen thousand lay midwives. As reported by an international news agency, Colom explained that this five-month program would "provide these midwives with training in the basics of gynecology and obstetrics, including how to identify complicated pregnancies and avoid preventable deaths. . . . For each high-risk pregnancy the midwives refer to a doctor, the government will pay them $20" (MSNBC 2008).[1]

Commenting on the training initiative was Jackeline Lavidali, the director of Guatemala's reproductive health program: "If we're able to get these women to see a doctor, high-risk cases could be identified and we could take steps to prevent them" (MSNBC 2008). However, a contradiction exists between the two statements. The president's statement assumes the midwife can be taught to recognize high-risk cases, which has been the focus of many of the internationally funded and sanctioned midwifery training programs (Kruske 2004; Mangay Maglacas and Simons 1986). But Lavidali's statement implies that only a doctor can identify high-risk cases, presumably in a prenatal exam, and that the midwife cannot be depended on or trusted to identify high-risk cases—or, if she does, she will not refer them. Moreover, Lavidali's assertion assumes risk to be preventable. Although treatable, some risk conditions are not predictable, much less preventable. Lavidali's assumptions about risk and risk prevention may also reflect the general attitude of biomedical personnel in Guatemala toward the midwife.

The view promoted by WHO is that pregnancy itself is a risk (see Dudgeon, this volume). In this chapter, I argue that the subtext of the new WHO Safe Motherhood policy, as it has been carried out in Guatemala, is that the midwife is the greatest risk factor in the reproductive process and to blame for the country's high mortality rates. The midwife's beliefs and practices, including not referring high-risk cases to the hospital, become the scapegoat for the high mortality rates; the improvement of these rates entails her removal or replacement (WHO 2009). The basic assumption is that if the midwife is trained to recognize risk factors in pregnant women and complications during delivery and refers these to the hospital or medical facility for delivery, the infant and maternity mortality rates will decrease. In examining the issue of reproductive risk and the role of the midwife, as well as the problems of the training programs and WHO's Safe Motherhood policy, this chapter explores three interrelated criteria used for the evaluation of midwives: (1) infant and maternal mortality rates; (2) reproductive risk factors, as well as the concept of risk (what is defined as high risk and by whom?); and (3) hospital referrals.

Methods

This chapter is based on ethnographic research in two locations in southern Guatemala over the last forty-two years. My first period of ethnographic fieldwork research took place for one year, 1968–1969, in the K'iche' Maya highland village of Novillero, an *aldea* (hamlet) of the town of Santa Lucia Utatlán, where I returned for briefer fieldwork visits throughout the 1970s and in 1996. I also conducted in-depth fieldwork on a sugar and coffee plantation, Finca San Felipe, at varying intervals from 1974 to 2010.[2] I gathered information through participant-observation, interviews with mothers that included their reproductive histories and data on illness and health-seeking behavior, intensive interviews and observations of *comadronas* (traditional midwives), shamans, and other healers, and observations of midwifery training sessions in Novillero and the city of Retalhuleu.

Definitions: Who Is a Midwife?

Both the training programs of the Ministry of Health's National Reproductive Health Program and the president's initiative of new midwifery training programs recognize that the majority of births in Guatemala are attended by comadronas, who also provide important social, emotional, physical, and ritual support to the laboring woman and her family, and that there is a lack of effective infrastructure and of a referral system to medical facilities, especially hospitals. Officials acquiesce. "If we want to have an influence on maternal mortality, we have to work with the TBAs," says Alejandro Silva of the Guatemalan Health Ministry's National Reproductive Health Program (Repogle 2007:177). This realistic policy comes at a time when WHO has come out against funding such programs in favor of eliminating them and training what it calls "skilled attendants," claiming that training TBAs has failed to lower the maternal mortality rate and therefore no longer deserves support.

WHO defines a TBA as "a person who assists the mother during childbirth and who initially acquired her skills by delivering babies herself or through apprenticeship to other TBAs" (Verderese and Turnbull 1975:7). In contrast, a "skilled attendant" is "an accredited health professional—such as a midwife, doctor or nurse—who has been educated and trained to proficiency in the skills needed to manage normal (i.e., uncomplicated) pregnancies, childbirth and the immediate postnatal period, and in the identification, management and referral of complications in women and newborns. Traditional birth attendants, who are not formally trained, do not meet the definition of skilled birth attendants" (WHO 2009:1).

WHO considers TBAs insufficiently skilled to "manage normal deliveries and diagnose, manage, and refer obstetric complications" (USAID 2010) and uses the term "midwife" to refer to a person who has some formal biomedical training in obstetrics and is officially licensed. These statements reflect a shift in policy toward midwives from supporters of to replacements for TBAs or traditional midwives (Kruske 2004). Earlier programs emphasized upgrading the midwife's knowledge by teaching hygienic practices, such as washing hands and cutting the cord with sterile scissors. In the 1980s, training shifted to recognizing the risk factors and danger signs for which midwives should refer patients for preventive care at prenatal clinics and for delivery at hospitals with skilled personnel. Following this policy, WHO's Safe Motherhood campaign states: "TBAs fall outside this definition" of skilled attendant, because "they lack the capacity to manage obstetric complications" (ibid., 308).

Anthropologists have criticized the term "traditional birth attendant" as ethnocentric, medicocentric, and political, as these midwives often do more than attend births (Cosminsky 1983; Glei, Goldman, and German 2003; Pigg 1997). They also provide prenatal and postnatal care and often perform important ritual and so-cial roles. The same criticisms can apply to the term "skilled birth attendant" as dis-tinct from "comadrona." This differentiation implies that traditional midwives have no skills, as opposed to acknowledging that their skills might be different from the biomedical ones taught to "skilled birth attendants." In addition, the assumption "that they lack the capacity to manage obstetric complications" (Kruske 2004:308) is condescending, as it implies they cannot be taught such obstetric management. In this chapter, I use the term "midwife" or "comadrona," the Spanish term used throughout Guatemala.[3] I use the term "TBA" when referring to literature that uses that term.

Setting

The plantation Finca San Felipe has a resident population today of about 310, compared to 690 in 1976, of Mayan Indians (whose parents or grandparents mi-grated from highland towns) and Ladinos (persons of non-Indian or mixed an-cestry or culture) from nearby coastal towns. Today, everyone speaks Spanish and wears Western dress, yet many still identify themselves as "naturales," the local Spanish word for indigenous Maya. Housing is provided by the plantation; most homes are poor and small, constructed of wood boards with corrugated metal roofs and dirt floors. They are often overcrowded and reflect the general poverty of the population. Environmental sanitation is very poor. Until around 2005 there was no electricity or running water, and there are still few latrines. Women commonly had nine to twelve children, but their children are now having only three or four, partly as the result of economic changes and the increased availability and accept-ability of contraception and family planning. Child malnutrition has been and still is prevalent.

More than 80 percent of the births on Finca San Felipe and in the surround-ing areas take place in the mother's home, attended by a comadrona. Through-out the 1970s and 1980s, one midwife, Doña Maria, delivered most of the babies on Finca San Felipe. Even though she was considered a Ladina, she married a K'iche'-speaking Maya and experienced all the signs of divine calling, such as hav-ing dreams, finding special objects, undergoing serious illness, experiencing bodily twitches, and being accompanied by the spirits of dead midwives who would advise her during a birth (see Dudgeon, this volume). She also became a shaman and used divining seeds and the ritual Maya calendar. One of Doña Maria's daughters, Doña Siriaca, started a midwifery practice in the 1980s. Since the 1990s, she has handled most of the deliveries, as Doña Maria became ill and died in 1997. Doña Siriaca did not receive the kinds of divinatory signs her mother did, although she does experience bodily twitches that indicate someone is going to call her for a birth, and she believes God is in her hands, guiding them during massages and the birth. I interviewed two other midwives—Doña Maria's sister-in-law, who was no longer practicing, and a midwife who lived in the neighboring hamlet but occasionally de-livered mothers on the *finca*. The nearest hospital, the National Hospital, is located

12.5 kilometers away in the department's capital, Retalhuleu. Some people use a private Catholic hospital, San Cayetano (now called Hilario Galindo Hospital), in the town of San Felipe. There are also public health centers in San Felipe and Retalhuleu where women can go for prenatal care.

In Santa Lucia Utatlán, 97 percent of the births are still assisted by comadronas (Guatemala 2005). Several midwives were practicing in and around Novillero, and I collected information during various fieldwork periods primarily from three K'iche'-speaking Maya midwives, all of whom had experienced signs of divine calling, and one Ladino midwife. Housing is primarily of adobe with tile or tin roofs and dirt floors, although some poorer ones have wattle-and-daub walls with thatched roofs. Until the mid-1990s, there was no electricity or running water, and few latrines. People have small corn plots, and many migrate seasonally to coastal plantations. Since the 1980s, migration to the United States has increased, resulting in improved housing and material conditions from remittances. The closest hospitals are either in Sololá or in Quezaltenango, both about an hour away by road. A Catholic mission–run clinic has provided basic health care services in Novillero since the 1960s and, at least until 2000, was also running a health promoter program and a midwifery-training program. In the 1970s, a public health clinic opened up in the town center of Santa Lucia.

To practice legally in Guatemala, comadronas must have a license. To get a license requires attending a training course offered or approved by the Ministry of Health. Comadronas are also supposed to attend monthly sessions at a local health center, where they make monthly reports and receive birth registration forms. These are all mechanisms of control over the midwives, as is the threat of having their licenses revoked if they do not comply with the regulations. Midwives who have not had biomedical training are legally prohibited from attending births.

Doñas Maria and Siriaca both have licenses, as did other midwives practicing on the finca or in the surrounding areas. However, in Santa Lucia Utatlán, some had their license but others did not—especially the older ones. Nonetheless, they still practiced, because some of these midwives believed they had a divine calling to practice and God would punish them with illness or death if they refused to help someone who requested their assistance (Cosminsky 1982).

The Guatemalan government also requires a licensed midwife's signature and official seal on the birth registration form if a baby is not born in a hospital. This means that if a baby was delivered by the mother herself, other family members, or an unlicensed midwife, the parents have to find a midwife who will obtain and sign the form for them. Some unlicensed midwives have informal agreements with trained midwives who are willing to sign the appropriate form. However, licensed midwives are told not to sign and give out the forms, and they put themselves at risk should the infant or mother develop a problem. Doña Siriaca has agreed at times to sign forms for certain unlicensed midwives but not for family members who deliver babies, since these births might present more problems. In this way, she bridges the gap between the biomedical system and the traditional one. Although she is in a subordinate position to the medical personnel, she is in a superior one to the unlicensed midwives, who are in a dependent and subordinate relationship to her (Cosminsky 2001). Such regulations, aimed at imposing greater supervision and control over the midwives, exacerbate the problem of underregistration of births and deaths.

Additional regulations introduced by the Ministry of Health pertain to the age and health of the mother; these prohibit midwives from attending births by first-time mothers, women under sixteen or over thirty-five, women with a breech or transverse presentation, and women with a previous cesarean. Comadronas remained uncertain as to whether there were legal restrictions in place to ensure the referral of these purported risk scenarios, but midwives were quite concerned that if they delivered a mother with such purported risk factors, they would be legally responsible if problems arose with the delivery. In addition, the midwife's role is increasingly being attenuated and reduced, as some of the training programs under the Guatemalan health reform or SIAS are emphasizing the training of new, young, literate midwives who are more easily medicalized and integrated into the national health care system (Maupin 2008).

Mortality Rates as an Evaluative Criterion

Training programs for midwives have been based on the assumption that such training will result in lower infant and maternal mortality rates. Consequently, these rates have been used as criteria to measure the effectiveness of the training. "For senior policy makers, however, success was focused on one indicator—the ultimate reduction in mortality rates" (Kruske 2004:307). But "training programmes for traditional birth attendants have failed to reduce maternal mortality in the past," according to WHO. "The short trainings were not adequate to teach an otherwise unqualified person the critical thinking and decision-making skills needed to practice" (2009:3). The logical conclusion would be to change the training. Instead, the onus is put on the midwife as being unqualified, and the conclusion is not to improve the training but to train someone else. According to Safe Motherhood, mortality rates have not dropped after training; therefore, training midwives is deemed unworthy of the expense. The underlying assumption is that the midwives' practices, their perceived inability to recognize purported high-risk cases, and their failure to refer at-risk mothers to hospitals are the cause of these mortality rates.

Before blaming the midwives, maybe we need to ask about the causes of maternal and infant mortality. Studies have concluded that the main causes of maternal mortality in Guatemala are hemorrhage, infection, malpresentation, hypertension, and unsafe abortion (Franco de Mendez 2003). Can training of midwives have an impact on these causal factors? And if so, what kind of training would that be? In addition, recent reports indicate that in Guatemala infant mortality rates have declined from 39/1,000 live births for 2000–2005 (PAHO 2007) to 26.9/1,000 live births (CIA 2010), and maternal mortality rates have fallen from 190/100,000 live births from 1995 to 1999 to 153/100,000 live births in the 2000s (Franco de Mendez 2003; PAHO 2007; Repogle 2007). Moreover, are there factors other than the TBAs that may influence mortality rates, including the training program, and structural factors such as poverty, poor sanitation, and lack of access to medical facilities?

"Deficient health infrastructure and budget . . . along with the country's high poverty and low education levels, all contribute to Guatemala's high maternal mortality rates" Repogle writes (2007:177). In a similar vein, Kruske argues that there was little understanding in WHO policy statements of the "importance of social factors, such as poverty, gender status, or lack of transportation, which influenced choices and behaviors in the presence of birth complications" (2004:307). Why not conclude that there is a need for more effective training or for improved environmental sanitation and other contributory factors rather than that a new category of "skilled attendants" needs to be trained and traditional midwives eliminated?

Another problem with the use of mortality rates as an indicator by which to evaluate training programs is the difficulty in the measurement of these rates. Underreporting, misclassification, and varied mechanisms of measuring maternal mortality result in widely differing rates (Kestler 1995; Kruske 2004). Similar problems exist with respect to infant and perinatal deaths (stillbirths and early neonatal deaths), which are commonly not recorded and are highly underreported. Since infant deaths are more frequent than maternal deaths, smaller samples are needed. This results in their more common use as an evaluative criterion for the training programs (Bergstrom and Goodburn 2001)—despite their potential for inaccuracy.

Reproductive Risk Factors as an Evaluative Criterion

The second consideration in evaluating midwives turns on the concepts of risk and risk factors. A woman classified by biomedical definition as at risk is considered to have greater chance of experiencing obstetric complications (Allen 2002:158). Here, we see a shift in the way that the term "risk" is conceptualized, from a statistical or epidemiological concept based on probability with either a positive or negative correlation to a purely negative understanding of risk as a predictor of danger or harm (Douglas 1990, 1992; Douglas and Wildavsky 1982) that attributes blame or accountability (Dudgeon 2008). In this shift, the term also becomes political. As Nichter states:

> Information about risk is typically presented to the public as "objective fact" backed up by statistics, which highlight correlations commonly misinterpreted by the public as causal relationships. . . . Knowledge about risk is far from neutral and often motivated by subtle and not so subtle social, political and economic forces. . . . The rhetoric of risk assumes a sense of determinacy which provides those in fields like public health with a "model of" as well as a "model for" action justifying as much as guiding recommendations (2001:101).

This rhetoric reinforces the blaming of the midwife for the problems encountered by the training programs and for the lack of improvement in the high mortality rates—whether she can be directly implicated or not.

Based on statistical analyses, WHO has outlined general risk factors that are purportedly mitigated through biomedical observation and care. These include personal factors such as age of mother (under sixteen or over thirty-five), parity, and previous birth complications including a cesarean section, high blood pressure, anemia, and pre-eclampsia; external factors like traditional practices, which, in the case of Guatemala, would include the midwives' practices of massage and use of the sweat bath; and unpredictable factors such as prolonged labor, malpresentation, hemorrhaging, and sepsis. While some of these conditions are undoubtedly life threatening, others lie in the realm of distant risk calculation and some can be reinterpreted as minimizing the potential dangers carried by other factors. For example, the midwife's use of massage—highly frowned upon by biomedical practitioners—may rectify fetal malpresentation, and a postpartum sweat bath may decrease bleeding and promote uterine healing.

Indeed, defining risk—and risk management—is a contested arena where the right to decide which risks are important depends on the political, social, and economic relationships within and between collectivities (Kaufert and O'Neil 1993). In Guatemala, pregnant women, physicians, midwives, the community, and the government vie for authority over reproductive interest. Midwives are told to identify and refer high-risk cases to the biomedical authorities for treatment. Above all, they are discouraged from attempting to minimize risk on their own.

Malpresentation is considered one of the main risk factors for both infant and maternal deaths. A hand or foot presentation and breech or transverse fetal position are biomedically defined risk factors necessitating a hospital referral that will usually end in a cesarean section. While midwives in both Novillero and Finca San Felipe do not deny the risks associated with malpresentation, they differ in their treatment and in the preventive measures they take to mitigate this risk *before* it occurs. Whereas biomedical practitioners view as a risk the practice of massage, both pre- and postnatal, midwives and pregnant women believe that *not* having a massage is a risk. The women among whom I conducted my research viewed prenatal massage as preventive of complications and as a treatment for pregnancy-related discomfort. Massage is believed to *accomodar* (accommodate) the baby and make it more comfortable, which in turn makes the pregnant woman comfortable. It also helps allay her anxiety and relieves any pain she may be experiencing.

It is also through massage that the midwife feels the position of the fetus and estimates its growth and time of delivery. She may also do an external version if there is fetal malpresentation. Midwives in both Novillero and Finca San Felipe described how they would carefully turn a baby "little by little" if they felt it to be in a position other than head down before the onset of labor. In cases of malpresentation during delivery, Doña Maria described how she would put oil on her hand and push the baby's hand or foot back into the woman while externally massaging the uterus to turn the baby into a head-down position. Preventive forms of external massage before the onset of labor and in situations requiring immediate attention are today done less frequently because of pressure from the biomedical profession to refer such cases to the hospital.

A midwife may also perform massage immediately after the birth of the baby to help expel the placenta and again about three days after delivery to relieve abdominal pain, reduce the risk of hemorrhage, and restore the uterus to its proper position—especially in cases of prolapse. Such massage is often accompanied by a sweat bath in the highlands or a herbal bath on the finca, which is believed to help heal the mother, restore the hot-cold balance to her body, cleanse her physically and ritually, and help stimulate the flow of her breast milk.

Both massage and postnatal bathing are measures of harm reduction, in that they are perceived as preventing complications and promoting healing. Nichter (2003) views the use of harm-reduction practices as an expression of agency that enhances a sense of self-control and reduces a sense of vulnerability for both mother and midwife, in that not doing these practices is perceived as a risk that might adversely affect the delivery or the recovery for the woman and her baby, upon which the midwife's reputation and practice depend.

Despite the negative regard many physicians and nurses have for massage, comadronas continue to perform it, albeit in a slightly modified form to accommodate medical authority and keep their own practice alive. When I returned to Guatemala in 2010, Doña Siriaca was charging separately for massages and the postpartum baths, as were other midwives, so that if the birth is in the hospital the woman can still have massages or baths from the midwife, and the midwife loses neither her reputation nor her financial security.

By 2010, Doña Siriaca had also adopted the discourse of risk that she learned from medical personnel during her review sessions, especially in reference to the restriction that midwives cannot attend primaparas because they are *alto riesgo* (high risk). That the doctor "lo prohibe" [forbids it] is believed by Doña Siriaca to mean she could lose her license, her kit, and the right to practice. She understands that she can provide pre- and postnatal care to first-time mothers, but that the delivery must be in the hospital. Even if such restrictions are not legal proscriptions, some midwives believe they are. Doña Siriaca's repeated use of the phrase "the doctor forbids it" raises questions about control and power in assigning blame and accountability. Moreover, midwives like Doña Siriaca are losing their skills because of their acceptance of medical authority. An unintended consequence is then the potential of heightened risk when a pregnant woman refuses to go to the hospital, leaving a comadrona to choose between tending to the pregnant woman—harking to her divine calling and community responsibility—or letting the woman deliver on her own. Doña Siriaca explained that if a "high-risk" pregnant woman refused to go to the hospital, she would have no choice but to deliver the baby. Depending on the circumstance, however, her skills might have atrophied, potentially adding to the risks that accompany malpresentation or many of the other complications she had been treating before medical technology redefined her heretofore life-saving skills as life threatening.

Interestingly, there are certain biomedical practices taught in the training course that Doña Siriaca perceives as a "risk" and refuses to adopt. Cutting the umbilical cord before the placenta is expelled goes against Maya sensibility, which holds that if the cord is cut first, the placenta will rise up inside the body and choke and kill the woman. She cited an example of a midwife who had recently followed this common medical practice, and the mother died. Doña Siriaca explained that in the hospital, the doctor uses clamps when he cuts the cord; this prevents the placenta from ascending into the body. Doña Siriaca, however, did not have such clamps and was not willing to risk the mother's life in favor of biomedical protocol. Her refusal was logical within the traditional image of the body as a tube in which organs can move up or down. Twenty-five years earlier, her mother had told me the same thing in almost the same words. Although the practice is discouraged by biomedical personnel, recent research has shown that waiting until the cord stops pulsing before cutting it maximizes the amount of oxygen going to the baby and is therefore quite beneficial (Grajeda 1997).

Risk Factors and the Larger Context

Sepsis is another of the risk factors mentioned for maternal mortality. In a study of a TBA training program in Bangladesh, Goodburn et al. (2000) concluded that training did not affect the incidence of postpartum infection, although it did increase TBAs' practicing hygienic delivery. The researchers concluded that "it may be that practicing a 'clean' delivery in itself does not prevent infection in an environment where every surface is contaminated" (398). They suggest it would be premature to recommend discontinuing TBA training altogether, but it might be better to divert scarce resources to interventions for which there is evidence of effectiveness in reducing maternal deaths, for example, the training of community midwives, and support for referral and essential obstetric services at first-level referral facilities.[4] Despite the findings that many TBAs changed their practices in accordance with the training and that maternal infection may be more attributable to larger hygienic impediments, the study's conclusions still reflect negative attitudes toward the TBAs, which influence policy recommendations.

In similar studies of a Safe Motherhood project in Quezaltenango, Bartlett and Bocaletti (1991) and Schieber et al. (1994) found that intrapartum asphyxia, birth trauma, prematurity, and neonatal sepsis were principal causes of neonatal death, and that significant risk factors linked to these deaths were maternal illiteracy, nulliparity, short interbirth intervals, and the use of traditional practices—including midwifery care—as opposed to modern medical services. While linking the midwife to infant death in important—and detrimental—ways, the illumination of factors irrespective of midwife involvement is significant to understanding how larger social and structural forces are at play in women's reproductive health in Guatemala—and in the fate of the midwife. A factor such as maternal illiteracy reflects the low rate of female literacy in Guatemala and can be changed only by government investment in female education. If the midwife referred all illiterate mothers to the hospital, the medical system would be inundated beyond capacity. However, the risk of inadequate hospital services is not mentioned in reviews of

Safe Motherhood as something the midwife can help to ameliorate. Instead, she is lumped with a traditional medical system that purportedly carries the risks associated with an underdeveloped and less than modern society.

Caplan (2000) points out that both Beck and Giddens view new kinds of risk as characterizing contemporary society, which they term "reflexive modernity" (Beck 1992) or "late modernity" (Giddens 1991). In such a framework, communities like those in Novillero and Finca San Felipe, as represented by the national government and international development agencies like WHO and USAID, are still "premodern." It is thus problematic to apply so-called new kinds of risk to non-Western or developing societies while ignoring the social and cultural characteristics that inform local understandings of risk. Caplan (2000) and Douglas and Wildavsky (1982) further argue that culture has been ignored in discussions of risk, and that both social scientists and scientists have treated causality in the external real world as distinct from the result of individual perception. Here, real knowledge has been allocated to the physical sciences, while illusions and mistakes are attributed to psychology and other social sciences. This view is apparent in a meta-analytic study of midwifery-training programs that concludes: "The real effects of TBA training on TBA and maternal behavior, if any, are likely to be small" (Sibley, Sipe, and Koblinsky 2004:1767). This raises the question as to what is meant by "real."

What are risk factors as perceived by the midwives and mothers, and how do these contrast or conflict with biomedical criteria for risk factors? Glei, Goldman, and German (2003) suggest that choice of care (midwife or hospital delivery) depends more on perception of risk than on the medical definition of risk. My research corroborates these findings to suggest that what the community identifies as risk factors do not necessarily coincide with those identified by national and international health policy makers.

Referrals as an Evaluative Criterion

The third issue is the use of hospital referrals as a criterion for evaluating midwives. "Referral is an essential component of health systems" (Sibley, Sipe, and Koblinsky 2004:1758). To where are the comadronas to refer high-risk cases or obstetrical emergencies? It has been estimated that Guatemalan hospitals can handle only about 20 percent of the country's births (Hurtado and Saenz de Tejada 2001). This figure has not changed over the past thirty years and is not likely to change much in the near future. If midwives referred mothers with all the risk factors that they have been taught—or even a small portion of the high-risk cases—the hospitals could not handle them. In addition, using the number of referrals as a criterion for evaluating the effectiveness of the midwife, her knowledge, or the training program ignores this circumstance: if the midwife recommends a hospital delivery, the decision is usually made by the pregnant woman's family, not the midwife or in many cases even the pregnant woman. That is, even if the midwife refers a woman to a hospital, she may not go. The medical personnel assume the midwife has more control or influence than she actually has, and that the pregnant woman has a decision-making role, whereas in actuality the decisions concerning the birth may be made by her husband and in-laws. As Douglas has observed: "Anger, hope, and fear are part of most risky situations and that a decision that involves costs also involves consultations with neighbors, family, and friends" (1992:12).

In such cases of noncompliance, the midwife may feel she must assist or attend the mother. As we have seen, many of the comadronas believe that they have a divine calling, and that if they do not honor it, they will be punished by God with illness or death. The midwife is not supposed to refuse to help someone. Thus, if she refers someone to the hospital, and the woman or her family refuses, the midwife is obligated to help, even though she may be legally liable if there is a problematic outcome.

Several studies that have examined the relationship between training programs and referrals have produced mixed conclusions. Although WHO and Safe Motherhood have stated that these training programs are a failure (as defined in terms of referrals of trained versus untrained midwives), other studies have reached different conclusions. Goldman and Glei (2003) in their study based on data from the 1995 Guatemalan Survey of Family Health found that trained midwives are more likely than other midwives to refer their clients to biomedical providers. Sibley, Sipe, and Koblinsky's meta-analysis of sixteen studies of the effectiveness of TBA training to improve access to skilled birth attendance for obstetric emergencies, which included two from Guatemala, produced mixed results: a "medium, positive nonsignificant association between training and TBA knowledge of risk factors and conditions requiring referral with small, positive, significant associations between TBA referral and maternal compliance and service use," along with the observation that since the training program was just one component of a package of integrated interventions, these results cannot be attributed to it (2004:1067).

One of the studies included in this meta-analysis focused on a training project in Quezaltenango, Guatemala, which included not only training for the midwives but also training for the health providers, mainly nurses, at the hospital to increase their understanding of the Maya medical system and culture in order to treat the comadronas more respectfully. Referrals increased for both trained and untrained midwives, and it was concluded that the main factor increasing the referrals was the change in attitude of the nursing staff (O'Rourke 1994). However, a report to the Guatemalan Ministry of Health and USAID, which concluded that the TBA training program did not increase referrals, has been used to justify discontinuing training programs for the midwives. The emphasis was on blaming the midwives, even though the change in attitudes and behavior of the nursing staff was found to be an important factor in referrals. Although the report did recommend "continuation of efforts to improve relationships between hospital staff and TBAs to make hospitals more family- and TBA-friendly in Quezaltenango as well as neighboring departments" (Bailey, Szaszdi, and Glover 2002:22), I do not know to what extent this has occurred—if at all.

Another review of TBA-based interventions to reduce maternal mortality, including the already mentioned program in Guatemala, found that six of the seven studies specified used referral rates to evaluate the training, and that recognition of the signs of serious complications had improved referral practices. In the two studies in which the changes were significant, the TBA training program had been accompanied by enhancement of hospital facilities and emergency transport system (Ray and Salihu 2004:10). This has not occurred in any of the Guatemalan interventions that I know of. Another evaluation of this program in the Department of Quezaltenango, Guatemala, produced "very mixed findings with regards to the impact of training TBAs on the detection and referral of women with obstetric complications" (Bailey, Szaszdi, and Glover 2002:22). The mixed findings of these studies raise the question: is the number of referrals a useful criterion for evaluating a training program or the midwives?

Luisa's Story: Mortality, Risk, and Referral, or Death by Chocolate

Doña Siriaca told me a story that illustrates both the interrelationship of the factors of mortality, risk, and referral and the different perceptions of risk factors. A family came to get the comadrona at 3:00 a.m. A husband had beaten his pregnant wife, Luisa, while he was drunk, causing her to have the illness of anger. As a result, she went into labor earlier than expected. Luisa's mother gave her hot chocolate with egg because she thought she was "cold." When she arrived at the scene, Doña Siriaca determined that these substances had contributed to the already hot and dangerous imbalance of Luisa's body, and because Luisa had a cesarean section with her previous child, the midwife reasoned that the birth would be high risk. Doña Siriaca explained that she would not attend the delivery and advised Luisa's family to arrange for an ambulance to take her to the hospital. However, obtaining transportation at 3:00 a.m. on the finca to go to the nearest hospital in the town of Retalhuleu, 12.5 kilometers away, was not easy. Meanwhile, Luisa had terrible pain after drinking the chocolate, her stomach swelled, and, within ten minutes, both Luisa and her unborn baby died.

The family threatened Doña Siriaca, blaming her for the deaths. However, they had not consulted Doña Siriaca earlier in the pregnancy. When Doña Siriaca told the story to the doctor, he said it was not her fault, but the fault of the husband who had hit the woman, causing her to have anger and premature labor. According to Doña Siriaca, the doctor did not attribute the death to a biomedical cause. Doña Siriaca had felt that she was in a vulnerable position and had found it necessary to appeal to the doctor for support, so she wouldn't be legally accountable in case the family threatened her or took her to court. Looking for the doctor's authority to validate her actions, however, reinforces her subordinate position in relation to the biomedical one and reveals how her own confidence is being undermined.

From Doña Siriaca's point of view, a number of interrelated risk factors were involved. One was domestic abuse in the form of the husband's drunkenness and his beating of his wife. Drinking is a big problem on the finca and often results in domestic violence. It is also a common cause of *enojo* or *colera* (anger illnesses). According to local beliefs, emotions should be kept in balance, as experiencing strong emotions such as anger, fright, and sadness can cause illness, miscarriages, premature labor, and other obstetrical complications. Strong emotions also reflect a conflict or disturbance of balance in social relations, which can likewise cause illness.

Anger also causes an imbalance of the qualities of hotness and coldness. As is the case in much of Guatemala, people on Finca San Felipe and in Novillero believe in the hot-cold principle of humoral medicine. Pregnancy is considered a hot state, the heat of which increases near delivery. Anger is a hot illness; thus, an angry body is in an imbalanced state of too much heat. This imbalance in Luisa was further exacerbated by drinking the hot chocolate, which is considered a hot substance.

Doña Siriaca was also following her biomedical training by telling the family they should go to the hospital because of the premature labor and the previous cesarean. However, there was nothing she could do about the lack of transportation, a reality that is often ignored by the medical profession. From the biomedical perspective, the main risk factors were the previous cesarean section and the preterm labor caused by the beating. It is not clear from Doña Siriaca's story whether the family had not consulted with her before, since they intended to go to the hospital for delivery because of the earlier cesarean section, or whether the husband's drunkenness caused a delay in seeking help. Any or all of these factors may have been involved in their decision, and Doña Siriaca could do nothing about any of them.

Hospital Deliveries and Risk Perceptions

Many people on the plantation view a cesarean surgery as a risk rather than a solution. According to local beliefs, a cesarean section may cause complications with recovery and with future pregnancies, as well as infection. These may also have been factors in Luisa's death. Berry (2008) points out in her study in Sololá, Guatemala, that many women think a cesarean delivery will affect future fertility. Such ideas may be reinforced by medical personnel, as in the warning given to a seventeen-year-old new mother on the finca who had a cesarean delivery with her first child. She was told that she had to have the cesarean section because her body was too small and narrow, and that she should not have any more children because it would be too "risky." For a newly married young wife, this message can be devastating, with psychological implications as well as implications for her relations with her husband and in-laws with whom she was living. Two years later she had another child successfully delivered with the midwife.

Other factors perceived as harmful in the hospital are restriction of food intake before the surgery, violations of the hot-cold principle in food served in the hospital, bathing in cold water, eating in social isolation, limited visiting hours, and not allowing husbands or other relatives to stay before, during, or after the birth. This last factor is in contrast to home births, at which the husband is supposed to be present if possible. Reluctance to go to the hospital may also be the result of other factors, including the expense, lack of transportation, fear (especially of surgery), the value placed on modesty, and concern about care for other family members (Berry 2008; Cosminsky 2001). Additional factors may include severity of the condition, perceived quality of care, perceived risk and local understanding of cause, and the value placed on women's lives (Sibley, Sipe, and Koblinsky 2004). Hospital deliveries, including cesareans, entail expense in transportation costs. When I conducted fieldwork in 1996, a hired car or taxi cost Q50 (US$8) each way—if one is available—and a cesarean cost an exorbitant Q320 (US$53).[5] Other problems are possible infection and the long recovery period from a cesarean, which may be an extra burden for the mother and her family.

Since the majority of hospital deliveries from the finca occur because of complications that the midwife has referred, such as malpresentation, they often result in cesarean deliveries. This likely outcome in turn increases people's reluctance to go to the hospital because of their fear of surgery. As Doña Maria explained, even when she tells a mother to go to the hospital for a breech birth or other complication, she says: "I won't go. If I die, I die here." Some are concerned that they could die on the way to the hospital because of the bumpy ride on the rough road. Yet in such cases, if something did happen to the mother or the child, the medical profession would blame the midwife for not "referring" her to the hospital and for attending the delivery. Moreover, the midwife can be held legally responsible and thus fined or jailed, especially if the family presses charges—as was Doña Siriaca's fear.

When I was accompanying Doña Siriaca on her visits to her clients, three women said their doctor told them during their routine prenatal examinations that they would need a cesarean section. When Doña Siriaca examined them, she said their babies were fine and in the proper head-down position. In each case, she took my hand to have me feel where the head was, indicating the position of the baby and thus validating her knowledge (Cosminsky 2001:368). Cesareans, even more than regular hospital deliveries, are an exertion of biomedical power over the midwife and the pregnant woman, exemplifying the contestation over authoritative knowledge (Jordan 1997).

According to PAHO (1999), 25 percent of all births in Guatemala are by cesarean section. In at least one public hospital, the cesarean rate has reached 42 percent (Houston 2001). According to WHO advisories, cesarean sections should never exceed 15 percent, even in high-risk populations. Multiple factors could be contributing to the high numbers in Guatemala, such as the policies of the doctors and the hospital, the acquisition of new technology, more referrals of complications by the midwives, financial gain, and the perception that cesareans are an essential aspect of modern obstetrics and a solution for birth complications. Some of the women on the finca said they had heard that so many cesareans are done in order to give the new doctors practice. The increase in cesarean births in Guatemala needs to be explored in future research.

Mothers and midwives perceive hospital deliveries in general as risky, partly because they are concerned about inattentiveness on the part of biomedical staff. Margarita, a pregnant mother from the finca who was also suffering from tuberculosis, went to the prenatal clinic and was told she was considered high risk and should not have any more children. Therefore, she should deliver in the hospital so that after the birth she could have a tubal ligation. With the onset of labor, Margarita went to the district hospital. However, she ended up delivering the baby by herself under the sheets because no one came to help her. The nurse came when she heard the baby crying and scolded Margarita for not calling her. The new mother was so upset that she did not go through with the tubal ligation.

Margarita's story is distressing but not anomalous. At least two other women told me they delivered their babies by themselves in the hospital because of the lack of attention. Although these cases occurred in the national hospital in Retalhuleu, Berry (2008, 2010) discusses similar problems experienced by mothers in the hospital in Sololá, Guatemala. Although this inattentiveness may be related to ethnic and class differences in some cases, in others it may not be deliberate prejudicial behavior but a result of crowded conditions and inadequate medical services.

The assumption has been that hospital-based delivery will lower maternal mortality rates. However, when stratified by ethnic group, the maternal mortality ratio increased with the increasing percentage of hospital-based delivery. "In all health regions, maternal mortality ratios were higher for hospital than for home delivery. These findings most likely reflect late transfers to hospitals, inadequate levels of care, and low number of hospital deliveries" (Kestler 1995:30). For a comadrona, referring a patient to the hospital may also be a risk, because the midwife may be blamed for the mother's condition or problem rather than praised for referring the patient. This risk is highlighted by the descriptions provided to me by comadronas of their treatment in the hospital. Midwives reported being yelled at, ridiculed, humiliated, and scolded in front of their clients and their families (Foster et al. 2004:221). As Dudgeon has stated (2008, this volume), the midwife risks her professional credibility and personal integrity in interactions with biomedical health care providers.

Conclusion

The persistence of high infant and maternal mortality in Guatemala has resulted in a number of strategies aimed at improving these statistics. Because the majority of births are attended by traditional midwives, one strategy has been to develop training programs aimed at teaching midwives to use more hygienic practices, to recognize what biomedically are considered risk factors for obstetric complications and emergencies, and to refer those cases to the hospital or other medical facility. The effectiveness of these programs has been evaluated by using mortality rates and the number of referrals made by the midwives. When improvements in these statistics are deemed insufficient, the outcome has been blaming the midwife rather than raising questions about the use of mortality rates, the numbers of referred high-risk cases, or the way midwifery-training programs are conducted. Indeed, each of these, as well as their interrelationship, is problematic. For example, using the number of midwife referrals to hospitals as the criterion to measure effectiveness of a training program does not take into account the cases when the midwife makes a referral but the mother or family refuses to go to the hospital. The biomedical health providers assume the midwife has more authority than she has. It is often the family, especially the husband and in-laws, that makes the decision. Some of these studies do not take this factor into account and blame the midwife, even though she may actually have advised a hospital transfer. While referrals by a midwife may measure the effectiveness of the training program (which is questionable), they do not measure the effectiveness of the midwife.

That midwifery-training programs may not have had much impact on mortality rates also ignores the larger socioeconomic context. Rather than blame the midwives and conclude that a new type of "skilled birth attendant" must be trained who can recognize and manage obstetrical risks more effectively, training programs need to be redesigned to be more bidirectional and to integrate input from midwives. Comadronas such as Doña Siriaca show that they are willing and capable of recognizing biomedically defined risks and are changing some of their practices or instituting new practices accordingly. However, they make such changes selectively, in part according to their own perceptions of risk. Unfortunately, medical personnel are not interested in or willing to learn what the mothers and midwives perceive and define as risks.

Midwives are not to blame for high mortality rates, and it is shortsighted to end midwifery-training programs. I hope the Guatemalan government will continue these programs but develop more effective and culturally sensitive ones. However, no matter how much and what kind of training a midwife may have, unless it is part of an integrated program—one that includes family and community education and addresses such factors as poverty, poor housing, poor sanitation conditions, lack of potable drinking water, lack of access to medical facilities, illiteracy, and lack of consideration of cultural factors by medical personnel as risk factors themselves—reproductive health will not improve and the high mortality rates will continue in Guatemala.

Acknowledgments

I wish to express my appreciation to the finca owner and his family and to the people of the plantation, of Novillero, and of the surrounding hamlets for their cooperation and hospitality. I also thank my research assistant, Blanca Estela Garcia, for her invaluable assistance and support. Research in Guatemala has been partly supported by Rutgers University Research Council grants.

Notes

1. US$20 would be about Q150 in 2008 at an exchange rate of Q7.5 to US$1.
2. For reasons of confidentiality, pseudonyms have been used for places and people when it may possible to identify locales or individuals in this chapter.
3. The K'iche' term "*iyom*" often replaces "comadrona" in Novillero.
4. The term "community midwife" refers to a professional or biomedically trained mid-

wife who is part of a community-based maternity care program (Goodburn et al. 2000).

5. To appreciate the extent of these expenses, these costs need to be viewed from the context of the average plantation worker, who at that time was earning about Q17 per day ($2.10). Since the work is highly seasonal, it is difficult to estimate an annual income.

References

Allen, Denise Roth
    2002   Managing Motherhood, Managing Risk: Fertility and Danger in West Central Tanzania. Ann Arbor: University of Michigan Press.

Bailey, Patricia, Jose Szaszdi, and Lucinda Glover
    2002   Obstetric Complications: Does Training Traditional Birth Attendants Make a Difference? Pan American Journal of Public Health 11(1):15–23.

Bartlett, A., and M. Bocaletti
    1991   Intrapartum and Neonatal Mortality in a Traditional Indigenous Community in Rural Guatemala. Acta Paediatrica Scandinavica 80(3):288–295.

Beck, Ulrich
    1992   Risk Society: Towards a New Modernity. London: Sage Publications.

Bergstrom, Staffan, and Elizabeth Goodburn
    2001   The Role of Traditional Birth Attendants in the Reduction of Maternal Mortality. Studies in Health Services Organization and Policy 17:77–99.

Berry, Nicole
    2008   Who's Judging the Quality of Care? Indigenous Maya and the Problem of "Not Being Attended." Medical Anthropology 27(2):164–89.
    2010   Unsafe Motherhood: Mayan Maternal Mortality and Subjectivity in Post-War Guatemala. New York: Berghahn Books.

Caplan, Pat
    2000   Introduction: Risk Revisited. In Risk Revisited. Pat Caplan, ed. Pp.1–28. London: Pluto Press.

Casteñada, Xochitl Camey, Cecilia Garcia Barrios, Xochitl Romero Guerrero, Rosa Maria Nuñez-Urquiza, Dolores Gonzalez Hernandez, and Ana Langer Glass
    1996   Traditional Birth Attendants in Mexico: Advantages and Inadequacies of Care for Normal Deliveries. Social Science and Medicine 43(2):199–207.

Central Intelligence Agency (CIA)
    2010   The World Factbook—Guatemala. Washington, DC: U.S. Government.

Cosminsky, Sheila
    1982   Childbirth and Change: A Guatemalan Case Study. In Ethnography of Fertility and Birth. Carol MacCormack, ed. Pp. 205–30. New York: Academic Press.
    1983   Traditional Midwifery and Contraception. In Traditional Medicine and Health Care Coverage. Robert Bannerman, John Burton, and Ch'en Wen-Chieh, eds. Pp. 142–62. Geneva: World Health Organization.
    2001   Midwifery across the Generations: A Modernizing Midwife in Guatemala. Medical Anthropology 20(4):345–78.

Douglas, Mary
    1985   Risk Acceptability According to the Social Sciences. New York: Russell Sage
            Foundation.
    1990   Risk as a Forensic Resource. Daedalus 119:1–16.
    1992   Risk and Blame. New York: Routledge.
Douglas, Mary, and Aaron Wildavsky
    1982   Risk and Culture. Berkeley: University of California Press.
Dudgeon, Matthew
    2008   Risk and Reproductive Health in Guatemala. Presented at the American
            Anthropological Meetings. San Francisco, November 19–23.
Foster, Jennifer, Angela Anderson, Jennifer Houston, and Maya Doe-Simkins
    2004   Report of a Midwifery Model for Training Traditional Midwives in Guatemala.
            Midwifery 20(3):217–25.
Franco de Mendez, Nanci
    2003   Maternal Mortality in Guatemala: A Preventable Tragedy.
            Population Reference Bureau. www.prb.org/Articles/2003/
            MaternalMortalityinGuatemalaAPreventableTragedy.aspx, accessed July 30, 2010.
Frankenberg, Ronald
    1993   Risk: Anthropological and Epidemiological Narratives of Prevention in
            Childbirth. *In* Knowledge, Power and Practice: The Anthropology of Medicine
            and Everyday Life. Shirley Lindenbaum and Margaret Lock, eds. Pp. 32–54.
            Berkeley: University of California Press.
Giddens, Anthony
    1991   Modernity and Self-Identity: Self and Society in the Late Modern Age.
            Cambridge: Polity Press.
Glei, Dana, Goldman Noreen, and Rodriguez German
    2003   Utilization of Care during Pregnancy in Rural Guatemala: Does Obstetrical Need
            Matter. Social Science and Medicine 57(12):2447–63.
Goldman, Noreen, and Dana Glei
    2003   Evaluation of Midwifery Care: Results from a Survey in Rural Guatemala. Social
            Science and Medicine 56(4):685–700.
Goodburn, Elizabeth, Mushtaque Chowdhury, Rukhsana Gazi, Tom Marshall and Wendy
Graham
    2000   Training Traditional Birth Attendants in Clean Delivery Does Not Prevent
            Postpartum Infection. Health Policy and Planning 15:394–99.
Grajeda, Ruben, Rafael Escamilla, and Kathryn Dewey
    1997   Delayed Clamping of the Umbilical Cord Improved Hematologic Status of
            Guatemalan Infants at 2 Months of Age. American Journal of Clinical Nutrition
            65(2):425–31.
Houston, Jennifer
    2001   Final Report: Midwives for Midwives. Behrhorst Partners for Development,
            Antigua, Guatemala. Unpublished manuscript.
Hurtado, Elena, and Eugenia Saenz de Tejada
    2001   Relations between Government Health Workers and Traditional Midwives in
            Guatemala. *In* Mesoamerican Healers. Brad Huber and Alan Sandstrom, eds. Pp.
            221–42. Austin: University of Texas Press.

Instituto Nacional de Estadistica Guatemala
　2005　Estadisticas Vitales. Guatemala City: Instituto Nacional de Estadistica.
Johns Hopkins Project for International Education in Gynecology
and Obstetrics (JHPIEGO)
　2004　Mobilizing for Impact: Engaging Guatemalan Communities to Save Mothers.
　　　　www.jhuccp.org/resource_center/publications/center_publications/mobilizing-
　　　　impact-engaging-guatemalan-communities-s, accessed June 11, 2010.
Jordan, Brigitte
　1997　Authoritative Knowledge and Its Construction. *In* Childbirth and Authoritative
　　　　Knowledge: Cross-Cultural Perspectives. Robbie Davis-Floyd and Carolyn
　　　　Sargent, eds. Pp. 55–79. Berkeley: University of California Press.
Kaufert, Patricia, and John O'Neil
　1993　Analysis of a Dialogue on Risks in Childbirth. *In* Knowledge, Power and Practice:
　　　　The Anthropology of Medicine and Everyday Life. Shirley Lindenbaum and
　　　　Margaret Lock, eds. Pp. 32–54. Berkeley: University of California Press.
Kestler, Edgar
　1995　Guatemala: Maternal Mortality in Guatemala. World Health Statistics Quarterly
　　　　48(1):28–33.
Kruske, Sue
　2004　Effect of Shifting Policies on Traditional Birth Attendant Training. Journal of
　　　　Midwifery and Women's Health 49(4):306–11.
Mangay Maglacas, Amelia, and John Simons, eds.
　1986　The Potential of the Traditional Birth Attendant. WHO Offset Publication no.
　　　　95. Geneva: WHO.
Maupin, Jonathan
　2008　Remaking the Guatemalan Midwife: Health Care Reform and Midwifery
　　　　Training Programs in Highland Guatemala. Medical Anthropology 27(4):353–82.
MSNBC
　2008　Shocked at Deaths, Guatemala Trains Midwives. www.msnbc.msn.com/
　　　　id/26793739, accessed June 13, 2009.
Nichter, Mark
　2001　Risk, Vulnerability, and Harm Reduction: Preventing STIs in Southeast Asia
　　　　by Antibiotic Prophylaxis, a Misguided Practice. *In* Cultural Perspectives on
　　　　Reproductive Health. Carla Obermeyer, ed. Pp.101–27. New York: Oxford
　　　　University Press.
　2003　Harm Reduction: A Core Concern for Medical Anthropology. *In* Risk, Culture,
　　　　and Health Inequality. Barbara Herr Harthorn and Laury Oaks, eds. Pp. 13–33.
　　　　Westport, CT: Praeger.
O'Rourke, Kathleen
　1994　The Effect of a Traditional Birth Attendant Training Program on Obstetrical
　　　　Practices and Perinatal Mortality in Rural Guatemala. Ph.D. dissertation,
　　　　University of Massachusetts.
Pan American Health Organization (PAHO)
　1999　Guatemala: Profile of the Health Services System. Washington, DC: Pan
　　　　American Health Organization.
　2007　Guatemala: Perfil del Sistema de Salud de Guatemala. Washington, DC: Pan
　　　　American Health Organization.

Panter-Brick, Catherine
  2002   Street Children, Human Rights, and Public Health: A Critique and Future
          Directions. Annual Reviews in Anthropology 31:147–71.
Perreira, Krista, Patricia Bailey, Elizabeth de Bocaletti, Elena Hurtado, Sandra Recinos de
Villagran, and Jorge Matute
  2002   Increasing Awareness of Danger Signs in Pregnancy through Community and
          Clinic-Based Education in Guatemala. Maternal and Child Health Journal
          6(1):19–28.
Pigg, Stacey
  1997   Authority in Translation: Finding, Knowing, Naming and Training "Traditional
          Birth Attendants" in Nepal. *In* Childbirth and Authoritative Knowledge. Robbie
          Davis-Floyd and Carolyn Sargent, eds. Pp. 233–62. Berkeley: University of
          California Press.
Ray, Alison, and Hamisu Salihu
  2004   The Impact of Maternal Mortality Interventions Using Traditional Birth
          Attendants and Village Midwives. Journal of Obstetrics and Gynaecology
          24(1):5–11.
Repogle, Jill
  2007   Training Traditional Birth Attendants in Guatemala. The Lancet 369:177–78.
Schieber, Barbara, Kathleen O'Rourke, Carmen Rodriquez, and Alfred Bartlett
  1994   Risk Factor Analysis of Peri-neonatal Mortality in Rural Guatemala. Bulletin of
          PAHO 28(3):229–38.
Schooley, Janine
  2009   Factors Influencing Health Care-Seeking Behaviours among Mayan Women in
          Guatemala. Midwifery 25(4):411–21.
Sibley, Lynn, Theresa Ann Sipe, and Marge Koblinsky
  2004   Does Traditional Birth Attendant Training Improve Referral of Women with
          Obstetric Complications: A Review of the Evidence. Social Science and Medicine
          59(8):1757–68.
United States Agency for International Development (USAID)
  2010   Before and After: Mayan Midwives Save Lives. Washington, DC. www.usaid.gov/
          stories/guatemala/ba_guatemala_midwives.html, accessed June 11, 2011.
Verderese, M. de L., and L. M. Turnbull
  1975   The Traditional Birth Attendant in Maternal and Child Health and Family
          Planning. WHO Offset Publication no. 18. Geneva: World Health Organization.
World Health Organization (WHO)
  2009   Making Pregnancy Safer: Skilled Birth Attendants. www.who.int/making_
          pregnancy_safer/topics/skilled_birth/en/index.html, accessed July 23, 2009.

CHAPTER 5

"They Don't Know Anything"
How Medical Authority Constructs Perceptions of Reproductive Risk among Low-Income Mothers in Mexico

Vania Smith-Oka

The Mexican state has promoted the concept of the modern woman with great enthusiasm, with low-income women the primary target. Many of these women are accused of engaging in risky and less than modern behavior, such as receiving prenatal care with midwives instead of physicians or not practicing family planning (see Gálvez, this volume, for contrasting prenatal practices among Mexican immigrants in the United States). By using health campaigns to further economic development, gender equality, and family planning, the state effectively promotes its own concept of modernity, good motherhood, and, ultimately, good citizenship. Using biomedical reproductive care is viewed as a necessary step toward achieving this modernity. Women who fall outside this norm of reproduction—through their perinatal or mothering choices—are perceived to be engaging in highly risky behavior and challenging the state's efforts at modernity. Responsibility and blame fall squarely on women who are perceived to risk their children's health by being disobedient to biomedical and state orders. They are considered bad mothers.

In this chapter, I explore the Mexican state's efforts to produce and reproduce good motherhood through women's engagement with biomedical reproductive care. I analyze local biomedical professionals' ideas of reproductive health and investigate the purported risks and actualized consequences borne by their female patients' perceived disobedience. This chapter reflects larger discussions of the structural processes and social arrangements that interact—in antagonistic and mutually supportive ways—to shape women's reproduction (Browner 2000:774). The confluence of institutional pressures and women's bodies produces many unintended consequences for the reproductive lives of marginalized women (Ginsburg and Rapp 1991; Smith-Oka 2009b; Van Hollen 2003). Medical authority is perceived as legitimate, privileged, and consequential, and to lie in direct opposition to other ways of knowing, which are dismissed or delegitimized (Jordan 1993, 1997). The use of technology by physicians legitimates their knowledge and authority and constructs "specific kinds of social, cognitive, and expressive order" in the interactions with their patients (Georges 1996). Davis-Floyd sees the use of technology in birth as part of a ritual that maps out a "technological view of reality onto the birthing woman's orientation to her labor experience" (1987:480). In this process the woman's beliefs, value system, and body become aligned with the beliefs and values held by a modern society.

Modernity has been defined by a number of scholars in a variety of ways. Comaroff and Comaroff speak about "many modernities" in which citizens of conquered societies struggled in various ways "to deploy, deform, and defuse imperial institutions" and in the process were themselves transformed through the coupling of local and global worlds (1993:xii). Giddens suggests that the historical period (AD 1500–1789) of modernity is marked by three key aspects: (1) the idea that humans can transform their world through intervention; (2) the revolutionizing of economic institutions, particularly industrial production, and an increasing role for a market economy; and (3) the transformation of political institutions, with the emergence of the nation-state and of mass democracy (1998:94). Beck (1992) finds that these changes bring about an increase in risks and hazards. He distinguishes between modernity, where agents become more individualized and free of structural constraints, and reflexive modernity, where risk becomes paramount and the circulation of "bads" or dangers is of central concern. Within the nation-state exist its associated institutions and forms of surveillance—all of which become very useful in the management of the population. In the modern birthing system, the movement of women through the process becomes central to the idea of modernity and, as Netz (2004) explores in his analysis of the history of barbed wire and modernity, the facilitation of motion as well as the prevention of motion are integral in understanding modernity. In the context of this chapter, then, who are the women who move easily and readily through the system? And, conversely, who are the women who, by their risky or noncompliant nature, grind the system to a halt, necessitating medical intervention to set the system in motion once again?

The Mexican government offers several welfare programs for its low-income population, each of them with the core intention of actively managing people's lifestyles so they can achieve better standards of living and become modern active citizens. One such program is Oportunidades, a cash transfer program that combines short- and long-term objectives of poverty alleviation (see Howes-Mischel, this volume, for other provisions of Oportunidades). Its aim is to tackle poverty by helping the poor to "cope, mitigate, or reduce their risk of falling into or being trapped in poverty" (Molyneux 2006:433). Specifically, it aims to improve human development by focusing on children's health, nutrition, and education. Based on the assumption that poor households do not invest sufficiently in their human capital and thus are caught in a cycle of poverty that is transmitted through the generations, Oportunidades establishes a relationship between the state and low-income mothers: the state transfers cash grants to the women in exchange for the health, nutrition, and educational enrollment of their children. In this exchange of money for compliance exists the essentialization of women as natural caregivers (Molyneux 2006) that primarily aims to resocialize women to fall in line with the Mexican state's expectations of motherhood. Any woman who falls outside this neat (and narrow) categorization might be accused of endangering her children's environment and of being a bad mother (see Tsing 1990). In effect, as shown by

Molyneux's (2006) work, the transfer of cash is made conditional on the women's good motherhood.

The mothers must be involved in the medical centers as patients and participants (Smith-Oka 2009b; Sridhar and Duffield 2006), where additional social engineering can take place. This program, along with other state programs, is implemented across the country without regional variations in services or funding. While Oportunidades began as a rural program, it has been implemented in identical manner among the urban poor in recent years.

Oportunidades emerged from the early twentieth-century Mexican nation-building drive, which strove to modernize the country economically and socially. Among the many things it targeted, social hygiene became of paramount importance, where negative and "backward" practices of the poor were to be replaced by modern and scientific behaviors (Stern 1999). These behaviors could best be implemented and controlled in medical settings. In the process, reproduction was moved from the domestic to the public domain, where perceived dangers and risks could be fully managed.

Davis-Floyd's concept of birth as a rite of passage (1992)—where ritual serves to bring order to natural processes—provides a useful framework for understanding how the physicians in my study strive to control risk. Birth is perceived to be extremely "unpredictable and uncontrollable" (Davis-Floyd 1992:2), and all the more so in the spaces between the structures. By "spaces" I literally mean the places outside the formal structured areas for obstetrical care, such as waiting rooms or hallways. These physical spaces are liminal, however, as they are not perceived as truly medical—even if they are physically part of the medical building. They are betwixt and between the existing and categorized medical structures (Turner 1967). Consequently, anything happening in these liminal spaces is classified as risky and needs additional medical intervention—through technology or language—to counteract the effect of risk and bring order back to the encounter. I draw upon Turner's (1967) and Van Gennep's (1960) ideas of liminality and Davis-Floyd's (1992) reframing of a rite of passage in birth to explain the interpretation of risk within women's reproductive activities.

Exploring Risk

Within the reproductive lives of marginalized women exists the label of risk. This label is created by the people and institutions possessing authoritative knowledge, who use it to exert power over the reproductive bodies of these women. Douglas (1990) has pointed out that "risk" originally had a neutral meaning, referring to the probability or mathematical likelihood of an event's occurring, combined with the degree of the losses or gains that would ensue. Over time, this disinterested understanding of risk has transformed into a central cultural construct in contemporary Western society, rife with political underpinnings, weakening its connection with the original calculation of probability (Hunt, Castañeda, and de Voogd 2006; Jacobs 2000). "Risk" is thus most definitely no longer a neutral term; rather, it has come to mean "danger." And as Douglas states: "Plain danger does not have the aura of science or afford the pretension of a possible precise calculation" (1990:4). It is this precision, this perceived science behind the term "risk," that makes it such a powerful concept in our current world context. Rapp shows us that risk is explained through scientific, mathematical, and statistical language—these are not neutral vocabularies. The medical understanding of this language is often markedly different from the language of the patients, creating a "tug-of-war of words" (1988:149). And, as Browner and Press (1995) inform us, "risk" rests on the assumption that modern life is filled with unpredictable dangers that can—or at least should—be minimized through human intervention.

The roles of language and culture play into risk as well, contributing to a racialized and class-based discourse. Beck (1992) argues that risk is distributed in a stratified and class-based society in an inverse way—wealth accumulates at the top of the structure and risk at the bottom. This distribution strengthens class stratification, with poverty attracting an abundance of risk. In a society like Mexico, where class and ethnicity are often intertwined, the distribution of risk will be similar among the lower classes and the indigenous groups. Thus, the discourse surrounding risk flows from top to bottom, as can be seen among Mexican medical professionals, where the definition and classification of what exactly entails risk takes place among the echelon of those with power and becomes enacted upon the ones with none. This is why, as Martin (1992) states and my research in Mexico suggests, there is an increase in the use of technology to control the behaviors of the populations who are not in a position to resist—and who are deemed to be inherently riskier. This increase occurs down the scale of class and race.

In discussions on risk in the medical field exists the idea of responsibility, wherein patients—preferably informed ones—are expected to deliberate carefully about the costs and benefits of certain behaviors and medical options by weighing them against their own preferences and values, finally coming to a decision about the course of action to be taken (Hunt, Castañeda, and de Voogd 2006). Similar to Maraesa's findings (this volume), physicians and patients often have widely divergent interpretations of what constitutes risk. This difference can lead to miscommunication, lack of informed consent, or perceptions of noncompliance (Hunt 1998).

Another key aspect of risk is blame. Though one might speak at length about risk factors and dangers, there also must be someone to blame if something does indeed go wrong (Douglas 1990). Blame goes hand-in-hand with responsibility. If an unfavorable event happens during a birth, for instance, blame can fall on the woman, the medical staff, or circumstances beyond the control of either. Yet mothers are often encouraged to engage in self-blame where society imposes "nearly total responsibility on [women] as prospective mothers for assuring a favorable birth" (Browner and Press 1995:309). If a woman did not engage in the expected appropriate behavior prenatally or during the birth, blame and responsibility will fall on her. A retrospective analysis of her actions during that time might elicit conclusions of disobedience and bad motherhood (Ellison 2003).

As part of the rhetoric surrounding the risk involved in women's reproduction,

I found in Mexico great importance placed on the type of health care women receive. Low-income women are encouraged to seek out reproductive care in clinics and hospitals, and are simultaneously discouraged from going to midwives (see Howes-Mischel, this volume, for a similar discussion of prenatal care advice and practices in Oaxaca, Mexico). This policy is enacted in government clinics and hospitals across the country and is enforced in the intersection of medical and social programs—such as Oportunidades.

The Field Sites and Research Methods

This chapter is based on ethnographic data I collected from 2004 to 2010 from two field sites in Mexico: the rural indigenous municipality of Ixhuatlán de Madero, where I have carried out ongoing research in the village of Amatlán since 2004, and a maternity hospital for low-income women in the city of Puebla, where I carried out a pilot study in 2008.[1]

Ixhuatlán de Madero lies in northern Veracruz, a few miles inland from the Gulf of Mexico in the rolling hills just shy of the Sierra Madre Oriental (Sandstrom 1991). The roughly six hundred inhabitants of the village where I did my primary research belong to the Nahua indigenous group, and while the majority of the older adults speak Nahuatl, the youth have lost much of their connection to their indigenous roots. Despite this, there remains an interest in traditional means of healing, which include *curanderos* (ritual specialists), *sobadores* (bone setters/massage givers), and midwives (Sandstrom 1991). There are five midwives in Amatlán, all well over the age of fifty. Their client base has decreased over the years, particularly with the introduction of clinics and hospitals and the Oportunidades program (Smith-Oka 2009b).

During my research I carried out participant-observation and interviewed fifty-two women, including the five midwives. These semi-structured interviews covered various topics, including women's enrollment in Oportunidades, their reproductive histories, and the health care–related changes experienced by the village. With the midwives I investigated more deeply traditional midwifery practices, their use of medicinal plants, and their response to changes in reproductive practices (Smith-Oka 2008). I also interviewed twelve physicians and nurses from the clinics and hospital of the region; our interviews covered topics such as their experiences with childbirth and family planning in the region, their use (if any) of Oportunidades in their practice, and their relationship with their patients.

The maternity hospital in Puebla lies within a larger government-run hospital for the city and its surroundings. Puebla is a city of more than two million people in central Mexico. The Hospital Público is part of the Ministry of Health system and is intended for very low-income populations. The female reproductive patients are cared for by a large staff of physicians and nurses in the three separate sections: outpatient and prenatal care, labor and delivery, and recovery and hospitalization. I carried out research at this hospital in 2008, which consisted of participant-observation of physician-patient interaction in all the sections, as well as during the labors and deliveries of various women. I also interviewed sixteen women about their birth experiences and eight physicians regarding their practices and philosophies. Additionally, I interviewed four midwives who have been professionalized at this hospital and whose practices range from indigenous rural village *parteras* to urban care as *empíricas* or *comadronas*.[2]

During my research on women's reproductive lives, various themes emerged that can help to elucidate the ways that the ideas of risk, modernity, blame, responsibility, and motherhood become part of interactions between physicians and their low-income female patients. These themes include medical professionals' concerns about midwife-assisted births, the authority in births that take place in clinical settings (Jordan 1997), and the general obedience to the accepted national norms of behavior.

Medical Concerns about Midwives

There is much concern with the role that midwives play in women's reproduction. The attitude of rural medical professionals toward midwives fluctuates between admiration for their abilities and repertoire of local knowledge and concern about their lack of biomedical knowledge and techniques. For Nurse Juliana, who has worked at a small clinic for more than thirteen years and who has seen the area change from one with a strong connection to indigenous medicine to one where biomedicine is becoming dominant, there is much to admire in midwifery practice: "They are very good; they can really detect multiple pregnancies, twinning, the [fetal] position, and they are good at attending the birth." Yet her admiration for the practice was tempered by the sort of training the midwives had; Nurse Juliana explained that the clinic allowed interaction only with midwives who had received training and government certification.

One of the midwives in Amatlán fell into this category of government-trained and -certified midwife: Lourdes, a hearty and energetic woman who managed her large household, made bread to sell, and worked as a *sobadora* (bone setter/massage giver) and *curandera* (ritual specialist) in addition to being a midwife. Lourdes was particularly proud of her certification in the city of Poza Rica. On various occasions she told me about her trips to the hospital where she was trained with other midwives, and how one physician in particular frequently told them that they "were like doctors." However, Nurse Juliana emphasized, "it's just that if they are not trained they do not know," thereby encapsulating the general medical belief regarding untrained midwives: if they are untrained, they do not have the important knowledge to manage birth and postpartum; thus, they carry a high risk.

In a similar vein, one can see Doctora Felipa's concerns with midwives:

There is always risk, and then onto that we add the fact that the [birthplace's] conditions are not the best, or if the midwife uses medicines that she is not trained to use. . . . In those cases the only thing that has worth is the experience they have to manipulate [the vaginal opening] because, wow, I have nothing but admiration for them. They do not allow it to tear. But it is their experience that has allowed them to do that. But from that to them having actual knowledge, that they don't.

Although Doctora Felipa has been working in rural Mexico for several years and expresses openness toward midwives (often allowing them to use the clinic's operating/maternity room for their patients), she does not permit midwives to attend the same births she attends, in order to retain full control over the birth. She believes risk can be fully controlled through the use of medical knowledge and action. As can be seen from her words, she admires many of the manipulative techniques used by the midwives, as well as their knowledge of local practices, yet she does not give their knowledge status equal to her own medical knowledge (Jordan 1997).

I found the same attitude among physicians in the city of Puebla, where, although they have a midwife certification program organized by the hospital itself, they do not encourage patients to go to certified or any other midwives. I was present at this hospital when a male physician arranged to transfer a laboring woman to the emergency ward. The doctor warned the woman, who was slightly dilated and had had a previous cesarean section: "Tell your husband that your uterus can tear, you can bleed out, and you and the baby [will] die." Turning from her, the doctor then said to me: "I prefer to tell them like that because if not, they think it won't happen, and they don't know [anything]. . . . In another hospital I received four midwife-caused ruptures; the uterus bursts and there the baby swims around in the abdomen. . . . Fortunately the kids, the babies, came out alive."

In this case the physician completely dismisses the necessary role that midwives play among low-income Mexican women, as well as any knowledge the pregnant women might have. His ideas and techniques become the authority in these contexts, and his orders must be obeyed if the women want to have healthy children. While there are certainly cases of midwife mismanagement of births, he groups all midwives and their practices into this same category of high risk and danger. This physician's conclusions harken to what Murphy-Lawless refers to as the extraordinary belief in obstetrics that "no birth is normal except in retrospect" (1998:8). And, as she shows in her work in Ireland, obstetrical mismanagement is not uncommon. Indeed, she points to how many dangerous practices in birth management become normalized over time—such as the breaking of the amniotic sac or artificial inductions, which carry their own risks yet remain part of the arsenal of normal medical practice. This physician was not an exception in this hospital, as the majority tended to view their female patients as exceptionally risky—from their prenatal care (diet or care from midwives), to their family planning (not enough, too many children, young/unwed/teenage mothers), to their mothering abilities (based on family size and the physicians' perceptions of motherhood).

The concerns with risk in midwife-attended birth often revolved around hygiene or emergency situations. As Nurse Juliana stated:

There are many dangers [that can kill the baby]. I have often seen the [midwives] so preoccupied with the expulsion of the placenta that they only

later clean the baby. And it should not be like that. Those are the risks. . . .
Sometimes they bring their patients here if they can't help them. And it is
important for them to see how a birth is managed in the clinic. . . . Yes,
for a midwife my concern would be hygiene. There is no ideal space for
birth [at their home]. And a birth requires lots of hygiene to prevent infections. Also, if a baby is coming out wrong, [or there is] lack of oxygen, the
midwife doesn't know how to act at that moment and there can be a death,
both maternal and of the baby.

For Nurse Juliana, as for the other nurses and the physicians, the only proper place
for birth was the clinic, where hygiene and sterility could be controlled. The clinic
also has medical equipment to deal with the entire processes of labor and birth, and
if an emergency were to arise, there were ambulances available to take the woman
to the hospital. For a woman giving birth at home with a midwife, an emergency
would require her to find private transportation, which might prove either too
expensive or unavailable. This reality creates additional risk that medical personnel
consider unacceptable. Nonetheless, when I pressed Nurse Juliana for statistical
evidence of the region's maternal and fetal death rates, she had to admit that in
the thirteen years she had been working in the region she had not heard of a single
death caused by lack of emergency care or because of a midwife-attended birth.
Such a discrepancy between belief and reality is problematic for all concerned, as
it creates a false notion of the risks involved in midwife-attended births and falsely
promotes physician-assisted births as the only safe alternative. This notion ignores
the strong evidence that there are significant benefits of midwifery-led care, such
as an increase of spontaneous labor, a reduction in pharmacological analgesia, an
increase in unassisted vaginal birth, a decrease in premature birth, and an increase
in breastfeeding (Jokhio, Winter, and Cheng 2005; Shorten and Shorten 2009).

None of the medical professionals in either Amatlán or Puebla were whole-
heartedly supportive of midwives. Though they acknowledged that midwives had
skills that could be used for checking and diagnosing their patients, they felt that it
was very risky for women to give birth with a midwife—whether that was at home
or in a clinical setting. Because of state policies such as Oportunidades that in effect demand that women (and their families) receive health care in medical settings,
women often have little choice but to accept that their reproductive care will come
from biomedical personnel, or, if they resist and give birth with a midwife, they are
perceived to be making bad choices that will affect both them and their children.
They are perceived as noncompliant and ultimately to be blamed for the risks inherent in their bad choices—whether these risks actualize or not. Indeed, a nurse
at the Puebla hospital said to me: "But they don't reflect upon the risk that each
pregnancy carries. They do not measure the consequences [going to a midwife] can
bring."

Authority in the Clinical Setting

All the medical professionals I interviewed considered the clinical setting the ideal place for birth. Here they could control for factors such as hygiene, they had the appropriate equipment and technology, and, very importantly, they had control over the birth and the woman. Doctora Felipa, a general practitioner who has worked in the region of Ixhuatlán since 1998, was particularly concerned about the various risks that come with the reproductive health of indigenous populations. She acknowledged that she is generally very supportive during what she deems a "normal" birth, but that in "risky" situations, she becomes very demanding and tells the women to push harder or they will kill their baby, explaining that she cannot be "soft" on these women or the baby's life will be at risk. If this threat does not bring about her desired result, Doctora Felipa brings in the husband and tells him to order his wife to help her and that, as a physician, she will not be held responsible for the risk to the fetus brought about by his wife's noncompliance, telling him: "Your child will die because [your wife] doesn't want to [help]."

The authority in the clinical setting lies firmly in the hands of the medical professionals. Doctora Felipa, in her concern for the health and well-being of the baby—and to reduce the purported risk of death for both mother and child—exercised her authority to demand the behavior she required from her patients. In such situations the fears and needs of the patients became secondary to the concerns and requirements of the physician. The authority of the physician stemmed from her authoritative knowledge, which both builds and reflects power relationships (Jordan 1997). Her authoritative knowledge is constantly recreated through discourse, as well as through its embeddedness in the "cultural authority" of medicine and physician status (Sargent and Bascope 1997:204).

For other physicians, however, authority was an end in itself. While the concerns for risk often underlay the behavior of the medical professionals, it was manifested as a very emphatic—even violent—exercise in the flexing of their authoritative and authoritarian muscles (Smith-Oka 2009a). This was particularly evident in Hospital Público in Puebla where the threat of a cesarean section was used on any woman who did not cooperate and follow medical authority: "If you do not cooperate we will do a cesarean" or "I will give you an injection in your spine if you do not cooperate [and allow me to do a vaginal exam]" are powerful examples of how physicians use their power to obtain the obedience and compliance of the female patients during the intense moments of their labor. Additionally, the use of technology as the weapon of choice creates a binary opposition—physician:modern versus patient:not modern—implying that if women wanted to be considered modern, they had to comply with medical authority and allow technology to shape their bodies.

Diana's birth experience illustrates the exertion of compliance and medical authority in a context of perceived risk during labor. Diana was twenty-three years old and experiencing her second pregnancy. Her labor progressed very fast, and the baby crowned while Diana was still on a gurney in the labor cubicle. As Diana strained and pushed with strong, rapid, and uncontrollable contractions, the staff surrounded her gurney and began to roll her down the hallway, repeatedly shouting at her to stop pushing because she was not yet in the delivery room. She was eventually wheeled into one of the operating/birthing rooms, which was still occupied by a woman who had given birth vaginally a few minutes earlier. Diana's gurney was rolled into a corner of the room, where she gave birth to her daughter. During this time the staff continued to chastise her for pushing when she was explicitly told not to.

Once Diana expelled the afterbirth, one of the residents began to carry out a vaginal exam to make certain that the entire the placenta had come out and there was no risk of hemorrhage or infection. The procedure was painful to Diana, and she squirmed under the physician's touch. This frustrated the doctor, who complained that Diana's actions compromised her ability to do a thorough examination. As the chief physician (also a woman) was present in the room to supervise and provide instruction for the younger physicians, the young female resident chose to exercise her authority over Diana by verbally chastising her for being difficult. Diana promptly burst into uncontrollable tears. A further examination that caused Diana to whimper and squirm in pain made the intern lose patience and threaten that either Diana cooperate and possibly receive a local anesthetic or continue to squirm, in which case she would receive a spinal injection to ensure her cooperation. At these words, Diana's body stiffened in fear and she very softly whimpered through her tears: "Examine me."

Diana's case illustrates how medical authority can use a discourse of risk to induce fear, thereby controlling the behaviors of pregnant and birthing women. According to medical rationale, Diana was at risk in two important ways: (1) she was birthing and pushing while not in the correct place, neither in the labor cubicle nor in the birthing room—she was in the hallway and, thus, in an in-between and liminal state that further augmented the risks associated with birthing in an inappropriate physical context (Turner 1967; Van Gennep 1960)—and (2) Diana was refusing to allow authority to examine her properly by squirming during a routine—and medically important—vaginal procedure.[3] While it turned out that Diana did not have any placental retention or discernable uterine abnormality in that immediate postpartum period, the concerns about the associated and projected risks prompted physicians to examine her in a very firm manner. Their fears and concerns gave them carte blanche to treat her roughly when she was perceived to jeopardize the thoroughness of the examination. The perceived risk justified the emergence of a strong and purportedly risk-reducing medical authority.

The Borders of Risk

As Diana's story exemplifies, the risks associated with birth have been constructed in such a way that anything digressing from the "normal" site of birth becomes a cause for concern. In the boundless spaces of ill-equipped hallways and unstaffed waiting rooms and hospital yards, medical authorities find risk more difficult to control and manage. The concept of liminality proposed by Van Gennep (1960) and Turner (1967) suggests how ritual—such as medical procedure and protocol—can return normalcy and structure to a purportedly risky reproductive encounter. One particularly poignant example occurred in one of the clinics in Ixhuatlán when Celeste, a teenage single mother-to-be, who was very embarrassed to give birth in the procedural—yet exposing—horizontal position, insisted on giving birth in a squatting, vertical position. The attending nurse told me the story later:

> She did not let us touch her or anything. She did not let us check to see how dilated she was. Finally the girl jumped off the bed and she ran to that post [indicating a post at the fence around the clinic], and she held onto it and squatted down and began to push. I told her that I would not attend to her there, and that if she did not come in and labor inside the clinic then she would have to go. She left and had her child along the road. It is very risky. That girl was very irresponsible.

In her retelling of Celeste's story, the nurse clearly defined the clinic's physical borders as the limits of her Hippocratic responsibility. Anything happening beyond the clinic's walls (and in direct opposition to medical order and medical control) was the patient's responsibility. Moreover, the boundless nature of the hospital yard evoked the liminality of an inherently dangerous and risky place of betwixt and between that is culturally significant (see Denham, this volume, for a similar cultural belief in Ghana, West Africa).

Because much of medical care is concerned with control (Davis-Floyd 1992), a situation such as Celeste's—where control is literally outside medical hands—serves to shine a very direct light upon these fears and concerns. Within the limen persons are structurally invisible; neither their former nor their soon-to-be new statuses are in existence. As Turner (1967) points out, much of the symbolism in the liminal space revolves around (structural) death: a loss of identity (a "woman" becomes a "patient"), of mobility (she is attached to intravenous fluids), and of control (she cedes complete control of her birth to the medical establishment). And it is perhaps the physicians' tacit acknowledgment of death and risk in the liminal space that marks their efforts to recapture control of a risky and liminal situation through an increase in medical technology and language.

As in Diana's birth experience, Celeste's anxiety to be outside the clinical walls meant that she was outside the controlled and controllable areas. To be outside the clinic meant to be in a dangerous and risky place where anything could happen. The pollution—physical and symbolic—embedded within Celeste's extraclinical birth existed because she was outside the normal defined category of "normalcy" (Douglas 1966). Her birth was neither clinical nor was it at home with a midwife. And, while the latter is not approved by the physicians, it is more acceptable because it exists as a classifiable place of birth. Celeste's birth location fell between classificatory cracks and so was (ritually) unclean (Douglas 1966; Turner 1967). Additionally, as Turner points out, within this liminal period the authority of the elder (or in this case, the physician/nurse) is absolute because it represents the axiomatic values of society in which are expressed "the common good" (1967:100).

By rejecting medical authority, Celeste was seen simultaneously to reject social values and society at large. In this way, Celeste was deemed irresponsible as a patient and mother; she disobeyed medical orders and thus her birth occurred at her own risk.

Obedience to Medical Power

Responsibility in the clinical setting goes hand-in-hand with cooperation and obedience, as happened when Estefanía, a sixteen-year old single mother-to-be, gave birth in the Puebla hospital. As she labored half-naked and frightened on the birthing table, about a dozen medical staff yelled conflicting instructions at her (to push, not to push, to hold her body a certain way, to hold her hands away from her lower quarters, to cooperate). At one point one of the physicians turned to me and said: "You see? A single mother and she does not want to cooperate. She's been that way since she came in. She does not want to help [us]. That is what they are like." It was not clear to whom the doctor referred as "they," whether young women, single mothers, or low-income women, but this term established a clear divide between herself as a physician and the women/patients to whom she attended—the former being a responsible, modern, biomedical knowledge producer in charge of her own (and others') reproductive faculties, the latter irresponsible, not modern, ignorant, and disobedient *re*producers of nothing of great importance. It was evident from this female physician's words that the women (from both worlds) lived in a system of stratified reproduction (Colen 1995).

After a particularly aggressive set of vaginal exams during which Estefanía cried out in pain, one of the physicians in charge impatiently pulled out his hand and, with a slashing motion over Estefanía's belly, said she had to be "cut open." He deemed that she was not helping the medical team, and that this was the expedient solution. And, judging by the attitude of the staff during her labor, this action was also partly punishment for Estefanía's perceived noncompliance. Despite the fact that she spent her time looking around desperately, asking the staff what she had to do and whether the birth was imminent, Estefanía did not meet the standards set for behavior—which extended beyond the hospital walls and into her sexual life—and so the medical professionals met even her entreaties to help and cooperate with distrust and even contempt. She was outside the "norm" and the "appropriate" forms of reproduction because of her age and marital status (Ellison 2003). This made her uncontrollable, dangerous, and therefore risky. The medical solution in this case was to control Estefanía by rendering her immobile through a cesarean section; then professionals could deliver the baby without interference from the noncompliant and socially aberrant laboring woman.

The system of stratified reproduction, where some women's reproduction is encouraged and supported while others' is prevented (Colen 1995; Ellison 2003), creates a situation that allows the questioning of women's very selves. As one of the head physicians in Puebla asked me when she learned I was an anthropologist researching women's reproduction: "Oh, won't you find out why they don't use contraceptives here? It is just that these [women] don't know. One explains and teaches them—and nothing. I think that their IQ is very low because they always have children. And [they are] such poor, marginalized populations, and they have tons of children. They don't understand."

This harsh sentiment encapsulates the beliefs of the medical professionals about their patients and their practices. Within this statement are also embedded several concerns the Mexican state has with a certain population's reproduction. First, these are low-income populations and they are reproducing too much by having many children. Second, their very intelligence is doubted; if they were not irretrievably stupid, they would reproduce responsibly. And third, such a combination of character traits—overly reproductive and stupid—is deemed a tremendous risk on several levels: (1) for the women themselves—too many children can weaken and debilitate the uterus, and there are too many mouths to feed and look after; (2) for the children—too many mouths to compete with, or not enough parental attention; and (3) for society—proliferation of children (and future citizens) who are not well adjusted; members of society who are too poor and uneducated; or ignorant women giving birth to ignorant children. This attitude matches a statement made by Doctora Felipa: "I think the [women] have become more aware, more conscious"—meaning that they now engage more readily with the national ethos of reproductive behavior.

Conclusion

Browner and Press (1995) demonstrate how medicine views life as both unpredictable and dangerous, factors that must be reduced through interventions. Because physicians consider birth an especially abnormal process (Murphy-Lawless 1998), it must be normalized in some way. Moreover, spaces of reproductive liminality (Van Gennep 1960), in which a woman lies between (Turner 1967) physical boundaries—and between ideological constructs of reproductive propriety—are of greatest concern for the medical professionals in Amatlán and Puebla. The inherent in-betweenness and ambiguity of this state of being translates into reproductive risk and the need for forceful medical control and exertion of authority.

Midwives are, likewise, not within the acceptable medical norm in Mexico. While midwives have a long history of existence in indigenous, rural, and low-income Mexican communities (Cosminsky 2001), they are not acceptable as potential managers of women's reproduction—especially birth. Birth is perceived as a liminal state, filled with many potential dangers during which the risks involved must be controlled as much as possible. Hence, there is an increase in medicalization and high use of intervention and technology during this period, further obviating the role of the midwife in the eyes of the medical establishment. Midwives are constructed as quaint remnants of a risky health tradition that either have to be changed through professionalization and certification, or removed entirely by encouraging women to go to clinics/hospitals through enrollment in programs such as Oportunidades.

In Diana's birth experience, transition was of paramount importance to the medical staff attending her. By being in labor, she was herself transitioning from one ideological state to the next—from girl to woman, not yet mother to *mamá*, and thus she did not belong to one particular structure at that point (Turner 1967:95). Additionally, she was laboring in the hallway—literally between two physical states, the labor cubicle and the operating/delivery room. A passage is not seen as a safe place to give birth, as events happening there cannot be controlled as readily through technology. The birth itself also took place on a gurney in a room where a woman had given birth a few minutes before. This compounded the purported risks of limited technological access with lack of hygienic control. This was an interstructural situation (Turner 1967:93)—a space between two firm structures where the only way to return to normalcy was through entering a known, nonrisky structure with the use of ritual as enacted through medical technology, language, and practice. In this way the medical reaction was to gain control by blaming Diana for their loss of control. The medical authorities consequently yelled at and chastised her for behaving in a way that was construed as uncontrollable and potentially dangerous to the reproductive project.

Apparent in all the women's birth experiences I have described are "deeply ingrained cultural assumptions about the categories of women who can legitimately lay claim to their sexuality, fertility, and maternity" (Ellison 2003:335). The cultural, social, and political-economic contexts in which physicians and patients exist shape the values and assumptions that underlie these categories (Hunt 1998:301). The axes of poverty, class, and gender (Farmer 2003) place low-income Mexican women in a position of little choice, which means they have to be obedient and good to survive in this medical setting.

Diana had absolutely no control over her laboring body because of the contractions, yet the physicians expected her to self-regulate or they would do it for her. Celeste was expected to labor in a position that exposed her, literally, to the view of others, a position she refused to accept. Because both women existed outside acceptable or normal behaviors for birth, the medical gaze was intensified to bring them back into the acceptable medical structure. Kleinman (2000) would argue that these situations promote a form of structural violence that constricts women's fertility and maternity.

Medical professionals often rely on technology to bolster their authoritative knowledge and to exert control over the management of pregnant women. Georges shows in her work in Greece how technology "provides a context for performing and reinforcing medical authority and, in doing so helps consolidate a growing . . . medical hegemony over women's reproductive experiences" (1996:170). The verbalized threat of spinal injections or cesarean sections can be an effective means of controlling women's bodies—and hence controlling the purported risks they embody. Additionally, the authority of experts such as medical professionals is persuasive because it "includes the veiled threat of powerful sanctions" (Irwin and Jordan 1987:319). In Mexico, women who challenge this authority are likely to have these sanctions unleashed against them.

Though Estefanía's and Celeste's births are markedly different in some ways—hospital versus extraclinical, high technology versus none at all—they share many similarities: because the women are both teenage, single mothers-to-be, they fall outside the purview of responsible reproduction. Neither had any control in the clinical setting (a factor that might have been exacerbated by their youth and inappropriate pregnancy), they were severely chastised for not cooperating, and they were held up as examples of risky behavior resulting in poor motherhood. Through these women's challenge of the medical establishment—through outright escape or through perceived willful noncompliance—they were also viewed as challenging the medical orders and the state, and ultimately seen as bad mothers.

The label "bad mother" signals a moral judgment by mainstream Mexico—embodied by medical professionals—whose historical roots lie in the opposition between indigenous and *mestizo* racial categories and in the social engineering colored by eugenics in early twentieth-century Mexico (Stern 1999).[4] The "empirical risk" (Ginsburg and Rapp 1991:316) of the integration of these racial categories lies in creating an ideal mixed race that will have the strong traits and values held dear by the emerging Mexican nation-state. A low-income woman's noncompliance is thus taken as an outright refusal to participate in the state social progress mandate rather than as an individual choice for a semblance of control in her own experiences with childbirth.[5]

To conclude, women who do not follow "appropriate" behaviors are labeled as risks, as bad mothers, and consequently, as disobedient citizens. Van Hollen's wonderful phrase "maneuvering development" is a particularly apt description of the situation in which these women find themselves (2003:166). The Mexican state creates various programs—Oportunidades, midwifery certification programs, and health campaigns promoting good motherhood—to maneuver their target populations into becoming modern subjects. As one of the health promoters I spoke with said: "We don't change [their] customs. We just come here to tell them where they are wrong." The women in my study have been classified as "less developed" and "less modern." Thus, their minds must be reformed and, most particularly, their bodily practices must be transformed. Not only do the women I have described have no claim to their fertility and maternity during their birthing experiences, they also can be—and arguably must be—physically and emotionally controlled and manipulated during this experience through intervention, as well as through verbal assaults of choice, responsibility, and blame.

Acknowledgments

This research was made possible in part by support from the Institute for Scholarship in the Liberal Arts, College of Arts and Letters, University of Notre Dame, and from the Kellogg Institute for International Studies, University of Notre Dame. I am indebted to the kindness of the women, physicians, nurses, and midwives who generously allowed me into their lives. I am also grateful for the thoughtful comments of the anonymous reviewers, who helped strengthen this paper. Many thanks go to my two student assistants, Caitlin Monesmith and Kirsten Prabhudas, and to Rahul Oka for inventive solutions to academic questions. A very important thank-you goes to Lauren Fordyce and Amínata Maraesa, whose countless hours of hard work have made this important project possible—and worthwhile.

Notes

1. I have used pseudonyms for places and people where there is a possibility of identifying actual persons with whom I conducted research.
2. All these terms mean "midwives." *Partera* is the general term for midwife. *Empíricas* is an unusual term physicians routinely use to refer to midwives; it literally means "empirical [women]," who gain their knowledge through practice, not formal education. *Comadrona* is another term used for midwife; its root is *comadre*—the term for fictive kinswoman.
3. It is a routine procedure after any medical birth to make certain that the placenta has come out entirely, as a retained placenta can result in infection, hemorrhage, and death (Magann et al. 2005).
4. *Mestizaje* in Mexico is intimately tied to state development and nationalism that originated at the beginning of the twentieth century after the Mexican Revolution. *Mestizo* (the product of miscegenation between indigenous and European lineages) was seen as the superior race, which would integrate the positive traits of indigenous life while eradicating the ones seen as backward and as stumbling blocks to modernization.
5. This label of noncompliance completely bypasses middle- and upper-class women, because they do not receive monetary support from the government.

References

Beck, Ulrich
    1992   Risk Society: Towards a New Modernity. London: Sage Publications.
Browner, Carole
    2000   Situating Women's Reproductive Activities. American Anthropologist 102(4):773–88.
Browner, Carole, and Nancy Press
    1995   The Normalization of Prenatal Diagnostic Testing. *In* Conceiving the New World Order: The Global Politics of Reproduction. Faye Ginsburg and Rayna Rapp, eds. Pp. 307–22. Berkeley: University of California Press.
Colen, Shellee
    1995   "Like a Mother to Them": Stratified Reproduction and West Indian Childcare Workers and Employers in New York. *In* Conceiving the New World Order: The Global Politics of Reproduction. Faye Ginsburg and Rayna Rapp, eds. Pp. 78–102. Berkeley: University of California Press.
Comaroff, Jean, and John Comaroff
    1993   Introduction. *In* Modernity and Its Malcontents: Ritual and Power in Postcolonial Africa. Jean Comaroff and John Comaroff, eds. Pp. xi–xxxvii. Chicago: University of Chicago Press.

Cosminsky, Sheila
  2001   Maya Midwives in Southern Mexico and Guatemala. *In* Mesoamerican Healers.
          Brad Huber and Alan Sandstrom, eds. Pp. 179–210. Austin: University of Texas
          Press.
Davis-Floyd, Robbie
  1987   The Technological Model of Birth. Journal of American Folklore
          100(398):479–95.
  1992   Birth as an American Rite of Passage. Berkeley: University of California Press.
Douglas, Mary
  1966   Purity and Danger: An Analysis of Concepts of Pollution and Taboo. New York:
          Routledge.
  1990   Risk as a Forensic Resource. Daedalus 119(4):1–16.
Ellison, Marcia
  2003   Authoritative Knowledge and Single Women's Unintentional Pregnancies,
          Abortions, Adoption, and Single Motherhood: Social Stigma and Structural
          Violence. Medical Anthropology Quarterly 17(3):322–47.
Farmer, Paul
  2003   Pathologies of Power: Health, Human Rights, and the New War on the Poor.
          Berkeley: University of California Press.
Georges, Eugenia
  1996   Fetal Ultrasound Imaging and the Production of Authoritative Knowledge in
          Greece. Medical Anthropology Quarterly 10(2):157–75.
Giddens, Anthony
  1998   Conversations with Anthony Giddens: Making Sense of Modernity. Stanford,
          CA: Stanford University Press.
Ginsburg, Faye, and Rayna Rapp
  1991   The Politics of Reproduction. Annual Review of Anthropology 20:311–43.
Hunt, Linda
  1998   Moral Reasoning and the Meaning of Cancer: Causal Explanations of
          Oncologists and Patients in Southern Mexico. Medical Anthropology Quarterly
          12(3):298–318.
Hunt, Linda, Heide Castañeda, and Katherine de Voogd
  2006   Do Notions of Risk Inform Patient Choice? Lessons from a Study of Prenatal
          Genetic Counseling. Medical Anthropology 25:193–219.
Irwin, Susan, and Brigitte Jordan
  1987   Knowledge, Practice, and Power: Court-Ordered Cesarean Sections. Medical
          Anthropology Quarterly 1(3):319–34.
Jacobs, Linda
  2000   An Analysis of the Concept of Risk. Cancer Nursing 23(1):12–19.
Jokhio, Abdul, Heather Winter, and Kar Cheng
  2005   An Intervention Involving Traditional Birth Attendants and Perinatal and
          Maternal Mortality in Pakistan. Obstetrical and Gynecological Survey 60:641–42.
Jordan, Brigitte
  1993   Birth in Four Cultures: A Crosscultural Investigation of Childbirth in Yucatán,
          Holland, Sweden, and the United States. Prospect Heights, IL: Waveland Press.
  1997   Authoritative Knowledge and Its Construction. *In* Childbirth and Authoritative

Knowledge: Cross-Cultural Perspectives. Robbie Davis-Floyd and Carolyn Sargent, eds. Pp. 55–79. Berkeley: University of California Press.

Kleinman, Arthur
  2000   The Violences of Everyday Life: The Multiple Forms and Dynamics of Social Violence. *In* Violence and Subjectivity. Veena Das, Arthur Kleinman, Mamphela Ramphele, and Pamela Reynolds, eds. Pp. 226–41. Berkeley: University of California Press.

Magann, Everett, Sharon Evans, Maureen Hutchinson, Robyn Collins, Bobby Howard, and John Morrison
  2005   Postpartum Hemorrhage after Vaginal Birth: An Analysis of Risk Factors. Southern Medical Journal 98(4):419–22.

Martin, Emily
  1992   The Woman in the Body: A Cultural Analysis of Reproduction. Boston: Beacon Press.

Molyneux, Maxine
  2006   Mothers at the Service of the New Poverty Agenda: Progresa/Oportunidades, Mexico's Conditional Cash Transfer Programme. Social Policy and Administration 40(4):425–99.

Murphy-Lawless, Jo
  1998   Reading Birth and Death: A History of Obstetric Thinking. Bloomington: Indiana University Press.

Netz, Reviel
  2004   Barbed Wire: An Ecology of Modernity. Middletown, CT: Wesleyan University Press.

Rapp, Rayna
  1988   Chromosomes and Communication: The Discourse of Genetic Counseling. Medical Anthropology Quarterly 2(2):143–57.

Sandstrom, Alan
  1991   Corn Is Our Blood: Culture and Ethnic Identity in a Contemporary Aztec Village. Norman: University of Oklahoma Press.

Sargent, Carolyn, and Grace Bascope
  1997   Ways of Knowing about Birth in Three Cultures. *In* Childbirth and Authoritative Knowledge: Cross-Cultural Perspectives. Robbie Davis-Floyd and Carolyn Sargent, eds. Pp. 183–208. Berkeley: University of California Press.

Shorten, Allison, and Brett Shorten
  2009   Independent Midwifery Care versus NHS Care in the UK: A Need to Balance Risks, Benefits, and Choice. British Medical Journal 338:1454–55.

Smith-Oka, Vania
  2008   Plants Used for Reproductive Health by Nahua Women in Northern Veracruz, Mexico. Journal of Economic Botany 62(4):604–14.
  2009a   Conceiving Right(s): Exploring the Connection between Medical Violence and Women's Reproductive Rights in Mexico. Paper presented at the American Anthropological Association. Philadelphia, December 2–6.
  2009b   Unintended Consequences: Exploring the Tensions between Development Programs and Indigenous Women in Mexico in the Context of Reproductive Health. Social Science and Medicine 68(11):2069–77.

Sridhar, Devi, and Arabella Duffield
  2006   A Review of the Impact of Cash Transfer Programmes on Child Nutritional Status
          and Some Implications for Save the Children UK Programmes. United Kingdom:
          Save the Children.
Stern, Alexandra
  1999   Responsible Mothers and Normal Children: Eugenics, Nationalism, and Welfare
          in Postrevolutionary Mexico, 1920–1940. Journal of Historical Sociology
          12(4):369–97.
Tsing, Anna
  1990   Monster Stories: Women Charged with Perinatal Endangerment. *In* Uncertain
          Terms: Negotiating Gender in American Culture. Faye Ginsburg and Anna Tsing,
          eds. Pp. 282–99. Boston: Beacon Press.
Turner, Victor
  1967   The Forest of Symbols. Ithaca, NY: Cornell University Press.
Van Gennep, Arnold
  1960   The Rites of Passage. Chicago: University of Chicago Press.
Van Hollen, Cecilia
  2003   Birth on the Threshold: Childbirth and Modernity in South India. Berkeley:
          University of California Press.

CHAPTER 6

Local Contours of Reproductive Risk and Responsibility in Rural Oaxaca

Rebecca Howes-Mischel

> For a safe pregnancy, attend your consultation. Care for yourself and care for it!
> —Mural outside a small community clinic in Oaxaca

> You are the ones who love your children because you came to this nutrition talk; you are the ones who care about your children's health.
> —Angelica, community clinic director

The two messages about good reproductive health that introduce this chapter, the first from a mural outside a small community health clinic in rural Oaxaca, Mexico, and the second by the clinic's director, remind women that they are responsible for their children's healthy futures. Further, they suggest that this responsibility involves specific forms of care practices learned at the clinic and, implicitly, that failure to follow these biomedical dictates leaves women open to external blame and censure. Love, safety, caring, and responsibility are all central elements in these instructions for good motherhood. In the first example, safety is the key message, as passersby—women who are potentially represented by the mural and their surrounding community members—are instructed to associate pregnancy with an unnamed risk that they may avoid with simple biomedical compliance. In the second quotation, the director implicitly invokes the specter of irresponsible and unloving women who do not care for their children: the women who did not come to the talk or participate in the clinic's activities and who are not concerned with their children's health. These institutional narratives about reproductive responsibility closely align it with narratives about a particular kind of risk that may be mitigated by clinical compliance. In these examples, public health messages about rural women's pregnancy in Oaxaca reiterate a narrative through which ever-present and amorphous risks must be managed in particular ways. Medical personnel frame these self-care practices as requiring clinical instruction to conjoin women's ways of acting in the best interests of their future children with their care of the body.

Women in Oaxaca's Tlacolula Valley echoed this emphasis on their own behaviors, as well as the association between institutional discipline and reproductive safety, in their narratives about how to be a good pregnant woman. During a lull at a wedding early on in my fieldwork, I asked Rosa, "So where is the best place to have your baby?"[1] An older woman with four children and seven grandchildren, she replied with a laugh: "Before, it used to be just a woman and her mother and the midwife, and women were strong. You just held on to the *rebozo* [a traditional and multipurpose shawl] and that was all you had. But now, now it's best to go to the clinic, it's safer, it's more modern, it's better for the mother and baby." In her answer, she aligns modernity, safety, and maternal love with clinical care. Her discursive construction echoes Fraser's (1995, 1998) argument that women in traditionally disenfranchised populations seek biomedical intervention as part of a project of modernity from which they have heretofore been excluded. Litt similarly typifies medical normativity as "a kind of gateway between the 'old fashion' and the 'modern'" that has further entrenched ethnoracial divisions among marginalized women in the United States (2000:3). Despite feminist critiques of biomedical hegemony over reproduction, I again and again heard the aspiration for a highly biomedically driven prenatal and birth process among the rural Zapotec women with whom I did fieldwork. Not only did they all expect and anticipate a clinical birth whose trajectory the doctor would direct, but also they desired one.[2] Further, women articulated a close association between their bodily care regimes and the health of their fetus similar to the connections outlined by medical personnel (cf. Gálvez, this volume). Discussing the need to make sure that in their own diet "he [the fetus] has enough but not too much," they drew an immediate connection between a woman's ways of acting on her body and her child's best outcomes.

In both these sets of narratives—those expressed by medical personnel and those by women in their homes—the pregnant body is the site through which future safety is ensured. However, in their quotidian narratives the logic that associated maternal behavior and fetal development also underpinned nonbiomedically authorized practices. In this chapter, I analyze how associated but different logics of health may motivate similar practices of bodily discipline. Seeking to make sense of the relevant terms through which prenatal health is managed and pregnant bodies disciplined, I consider how both women and doctors articulate a similar desire for biomedical intervention but through different projects of modernity. While public health institutions draw together tropes of risk and responsibility to motivate specific bodily practices and frame women's bodies as requiring their intervention, women talk about safety, love, and modernity and frame their bodily practices within a long-standing logic of care. This gap between medical personnel's and women's constructions of medical compliance highlights what is missed in public health interventions when oft-heard and off-handed comments like "I just do what the doctor tells me" are taken at face value.

During nine months of fieldwork in and around public health clinics in the central valleys of Oaxaca in 2008, I came to realize that this gap I observed between a public health and a local rationality of pregnancy might be best glimpsed not by an attention to practices but rather to the rationalities that underlay them. I spent the majority of this research time with medical professionals and other public health figures, recording and observing prenatal exams (and other medical encounters) in a regional rural public hospital and a smaller community health clinic. I quickly realized that questioning women inside or around biomedical sites yielded monosyllabic responses that closely mirrored institutional ones; either pregnancy was not a subject about which they were interested in speaking, or I was too much like an institutional figure. To gain a fuller picture of the quotidian experiences of prenatal life, I supplemented this data by participating in community life in a neighboring and medium-sized Zapotec town that mirrored the hospital's demographic profile. It was here that I heard women speak at length about pregnancy, health, and child rearing. Initially these women responded negatively to my inquiries about nonbiomedical practices, family lore, or any other cultural practices, reiterating, "I just do what the doctor says, nothing special." Yet, over the course of research, I began to hear other narratives in side conversations at weddings or as I eavesdropped during a lull at a new roof celebration—narratives about giving in to fetal demands, about protecting against physical deformities, and about following customary mandates that stemmed from another logic of health and the gestating body. It is these narratives that hint at another vision of prenatal health—a vision that aligns closely with the biomedical model, while not fully replicating it.

A Disordered Population and Risky Bodies

In rural Oaxaca, narratives of responsibility and blame play out against a political and public health backdrop in which indigenous reproduction is often represented as structurally disordered and dangerous. Located in southwestern Mexico, Oaxaca is typified in the national imaginary as "the indigenous state" through simultaneous representations of indigenous communities as bearers of a national cultural heritage and as culturally different, caught in a static historical present (Alonso 1994, 2004). Over the last century, Oaxacan health has been a target for international and national interventions premised on modern hygiene practices (Birn 1998). Its current position atop national indices of poverty, malnutrition, and maternal mortality frames state interventions in terms of these modernizing projects, bringing Oaxaca into alignment with the rest of modern Mexico, and Mexico in turn with the rest of the developed modern world.[3] In the domain of reproductive public health, it is the maternal mortality statistic that looms largest. Oaxacan maternal mortality rates are thus materially real (see Sesia 2005 for a discussion of the deaths not included in the official statistics) and symbolically potent, as I argue that contemporary public, rural, and reproductive health care operates under its shadow.[4]

The goals and practices of public health institutions are intimately intertwined with an acknowledgment of maternal mortality, and their work is animated by an urgency to decrease it. These public health professionals, charged with ensuring and producing healthy populations, act within a double bind of reproductive responsibility. They are responsible both to the communities they serve and, more importantly, to national and international institutions who assess their work based on abstracted epidemiological statistics. Risk in this context operates at the scalar level of both population and individual; it both frames the institutional context of Oaxacan prenatal care and reflects individual medical professionals' need to make this risk manageable for their own work. Thus, while some public health professionals described the context of reproductive risk to me in structural terms of geographic and resource obstacles, they instructed pregnant women in self-care regimes in ways that obviated this context, invoking instead a sort of neoliberal vision of care of the self (Rose 2006) as *the* path toward ensuring healthy reproductive outcomes.

In my fieldwork, the maternal mortality statistic loomed large in the implicit and explicit reiteration of a public health category, *riesgo* (risk), and became a way to locate population-level concerns in individual bodily practices—practices that may be clinically managed. Yet the apparently obvious nature of the statistic as a clinical problem is challenged by representations like *Paso a Paso . . . hacia una maternidad sin riesgos*, a documentary film produced by Grupo de Estudios Sobre La Mujer Rosario Castellanos that presents a full, nuanced picture of the various structural, personal, and cultural barriers that may contribute to Oaxaca's maternal mortality rate.[5] Here, the structuring statistic is the accumulated product of: (1) communities high in the mountains whose only roads wash out in the rainy season, separating them from the nearest medical clinics; (2) women who get married and pregnant too young; (3) women who are forced to bear too many children; (4) domestic violence; and (5) clinic workers who explicitly and implicitly tell women that their bodies are dirty or uncared for. Following one woman's reproductive journey until her death in childbirth on a road en route to the clinic, the film suggests that improving reproductive health requires intervention at the community, institutional, and individual levels. In this representation, women are at risk for maternal mortality based on a lack of investment in infrastructure, racism, cultural patriarchy, and structural stratification, rather than based solely on their manageable self-care practices. It best reflects the extremes in the complicated matrix of forces that structure rural indigenous women's prenatal health by adding nuance, indicting structural forces, and offering a model for improving person-centered culturally competent care. With this multidimensional portrayal, it emphasizes that maternal mortality is something produced by failures at both the structural and the personal levels.

Medical professionals in the regional IMSS (Mexican Social Security Institution) public hospital in the Tlacolula Valley were acutely aware of this double valence. While the hospital is located within the metropole of the capital city—accessed by an easy forty-five-minute bus ride along the Pan-American Highway—it serves communities from both the valley and the surrounding mountains. Its family doctors see on average thirty patients a day, who in turn may spend a large portion of their day traveling for clinical care; time and resources are two things of which the medical personnel wish they had more.

Oaxaca's unique geographic features and the ensuing difficulties of poor rural health infrastructure were made material during my first meeting with Rodolfo, the clinic director. When I brought up the issue of maternal mortality and how the hospital addressed the complications of reproductive health, he drew me a map of where the hospital is located in relation to the communities it serves. Rodolfo began by explaining the constraints under which the hospital and its population operate: it is better equipped than others and therefore receives patients from far afield. Explaining the "difficult places" with a pen and paper, he told me: "This one is four hours away, this one six, if the road is not washed out by the rain, but that happens every spring. There is a hospital here, but it has no resources, or the doctors don't go, so they come here. In these communities in the mountains here, the doctor is not there on the weekends unless there is a fiesta, and so the people don't trust him," and so on.[6] As I peered closer, trying to copy the names of the communities and match the map that he was sketching to my mental map of the state, he returned to his earlier discussion of the major reproductive health problems faced by the hospital's target population: too many teenage pregnancies, too few women arriving at the hospital early enough in their pregnancy, and too many women too "ashamed" to acknowledge and take care of their prenatal health. Suddenly, he crumpled the paper slip and then opened it partially, explaining: "Y por eso, asi es Oaxaca" [And, therefore, thus is Oaxaca].

At first take I assumed that he was saying that Oaxaca was metaphorically trashed or unredeemable, or that the situation in which he too was caught was an impossible one. However, he continued with an anecdote about being called to task for Oaxaca's health statistics at a meeting of Mexican public health professionals "up north," where they questioned the roots of the disordered population instantiated by these numbers. I soon realized that he was also making a more literal point. The crumpled map mimicked the dense mountainous landscape that many patients must traverse by public transport to reach what he considered "good" medical attention. The creased paper represented how distances that seem close on an official flat map become more complicated in reality. "So," he continued, "when people in the North ask me what's wrong with Oaxaca, I say, this is Oaxaca." Gesturing at the scrunched paper, he said: "What can I do?"[7] The crumpled map became a way for him to describe how he too was caught within a national framing of Oaxacan reproduction as disordered. And how it was uncontrollable geographic and structural forces that contributed to "what's wrong with Oaxaca."

The contrast between a flat map and the topographically rendered one also metaphorically points to the complexity through which public health statistics work. While the clinic director's work is governed by his ability to produce good statistics—where good is determined by their ability to point toward Mexico's accomplishment of a certain kind of modernity—these statistics are produced from the messiness of individual lives and bodies. Tropes of risk and responsibility not only permeated public health narratives directed at patient populations, but also were the terms under which public health workers understood their own work.

Although risk is a general theme in the transformation of rural communities into modern, rationally organized, healthy populations (see Beck 1992 and Giddens 1990, 1991, for more general discussions about the close association between modernity and risk management), the specter of maternal mortality makes it ever more urgent in the context of reproduction. From the moment pregnant women enter the hospital, risk becomes a central theme for their encounters with bio-medical health care. Once a nurse has taken their vital statistics and they have waited (often for hours) for their appointment, the first element of the medical encounter between doctor and pregnant woman is the completion of the "Prenatal Monitoring, Reproductive Risk, and Obstetric Risk" questionnaire that assesses a woman's numerical "risk valuation." Distributed by the national public health service, these standardized forms give women points for every question they answer affirmatively.[8] At the end, the doctor tallies the points while announcing which conditions increase the woman's risk score (e.g., "she has one point because she did not finish high school, another four points because she had a cesarean section before") and assigns her a final risk number. The questions range from the date of her last menstrual period to her consumption of controlled substances and the outcomes of her previous pregnancies.[9]

During the majority of the active interview time, doctors address the number of years of schooling women have completed, their birth spacing, family-planning preferences, and marital status (the last two questions do not actually appear on the risk sheet).[10] In the initial visit, the doctor uses the woman's last menstrual period to determine the approximate gestational age and then instructs her on how to properly "count" the duration of her pregnancy.[11] Finally, the doctor outlines new nutritional and self-care practices, such as specific forms of exercise. The risk sheet then goes in the front of the woman's file. While the doctor adds her weight and fundal measurement at each visit, the risk score is not altered during the course of pregnancy; instead it represents her initial score as her permanent risk status.[12] During this risk assessment, rather than discussing biological or genetic risk, doctors encourage women to look to their individual lives as the site of risk production and alleviation. As their risk score operates as an indelible and orienting frame from their past, future daily practices are now their only space of risk remediation.

In this framing, risk is a condition that haunts individual women as they are slotted into a reproductive population that is materialized via epidemiological statistics. Doctors may tell women: "There is a risk, and we will keep checking"; rarely do they explain the particulars of that risk. Even in instances of a specific pathological concern, risk itself remains an open category. For example, Edeline, an eighteen-year-old accompanied by her two-year-old daughter, was referred to the obstetrical specialist because she was at risk for pre-eclampsia. Notably, Doctora Celia never really explained what pre-eclampsia is—offering only its indicator ("there's some protein in the urine"), some reassurance ("he's moving and that's good"), and a plan ("we're going to monitor for it and make sure that everything's okay"). In lived experience, risk is a category of bodily vulnerability without substantive information, or, as Doctora Celia says: "You have a risk for it, and it's very serious if you have it. It's a risk for both you and the baby." What is important for her is not that Edeline learns about pre-eclampsia as a disease qua disease, as might be expected in an informed-consent model of bioethics, but that she learns how to understand the management of pre-eclampsia in her own body. Operating as a capacious category in which other kinds of concerns about the body, population, and modernity are intertwined, risk in public health talk in Oaxaca becomes a way to discuss certain forms of responsibility (individual) and not others (structural) (see Smith-Oka, this volume).

Responsibility

During an orientation meeting I had with Angelica, the director of the community health clinic in an outlying Oaxacan neighborhood, she commented that this community had a higher rate of pre-eclampsia than she had expected: "It's something we see a lot, women get sick. It makes the care hard and there's risk, you see." This community is located alongside the Oaxacan municipal trash dump and is largely populated by intrastate migrants who have moved closer to the city in the absence of economic opportunities in the rural highlands. As one nurse explained to me: "This is a little Oaxaca. We have people from everywhere, but there's no community, you see. People are just trying to get ahead." Only the central street is paved, and the built landscape reflects its relative newness and marginal economic status; there is little coordination to the cinder-block houses guarded by chicken-wire and sheet-metal fences, birds circle above the nearby massive trash heap, and I always left the community feeling sick from the kinds of dust I had taken into my body. With these considerations in mind, I asked the director whether she thought there was something in the community that led to this epidemiological pattern. Could it be something in the economic or, more importantly, environmental context that made pregnant women especially sick? "No," she countered. "No, I think that it's just that the people here, they're lazy. They want so much from us. But they don't do the work to take care of themselves, and then there's only so much we can do. They just want so much." Actively resisting my question about structural and environmental causal factors, Angelica tied together risk and personal responsibility to individualize the reproductive disorder: they do not "take care enough."

First articulated by Rodolfo, the public hospital's director, the issue of being called on to account for Oaxaca "up north" was a constant narrative thread running through public health professionals' discussions about the frustrating nature of managing a community's health. Public health in Mexico is organized in a heavily top-down and centralized manner, with public health care a national right in which the government takes an interest via state and national programs.[13] As Julie, a social worker, told me one afternoon, community public health professionals are often called on to justify negative health outcomes in their communities up the bureaucratic ladder. In this instance, an outbreak of dengue fever had been diagnosed in her community. She was obligated to report it to the state public health office, where officials asked her what she was doing wrong—what had happened in this community to produce dengue? Rather than offering an explanation about the community's environmental hazards located next to the dump, the lack of paved roads, or the absence of state provided antimosquito powder, she lay the responsibility on the community's health committee: "I told them to sweep the streets, to organize the community to sweep the streets, but they didn't and now they have dengue. And I'm in trouble." Her frustrated analysis of the problem reflects a top-down reframing through which risk and responsibility become located not at the structural level—as being geographic or material resource–driven problems—but in the inaction, or inappropriate actions, of individuals at the local level. In this double bind in which medical professionals find themselves, they are called to account by external pressures but without the resources or ability to address what they may see as key factors in the structural production of this disordered population. Disciplining individual bodies (Foucault 1997[1977]), however, *is* something within their power.

Making do within this quandary, medical professionals emphasize interventions that appear most controllable—ones that reframe risk as located not in large structural conditions, but in individual bodies and personal practices. Responding to the question, "What's wrong with Oaxaca?" the hospital director cannot flatten the mountains or build better roads. But he can get more women enrolled in biomedical prenatal care and on a trajectory of relating to their pregnant bodies within a bioscientific frame. In response to this external censure, when it comes to prenatal health, public health institutions emphasize to the communities they serve that increased clinical attendance is the only pathway toward better outcomes. Once pregnant women are in the clinic, medical professionals encourage them to learn particular regimes of *autocuidado* (self-care) deemed essential for managing and mitigating risk. Again, the specter of maternal mortality statistics influences the way that risk is conceptualized in this context, and it becomes a guiding trope for institutional narratives about reproduction; clinic attendance is held up as a sort of magical first step to reducing this statistic.

A nurse told me as we walked around a community looking for women who had missed prenatal appointments: "The most important thing is that they come into the clinic; if they don't, we don't know what they might be doing, and then bad things could happen."[14] She does not outline the benefits of a biomedical plan of action, but rather presents surveillance by itself as enough to ensure that "bad things" don't happen. While this is not to say that early detection of potentially dangerous prenatal conditions is not a central part of standard care, her ambiguous reference to "bad things" suggests that this intervention is not framed solely in those terms. In this construction, risk becomes manageable as populations become manageable, and as individual practices are brought under the clinic's surveillance. It is thus part of the institutions' responsibility to socialize women into a sense of responsibility predicated on a specific form of self-care—a set of self-care practices that women in turn learn from the institution.

Governance

Central to contemporary analyses of reproductive risk and responsibility is a form of bodily governance closely associated with the cultivation of a neoliberal sensibility. As Foucault (1978, 1979) presciently argued, the central concern of the modern state is the administration of and management of populations, as incarnated in individual bodies and dispositions. Under contemporary regimes of governmentality, citizens are encouraged to think about and act upon themselves as "modern" in ways that mirror state concerns in their own desires; in these ways, "government is intimately involved in making modern subjects" (Inda 2005:10). As Rose (2006) lays out in his presentation of "biological citizenship" (see also Rose and Novas 2005), this modern self-enterprising subject engages in bodily projects that minimize and privatize risk by attention to lifestyle. Acting as an appropriately modern subject therefore involves acting as an autonomous, self-regulating individual who polices herself by incorporating a discourse of risk into her "techniques of the self" (Foucault 1988). Risk avoidance, or risk management, becomes part of a larger moral enterprise of self-governance as a modern citizen in ways highly tied to the biomedical body. Rose's (2006) theoretical frame, however, both assumes and requires access to technomedical ways of knowing the body—relying on the ability to estimate a somatic future and then to act according. As routine reproductive risk is conceptualized in late modernity, the possibilities and promises of technology are writ large, both as sources of information and as corrective tools (Rapp 1999).[15] In the regional public hospital, these technological tools were largely absent or were restricted to emergency scenarios (e.g., the sole ultrasound machine was located in the emergency room). The technologies of prenatal exams were limited to fetal stethoscopes, measuring tapes, and doctors' manual fetal assessment and expert knowledge base. While these are all basic technologies, they rely on skilled haptic engagement and offer readily apparently diagnostics, unlike those from the highly mediated technologies Rose (2006) and Rapp (1999) discuss, such as ultrasound, amniocentesis, and other genetic tests. Thus, entering the biomedical clinic does not offer these women access to the kinds of interventions commonly associated with neoliberal forms of understanding, and thus reducing, reproductive risk.

In the absence of readily available medical technology, the narratives about reproductive health encourage women simultaneously to view medical attention as essential for their own risk reduction and to construct a sense of personal control over prenatal health in ways unmoored from specific technological information. The initial obstetric risk questionnaire itself appears to act as a form of medical technology—one that encourages women to conceptualize themselves as pregnant subjects in the particular terms of their sociomedical histories. It then also frames women's quotidian activities as the sites of responsibly acting on risk. Within this model, modern responsible subjects are ones who comply with doctors' instructions about how to organize their intimate lives against risk. Much of this instructional work circled around reinscribing basic and mundane wisdom as "medical" by making those things, such as breastfeeding (usually glossed as "most natural"), into modern medical practices.

One afternoon during a mandatory workshop for pregnant women in a small community within the hospital's catchment area where medical personnel set up a temporary biweekly clinic, Bianca, the nutritionist, paused in her presentation to comment that "the breast promotes the love for the mother." [16] Using a semi-

Socratic method, she then asked: "So why do we breast feed?" In the face of her participants' silence, she continued: "Because, if you do this, your baby won't be sick." She had started the session by stating: "It's important that we learn this stuff. Many times we don't plan for children, so we aren't as healthy as we can be. We have too many children or too close together. That's why we have these workshops to learn how we can be as healthy as possible, right?" Her explicit goal centers on making women into better mothers by advocating quotidian changes in their diets and child-raising practices. Notably, these are all things that are more commonly associated with "folk knowledge" practices (Lindee 2005). Tying this instruction to a governmental public health program, she aligns her guidance about how to offer a child the breast with the larger projects of a neoliberal modernity that center on personal responsibility and self-maximization. Returning to her first point, she concludes: "And so, when we do this, we show them love and then there is less risk."

It is telling that Bianca does not position herself only as an infallible external authority but also adopts a collaborative posture of "we." Rhetorically eliding a medical/layperson distinction, she aligns her own health with that of the women by referencing an imagined universal connection of mothers. Invoking a shared project or desire ("we all want to be as healthy as we can be"), she positions her own project of biological citizenship alongside theirs ("many times we aren't as healthy as we could be"). Her impressive rhetorical performance of embodying a shared experience calls attention to a constant negotiation over claims to "we" as national health programs try to enroll community members as active stakeholders.

Self-care bodily practices are ways for individuals to demonstrate their responsibility and maternal love to minimize risk. Yet, in Oaxaca, glossing them as modern and associated with a national health agenda frames biological citizenship differently than that of Rose's (2006) neoliberal subject. Rather than serving as the ground on which to articulate a new form of empowered citizenship, as Rose (2006) suggests, I argue, the internalization of these didactic messages about risk and self-care regimes reflects a mode of organizing the self in response and accommodation to the state's demands on its modern citizens. Rather than risk being located in the specific somatic condition of an individual, as she enters biomedical modes of governance an individual woman is automatically slotted into an established somatic population: as a rural, indigenous Oaxacan woman, she is automatically at risk of maternal mortality. This external subjectification process then orients her to a large potential risk that is not tied to any specific condition located in her body—in effect, the trickle down of maternal mortality. In these lived experiences, risk operates as both a structuring and an empty category in this unmoored state, bringing women into new forms of subjectification through their biomedical governance. It is then from this governance that they can form a new sense of biological citizenship. Across this process of finding, labeling, and teaching about risk potentials, the institutional narrative centers on individual self-care practices: come to the clinic, follow medical dictates, and learn to orient to your body through them.

Modern Subjects and Safe Bodies

If an open and amorphous category of risk, located simultaneously in populations and in individual bodies, structures the public health institutional focus, it was not the way that individual women addressed how to care for their future children. While public health officials were consumed with the overdetermined maternal mortality statistics, no woman I talked with offered a personal experience with what Maraesa (this volume) calls an "embodied recognition of the fatalities." Rather than using a discourse of risk premised on epidemiological statistics, they employed one of safety. For example, when I asked one woman about her preferred birth plan, she replied: "I don't know, the doctor hasn't told me." "But do you have a choice?" I queried. "No, just what he tells me, that's more safe." On one level, there is little difference between her emphasis on safety and the medical discourse on risk; both lead to similar kinds of self-care practices that privilege the medical model. Yet, similar to Nichter's discussion of the difference between "vulnerability" and "risk" in harm reduction programs, the former refers to an actual feeling grounded in her subjective experience and the latter to an amorphous "hazard, chance, or uncertainty" (2003:14). While it may be arguable that "safety" necessarily has a clearer referent in people's lives than the way that "risk" has been framed here, it is a term that implies a positive and proactive orientation to health, whereas "risk" implies a negative and unstable one.

Even as women constantly reiterated, "I only do what the doctor told me," in side comments and informal conversation they presented a more nuanced picture of bodily governance that drew on nonbiomedical frameworks of self-regulation and responsibility. As one woman explained to me: "When I was pregnant with her, I had these cravings for beer, and I didn't drink any. But I had these cravings, and when she was born, her mouth was open like this. And she still does that [she opens and closes her mouth repeatedly in a pucker], and she reaches for it and cries when I drink beer." She turned to her pregnant cousin-in-law sitting next to her and continued: "So pay attention. When you have these cravings, maybe a little, it can be good." Another woman chimed in: "You have to be careful—he [indicating her sleeping son] was born with these rashes on his arm, all blotchy like this when he came out. And I think it was because I was so angry for no reason when it was almost time to have him, so that was the rash." I repeatedly heard these kinds of explanations in which maternal behavior was materially manifested on their children's bodies; such as a story of a pregnant woman who ate too many berries, which led to her child's recurring skin rashes as a toddler.[17] Employing a form of haptic or embodied knowledge, they outlined the relationship between their self-care practices and their fetuses' responses, for example: "When I eat chilies he kicks a lot, so I think it's not good for him. So I try not to eat them because it must not be good. But I then had just a sip of beer, just a little, and he was quiet. So I think a little is good, that he wanted that." This directly causal model meshes well with the neoliberal forms of maternal responsibility, as again it is the woman's adherence to the prescribed regime that produces the fetus's (and then the child's) health condition.

Yet a different rationality of the body is at play to produce these kinds of responsibility, one that mirrors but does not reproduce those emphasized by public health professionals.

Francisca, a Zapotec woman in her fifties, described getting very sick shortly after giving birth to her son, but not her daughter, to illustrate that according to this logic there are clear causes and effects associated with adherence to proscribed practices:

> It was the summer and I was so hot, and they told me to wrap up tight
> in my *rebozo* to hold all the heat in, but it was so hot and I thought just
> for a little I could do it. And so I didn't wrap up tight and I got *aire* and
> I got sick, so sick, because I didn't wrap up tight. But with my daughter I
> wrapped up tight and I didn't get sick.[18]

As Francisca explains, following traditional self-care routines results in safety from ill health in the same way that following medical dictates results in safety from adverse outcomes.

Even as Francisca is drawing on a radically different and humoral vision of the body in which its porousness and susceptibility to temperature is at the heart of etiological explanations, it is one that aligns well with the way that public health is tied to individual practices. Women look to their bodily practices, largely nutritional, as the sites at which they have control over shaping the future—giving them a sense of control and opening them up to accusations of being inappropriately healthy. Further, we see a sort of self-disciplining that emphasizes the intimate as the site of this work rather than larger structural or supernatural forces. In both rationalities, women can produce health, or prevent ill health, by following discrete and knowable dictates for acting on the body. Self-care practices and health risks are directly connected in these explanations, although when asked directly, few women would characterize these practices as "medical" and often brushed them aside with a comment that "these are just beliefs that we have," or "I just do what the doctor tells me."

Conclusion

Medical pluralism is an old story in medical anthropology (see Baer, Singer, and Susser 1997; Leslie 1980; Pelto and Pelto 1997), and, as Root and Browner cogently explain, women's pregnant subjectivities are formed in complicated responses to medical hegemony and their own "subjugated knowledge" (2001:217). What I further suggest is somewhat novel is the self-conscious reference to modernity that takes place within these narratives of plurality. Rosa stated, as we saw at the opening of this chapter, safety is related to modernity; the assessment of clinic-based pregnancy management as "more safe and more modern" was one I heard constantly among women in Oaxaca and first-generation Oaxacan immigrants in Southern California. However, I do not want to dismiss the power of the other ways through which they made pregnancy healthy and manageable. Instead, I want to suggest that a complicated form of acknowledgment and occlusion is in play as they shape a model for modern and Oaxacan prenatal health. Although discussions of the intricacies of global reproductive health (see Inhorn 2003; Mitchell and Georges 1997; Press and Browner 1997) often emphasize the associations between modernity and technomedicine, clinical prenatal health for most rural Oaxacans is largely devoid of the mystique of highly technologically mediated encounters. Instead, doctors manually feel for the fetal body by probing the fundus, listen to its heartbeat with a basic aluminum fetal stethoscope, and stress dietary practices as a means toward producing good health—all practices that would not be out of place in a prebiomedical midwife-assisted prenatal experience. Thus, without contradiction, women can both discursively emphasize the association between modernity and biomedicine and act according to nonbiomedical models. By dismissing these alternative practices as beliefs—even as they still practice them—and emphasizing the importance of modern modes of engaging with their health, these women are demonstrating a particular form of modernity aspiration that melds tradition with scientific frames of action. It further obviates the perhaps failed promise of their local technomedicine in which women's biomedical encounters involve the governance of modernity but not the access to its technological fixes.

What I want to highlight in the construction of reproductive risk in Oaxaca is that as it is constructed, both sociomedically and locally, women's individual self-care practices are targeted as the site for the enactment of responsibility. Rather than existing as competing forms of authority over women's bodily practices, biomedical and local productions of responsible prenatal health are melded in women's practices, and women use the trope of safety as opposed to that of risk to sort out ostensibly competing logics of the body and care. As their narratives express an alignment of both frameworks of responsibility and governance, they shed some light on the ease of the adoption of a medicalized neoliberal orientation toward the care of the self; women are compliant in the face of different—but not radically so—practices and modes of governance. Further, being safe involves adding biomedical regimes to their existing ones in a value-added model in which the two do not conflict. This pragmatic uptake is further eased as, in practice, medicalized routine prenatal care in rural Oaxaca invokes the modernity of technomedicine without an accompanying radical reorganization of pregnancy management. Thus the local contours of risk, responsibility, and modernity orient women toward new and possible conceptions of themselves as modern biological citizens, achieved in part through compliance with biomedical norms.

Acknowledgments

I am grateful for the mentoring and support of Rayna Rapp, Emily Martin, and the New York University Ethnography and Science Studies Working Group, whose thoughtful commentary helped refine my early thinking for this piece. I am especially appreciative of the Wenner-Gren Foundation, which funded the eighteen months of research on which this paper relies (Grant # 7615).

Notes

1. I have given pseudonyms to all individuals whose names appear in this chapter.

2. While there may be no "outside" of biomedical discourses given its hegemonic claim to defining the terms of health and bodily conditions globally, there are contemporary moves in Oaxaca (and Mexico more generally) to bring back traditional midwifery practices (Davis-Floyd 2001). However, the Zapotec women with whom I spoke did not express a nostalgic desire for these more woman-centered models of care. Instead, they drew a direct historical lineage from the midwife's services to those offered by the clinic—one was just a more "modern" version of the other.

3. I argue that maternal mortality is one index of national modernity, given its etiological connotation as a disorder of resources rather than of disease (Loudon 2000).

4. In 2003 Oaxaca's maternal mortality rate was 89 per 100,000 live births, while that year's national rate was 63 per 100,000 live births (cited in Sesia 2007:40).

5. The Study Group about the Woman, Rosario Castellanos, is the largest feminist center in Oaxaca City. The eighteen-minute film *Step by Step . . . Making Motherhood without Risk* (English translation) was funded in part by the UN Population Fund (UNPFA) as part of a multiagency project to reduce maternal mortality. International NGOs have taken a keen interest in improving Oaxacan public health and fund many of the large-scale national NGO interventions. The joint UNPFA and WHO Safe Motherhood Initiative has collaborated with the Mexican health system in its community outreach and programmatic work, but policies around the practices of health delivery are set nationally.

6. The doctors he is discussing are mostly nonlocal medical residents completing their mandatory year of service. A centralized national office assigns this service placement, and most of the hospitals' family doctors/general practitioners are also residents completing this service. The majority of these residents come from medical school in Mexico City and are ill equipped and ill disposed to live in remote indigenous communities for a year. Anecdotally I was informed that many would leave at any possible opportunity, further funneling patients into the regional hospitals.

7. This gesture directly mirrors the apocryphal tale of Cortes's representation of New Spain to King Carlos V: "'Draw me a map of New Spain,' said his majesty Carlos V. . . . Legend has it that Cortes picked up a piece of paper, crumbled it between his hands and dropped it to the table. . . . 'That,' Cortes is said to have replied, 'is a map of New Spain'" (Marcus and Flannery 1996:9).

8. To the best of my knowledge, this questionnaire was developed by the Mexican public health system under the auspices of the Medical Benefits Department. The doctors worked with a version dated May 2000 that referred to the Health Ministry in Mexico City as its source. It is worth further research to explore the form's genealogy to uncover possible connections to materials developed by international NGOs as part of the joint UNPFA and WHO Safe Motherhood Initiative.

9. Notably, the questions about medical history ask only about that of the woman rather than including family histories, as might be expected in considerations of genetic or heritable risk.

10. Approximately a third of a woman's exam time with the doctor is occupied with the silent process of producing and cross-referencing paperwork.

11. Learning to "count" gestational age is central to the doctors' socialization of pregnant

women, as they want women to be attuned to specific markers in gestational development and, more importantly, to know when to come to the hospital to give birth.

12. Strikingly, the worry about conditions such as pre-eclampsia or gestational diabetes are also framed in the language of risk, but they are not added to this initial risk score.

13. Article 4 of the 1917 Mexican Constitution codifies both citizens' right to and responsibility for health: "All Mexicans have the right to be included in the Social Protection System for Health . . . irrespective of their social condition. . . . Beneficiaries have the following duties: to adopt behavior to promote health and prevent disease . . . ; to keep themselves informed concerning the mode of operation of establishments for access to medical services; to cooperate with the medical team by providing accurate personal information; to follow the recommendations, instructions, treatments, and procedures they have accepted; to inform themselves of the risks entailed and the various possible solutions and of consultation and complaint procedures . . . ; to make responsible use of the health services."

14. Nurses performed this exercise of finding "hidden women" regularly, and it has clear parallels to the one Maraesa (this volume) describes in Belize. Yet while Maraesa discusses these outreach attempts as marked by "a language of encouragement" that often ventures into scolding, the Oaxacan community clinic's nurses performed this task with a visage of respectful earnestness. This was not a small and intimate community like Toledo, and these relatively inexperienced nurses were not community members; here the language of encouragement did not contain the same coercive tones. Additionally, the high rate of instances in which "bad paperwork" often led them to women who were still enrolled in biomedical care diminished their certitude that the women were necessarily at fault.

15. In these theoretical models of biological citizenship, access to genetic probabilistic information is crucial, and citizen subjects are required to learn to understand and act in the face of potential health futures on the basis of this knowledge.

16. This workshop was ostensibly mandatory only for women receiving public benefits through the Oportunidades governmental program (see Smith-Oka, this volume). However, in practice medical professionals encouraged all pregnant women in the community to attend.

17. See Laderman (1983) for an in-depth discussion of associated illness, as well as Gálvez (this volume).

18. *Aire* is literally "air," and more commonly glossed as "evil air." It is a common Latin American folk medical term tied to humoral theories of the body, heat, cold and porousness (Foster 1976, 1993; Pedersen and Baruffati 1985).

References

Alonso, Anna Maria
    1994   The Politics of Space, Time, and Substance: State Formation, Nationalism, and Ethnicity. Annual Review of Anthropology 23:379–405.
    2004   Conforming Disconformity: "Mestizaje," Hybridity, and the Aesthetics of Mexican Nationalism. Cultural Anthropology 19(4):459–90.

Baer, Hans, Merrill Singer, and Ida Susser
   1997   Medical Anthropology and the World System: A Critical Perspective. Westport,
           CT: Bergin and Garvey.
Beck, Ulrich
   1992   Risk Society: Towards a New Modernity. London: Sage Publications.
Birn, Anne-Emanuelle
   1998   A Revolution in Rural Health? The Struggle over Local Health Units in Mexico,
           1928–1940. Journal of the History of Medicine and Allied Sciences 53(1):43–76.
Davis-Floyd, Robbie
   2001   La Partera Professional: Articulating Identity and Cultural Space for a New Kind
           of Midwife in Mexico. Medical Anthropology 20(2/3–4):185–243.
Foster, George
   1976   Disease Etiologies in Non-Western Medical Systems. American Anthropologist
           78(4):773–82.
Foster, George
   1993   Hippocrates' Latin American Legacy: Humoral Medicine in the New World.
           London: Routledge.
Foucault, Michel
   1978   The History of Sexuality. New York: Pantheon Books.
   1979   Governmentality. M/F: A Feminist Journal 1(3):5–21.
   1988   Technologies of the Self. *In* Technologies of the Self: A Seminar with Michel
           Foucault. Michel Foucault, Luther Martin, Huck Gutman, and Patrick Hutton,
           eds. Pp. 16–49. Amherst: University of Massachusetts Press.
   1997[1977] Discipline and Punish: The Birth of the Prison. New York: Pantheon Books.
Fraser, Gertrude Jacinta
   1995   Modern Bodies, Modern Minds: Midwifery and Reproductive Change in an
           African American Community. *In* Conceiving the New World Order: The Global
           Politics of Reproduction. Faye Ginsburg and Rayna Rapp, eds. Pp. 42–58.
           Berkeley: University of California Press.
   1998   African American Midwifery in the South: Dialogues of Birth, Race, and
           Memory. Cambridge, MA: Harvard University Press.
Giddens, Anthony
   1990   The Consequences of Modernity. Stanford, CA: Stanford University Press.
   1991   Modernity and Self-Identity: Self and Society in the Late Modern Age. Stanford,
           CA: Stanford University Press.
Inda, Jonathan Xavier
   2005   Analytics of the Modern: An Introduction. *In* Anthropologies of Modernity:
           Foucault, Governmentality, and Life Politics. Jonathon Xavier Inda, ed. Pp. 1–22.
           Malden, MA: Blackwell.
Inhorn, Marcia
   2003   Local Babies, Global Science: Gender, Religion, and In Vitro Fertilization in
           Egypt. New York: Routledge.
Laderman, Carol
   1983   Wives and Midwives: Childbirth and Nutrition in Rural Malaysia. Berkeley:
           University of California Press.

Leslie, Charles
  1980   Medical Pluralism in World Perspective. Social Science and Medicine
         14B(4):191–95.
Lindee, M. Susan
  2005   Moments of Truth in Genetic Medicine. Baltimore: Johns Hopkins University
         Press.
Litt, Jacquelyn
  2000   Medicalized Motherhood: Perspectives from the Lives of African-American and
         Jewish Women. New Brunswick, NJ: Rutgers University Press.
Loudon, Irvine
  2000   Maternal Mortality in the Past and Its Relevance to Developing Countries Today.
         American Journal of Clinical Nutrition 72(1):241S.
Marcus, Joyce, and Kent Flannery
  1996   Zapotec Civilization: How Urban Society Evolved in Mexico's Oaxaca Valley.
         New York: Thames and Hudson.
Mitchell, Lisa, and Eugenia Georges
  1997   Cross-Cultural Cyborgs: Greek and Canadian Women's Discourses on Fetal
         Ultrasound. Feminist Studies 23(2):373–401.
Nichter, Mark
  2003   Harm Reduction: A Core Concern for Medical Anthropology. *In* Risk, Culture,
         and Health Inequality: Shifting Perceptions of Danger and Blame. Barbara Herr
         Harthorn and Laury Oaks, eds. Pp. 13–33: Westport, CT: Praeger.
Pedersen, Duncan, and Veronica Baruffati
  1985   Health and Traditional Medicine Cultures in Latin America and the Caribbean.
         Social Science and Medicine 21(1):5–12.
Pelto, Pertti, and Gretel Pelto
  1997   Studying Knowledge, Culture, and Behavior in Applied Medical Anthropology.
         Medical Anthropology Quarterly 11(2):147–63.
Press, Nancy, and Carole Browner
  1997   Why Women Say Yes to Prenatal Diagnosis. Social Science and Medicine
         45(7):979–89.
Rapp, Rayna
  1999   Testing Women, Testing the Fetus: The Social Impact of Amniocentesis in
         America. New York: Routledge.
Root, Robin, and Carole Browner
  2001   Practices of the Pregnant Self: Compliance with and Resistance to Prenatal
         Norms. Culture, Medicine and Psychiatry 25:195–223.
Rose, Nikolas
  2006   The Politics of Life Itself: Biomedicine, Power, and Subjectivity in the Twenty-
         First Century. Princeton, NJ: Princeton University Press.
Rose, Nikolas, and Carlos Novas
  2005   Biological Citizenship. *In* Global Assemblages: Technology, Politics, and Ethics
         as Anthropological Problems. Aihwa Ong and Stephen Collier, eds. Pp. 439–63.
         Malden, MA: Blackwell.
Sesia, Paola
  2005   Maternal Mortality Under-Reporting in Oaxaca. Paper presented at the Annual

Meeting of the American Anthropological Association. Washington, DC, December 2.

2007   Reproductive Health and Reproductive Rights after the Cairo Consensus: Accomplishments and Shortcomings in the Establishment of Innovative Public Policies in Oaxaca. Sexuality Research and Social Policy 4(3):34–49.

CHAPTER 7

New Countryside, New Family
The Discourses of Reproductive Risk in Postsocialist Rural China

Qingyan Ma

After three decades of economic reform and a massive effort toward "modernization construction" (*xiandaihua jianshe*), China has become an emerging world power. Challenging the image of modernity, however, is the huge gap in reproductive health that exists between China's underdeveloped west and well-developed east. In the impoverished rural southwest region of China, exceedingly high rates of infant and maternal mortality sparked the creation of the Larger Shangri-la Project (LSP), involving multisector collaboration among local residents, NGOs, and official state family-planning agencies. Under the LSP, the National Population and Family Planning Commission of China (NPFPC) grouped together adjacent but administratively distinct territories across two provinces (Yunnan and Sichuan) and the Tibetan Autonomous Region because of their shared interest in ameliorating reproductive mortality rates. This resulted in the creation of an administrative area, the Larger Shangri-la Area.

The contrast in maternal mortality statistics between the Larger Shangri-la Area and China's eastern coast is astonishing. According to a report from Xinhua News Agency in 2005, the maternal mortality rate in Suzhou, a city on the eastern coast, was 24 per 100,000 live births, while in western China in Ganzi Tibetan Prefecture in Sichuan Province (part of the Larger Shangri-la Area) the rate was 1,119 per 100,000 live births—close to fifty times higher. This gap contradicts the state's promotion of "constructing a harmonious society" under the current Hu Jintao administration, and consequently was used to justify reproductive intervention by the Chinese state in the Larger Shangri-la Area.

One strategy proposed under the LSP for resolving the health gap between east and west was to increase hospital versus home births. Through the LSP, local residents were to be educated about the purported dangers associated with home birth and to adopt a belief in the biomedical definition of risk as it related to their reproductive practices. As a result, the current reproductive practices of the local people are the outcome of constant negotiation among public health experts, local officials, local health providers, and local residents. Moreover, the construction of risk, as differentially perceived by these multisituated and at times conflicting actors, becomes an arena for the political control of outlying populations. In a country well known for a eugenically motivated birth-planning policy (Anagnost 1995; Greenhalgh 2008), the LSP targets minority ethnic populations residing in the borderland in particular, encapsulating the state ideology toward Chinese nationalism, borderland security, and family planning.

This chapter examines the current reproductive practices of those ethnic groups (Lisu, Naxi, Tibetan, and Han) living in Weixi Lisu Autonomous County in northwest Yunnan Province—now a part of the Larger Shangri-la Area—and explores the discourses of reproductive risk as conceived by various parties influenced by their relation to biomedical knowledge and hierarchies of power. Focusing on how the Chinese state's intervention in reproduction and the promotion of hospital birth is challenged by poverty, class-stratified ecological residence patterns, and ethnic differences in Weixi County, this chapter looks at specific reproductive social policy as it is administered to a stratified population with varied understandings of risk.

As state-level reproductive interventions in People's Republic of China have historically been tied to political motive and rationale (Anagnost 1995; Greenhalgh 2008), such a multilevel construction of risk is analyzed in the context of postsocialist rural health care reform and population policy as articulated by the Yunnan Health and Development Research Association (YHDRA). This state-sanctioned NGO, made up of public health experts, governmental officials in charge of public health, and social scientists concerned with researching medicine and health, is responsible for initiating, implementing, and evaluating the LSP. This chapter looks at how the discourses of reproductive risk generated by YHDRA and articulated through the LSP impact the attitudes and actions of the minority ethnic populations of Weixi County.

Research for this chapter was conducted in the Weixi Lisu Autonomous County and in the capital city of Yunnan Province, Kunming, in the summers of 2007, 2008, and 2009, during which I interviewed public health experts from YHDRA, local village doctors, and obstetricians working in the county hospital and local villages. I also conducted participant-observation in meetings between the members of YHDRA and local state officials.[1] For several months pursuant to this research in China, I followed up on the progress of the project via YHDRA's website.

An Overview of Weixi County

The Larger Shangri-la Area incorporates nine counties of the adjacent territories of Yunnan Province, Sichuan Province, and Tibet Autonomous Region in southwest China, an area of 206,642 square miles with a population of 11,958,300. Among the nine counties, Weixi Lisu Autonomous County has the highest rate of maternal mortality. Located in the heart of the Larger Shangri-la Area and the Three Parallel Rivers of Yunnan Protected Areas in the southwestern Chinese borderland, Weixi

County, a land of deep valleys and high mountains, boasts stunning natural beauty and is a UNESCO World Heritage site. Its four ethnic groups (Lisu, Tibetans, Naxi, and Han) live along the mountain slopes. Farming provides more than 90 percent of the local residents with most of their income.

The ethnic differences in the "spatial division" (Hyde 2007; White 1997) of this area play a crucial role in shaping perceptions about hospital birth, as well as individuals' relationship with the state. These ethnic groups differentiate themselves based on identifying names, religious beliefs, modes of subsistence, histories, residence patterns, and internal tensions; they compete for natural resources, such as access to water and land, education, and health care. Those who live in the valley with easy access to transportation, education, and health care are usually those who historically have strong cultural, religious, and political influence in the local area. For example, the Han and Tibetans historically have been identified with large state societies and have cultural, religious, and political hegemony over their neighboring groups. The Naxi usually live halfway up mountain slopes, while the Lisu, who make up over 50 percent of the population, live higher up the mountains and have the least political influence and control. All the ethnic groups, however, are subject to the same state apparatus: the same local administrative unit, the same educational and medical resources, and the same state ideology, which on postsocialist China's development agenda prioritizes economic development over the needs of areas regarded as backward and remote. Nevertheless, these differently self-identified and identifiable ethnic groups in Weixi County have not constructed a homogenous Chinese identity; rather, their identities reflect a fragmented and hierarchized relationship.

Aside from the formal state practice that seeks to motivate the nation's population to share a common "imagination" as Chinese, other discursive practices contribute to the construction of the identities of the Weixi County populace (Anderson 1983). By the end of the eighteenth century, foreign missionaries had spread Catholicism and Christianity in the area, and many people in Weixi County, especially the Lisu, have since converted to Christianity. Tibetan Buddhism and Christianity thus coexist in the same village. These multiple cultural, religious, and ethnic identities are reflected in people's ideas of health, family, and childbirth.

It is within this social context that local reproductive practices are shaped and changed. Home births attended by female family members are traditional in the rural area of this region. The state points to official statistics that suggest that home births lead to high infant mortality and high maternal risk to justify its campaign to eradicate this tradition, pointing to the accompanying dangers of limited prenatal care, postpartum hemorrhage, infections, and heart failure. Home births also obstruct the state's power to monitor and control the number of births in one household. The Larger Shangri-la Project was introduced to transform local reproductive practices to reflect the modern and scientific standards of state expectations, including the state's birth-planning policy, which signifies long-term intrusion into the reproductive life of every Chinese citizen (Chen 2009).

Situating the Larger Shangri-la Project

Rates of high maternal and infant mortality often reflect the commonly uneven distribution of medical and other resources in peripheral regions of the world (Pinto 2008; Scheper-Hughes 1993), as well as in peripheral regions of nations. The worldwide spread of a universalized biomedical discourse about the safety of birth, along with a similarly standardized discourse of risk, has legitimized the shift from home to hospital births (Fraser 1995; Kaufert and O'Neil 1993, 1995; Murphy-Lawless 1999), and high rates of mortality often legitimate a state's medicalized intervention in childbirth (Morsy 1995). This type of intervention informs China's thirty-year birth-planning policy—a policy loaded with eugenic dimensions (Anagnost 1995; Greenhalgh 2003, 2008; Greenhalgh and Winckler 2005).

Foucault (1978, 1991, 1994) has identified a rise in forms of power no longer concentrated in governmental institutions of the state but increasingly dispersed throughout society in the disciplinary institutions of medicine, education, and the law. Through these power channels, governance spreads beyond the direct control of a nation's population to create rationalized schemes and programs with a variety of techniques and forms of knowledge that intimately tie the corporeal to the body politic (Foucault 1991). As knowledge of the body becomes closely related to overt juridical and administrative power, a structure of bodily dispositions is cultivated whereby policies become the vehicle for the implementation of modern power and the instruments of modern governance (Bourdieu 1992; Foucault 1978; Greenhalgh 2003; Shore and Wright 1997). In China, the LSP, a state policy, interrelates the power, knowledge, and interest of hierarchically situated parties though their reproductive discourses, behaviors, and practices by paying particular attention to where mothers choose to give birth.

In my case study of the LSP, hospital versus home birth has become a yardstick with which to measure the degree of modernity of a community, especially in areas historically marginalized in the country's political geography (cf. Fraser 1995). The LSP's emphasis on hospital birth conforms to and embodies the state's grander plan to develop the marginal, ethnic minority area. In its pursuit of modernity, the postsocialist Chinese state employs a development ideology that originates in Marx's unilineal evolution. Leys (2005) critiques development theory as too universal in its assumption that individuals make rational choices that maximize their utility. Similarly, the reproductive practices of ethnic minorities in Weixi County and the public health policies targeting these groups encompass broader issues of development and the governance of ethnic minorities in borderland China, revealing the uneven nature of people's positionality in responding to the LSP and to state governance at large.

The LSP is part of the New Countryside, New Family plan that the National Population and Family Planning Commission of China (NPFPC) implemented to improve the overall health of rural peasants throughout the country. The LSP is part of the New Cooperative Medicine policy proposed in the Sixteenth National Congress of the Communist Party of China in 2003, which aimed at providing rural peasants with the basic health care that had been suspended since the dismantling of collectivization in the early 1980s. Since 1978, the economic reforms that transformed the Maoist planned economy to the post-Mao market economy under the governance of a centralized state constitute a process referred to as "socialism with Chinese characteristics" (Greenhalgh and Winckler 2005). With these reforms, drastic changes have taken place in every social sphere. In the rural areas, the dismantling of the commune system led to a loss of support for the cooperative medicine implemented during the Maoist period (White 1998). In the following decades, rural peasants in China were more or less left on their own to pay for health care, while urban residents were still guaranteed a certain form of insurance. In many ways, China took on a more neoliberal attitude toward health policy.

In the marketization of postsocialist China, population policy has held a unique place. Since the founding of the People's Republic of China in 1949, how to govern the mass population has been a consistent focus of state policy. In the Maoist period, the emphasis was put on increasing the population while forcing people to remain in their rural or urban locales via a strict *hukou* (household registration) system (Potter and Potter 1990). After Mao's death in 1976, and with the early economic reforms in 1978, China recognized that its population was the largest of any nation—thus the growing state interest in population control. The postsocialist Deng Xiaoping administration emphasized controlling population growth and "raising the quality of the people" (Anagnost 1995). Reflecting this emphasis, the state instituted the urban one-child-per-family policy; in rural areas the policy has been more flexible. For instance, in Weixi County, each household could have two children, the exception being Tibetans, upon whom no childbearing limits were placed, in line with the minority policy.

Although health care in both rural and urban areas is largely neoliberalized, access to health care for peasants in the rural areas is much more difficult. Thus the health and well-being of the peasant classes symbolizes the deepening disparity between rural and urban populations and is viewed as a potential threat to social stability and the ruling party. As a result, state intervention is visible in various ways despite a neoliberalizing tendency. Public health policy and population policy are the most dramatic interventions. In 2003, in the aftermath of the SARS epidemic and a countrywide public health crisis, the Sixteenth National Congress proposed the New Cooperative Medicine, a revitalization of the Cooperative Medicine established under collectivization during the Maoist period. The New Cooperative Medicine exemplifies the Hu administration's effort to "construct a harmonious society" aimed at providing basic health care to rural peasants (Zhang and Liu 2007). In the following years, the New Cooperative Medicine was gradually expanded from trial areas to the entire countryside, including Weixi County, where this project began in 2006.

To participate in the New Cooperative Medicine, each peasant must pay ten yuan a year, for which he or she is given a certificate of participation in the program.[2] Taking the certificate to the clinic or hospital, individuals can receive a designated percentage of reimbursement from the state when they seek health care

Table 7.1. Reimbursement amounts paid by the New Cooperative Medicine in Yezhi town, Weixi County (in percentages)

	Inpatient	Outpatient
Village doctor	N/A	30
Township clinic	70	40
County hospital	60	N/A
Prefecture hospital	40	N/A
Out-of-prefecture hospital	35	N/A

Source: Data gathered during my 2008 research in Weixi County. The financing of New Cooperative Medicine varies in different parts of the country.

(see Table 7.1). Through the New Cooperative Medicine initiative, each person is eligible for health care benefits of up to 15,000 yuan per year.

Population policies, although initially intended to be independent of the New Cooperative Medicine project, often end up interwoven with it. The LSP, initiated by the NPFPC, thus required the collaboration of various state departments at the local level, as well as the involvement of the state-sanctioned NGO.

Discourses of Risk in the Larger Shangri-la Project

Discourses of risk play an important role in the Larger Shangri-la Project. The LSP was a three-year project (2007–2009) whose long-term aim was to change the "traditional" mode of life and reproduction to the "modern" and "scientific" one, thereby promoting the construction of a "socialist new family" and a "new country-side" in the country's "remote" and "multiethnic" areas.[3] The project focused primarily on lowering the rates of maternal and infant mortality. Several parties in the state/NGO/local hierarchies participated in this project: public health experts, policy makers, local officials, local health professionals, and local peasants. Each has specific knowledges and attitudes toward the mortality rates, specific positions in the power hierarchy, and specific discourses of risk in relation to the project. All these differentiations shaped LSP's practices and outcomes.

The State

The state, represented by policy makers and public health experts, was the initiator of the LSP. High rates of maternal and infant mortality in the Larger Shangri-la Area compared to low rates in inland China motivated its proposal. According to public health experts and policy makers, the widely accepted explanation of the high risk for poor maternal outcomes in the area was the low rate of delivery in hospitals. They argued that this low rate is related, first, to uneven economic development, as evidenced by personal income, education level, and infrastructural issues such as transportation, communication, and health facilities. Second, experts pointed to the demography of the Larger Shangri-la Area: predominantly Tibetans, Naxi, Lisu, and other ethnic minorities. Based on Marx's unilineal evolutionary agenda and the Han Chinese's long-term civilizing project (Harrell 1995), public health experts and policy makers regard high maternal risk as a result of these minorities' cultural, religious, and medical practices, traditionally regarded as backward and thus in need of improvement or eradication. Geography was cited as a third risk factor. The Larger Shangri-la Area lies in the country's "periphery," shares its borders with Burma, Nepal, and India, and is located far from China's central government. The central government argues that this distance complicates its goals in implementing health policies.

These purported weaknesses in policy implementation make the Larger Shangri-la a critical area, because of both its borderland location and its diverse demography, geography, and natural resources. Therefore, the state argues, particular interventions to alleviate maternal risk are necessary to reduce disparities in public health, as well as to promote the "New Countryside in the harmonious society" (Zhang and Liu 2007). I would add that by instituting these measures, the state also can continue to reinforce its control within the periphery, as well as motivate the ethnic minorities in this area to become more involved in the larger "civilizing projects of the state," such as education and economic development (Harrell 1995). I would also argue that the state hopes to succeed in advancing ethnic minorities' reproduction of "responsible Chinese citizenship" by emphasizing their maternal bodies.[4]

The health experts and policy makers involved in the LSP were members of the Yunnan Health Development and Research Association. YHDRA operates outside the official state sectors; most of its members have dual identities as NGO members and as government officials, public experts, and social scientists working for the state. Although the LSP was first proposed as a state project, YHDRA made the detailed plan of the project. In other words, YHDRA was the agency that performed the state's function at the local level. NGOs like YHDRA are often called GONGOs (GOvernment NGOs). These GONGOs receive funding and support, as well as subcontracted projects, from the state.[5] Moreover, the LSP required cross-sectorial collaboration across various county health bureaus, county treasury bureaus, county committees of minority affairs, and county population and family-planning commissions. None of the current governmental agencies can oversee such a collaboration; YHDRA's special identity made it the most appropriate choice. In addition, in the postsocialist neoliberal economy, the state has more need for GONGOs like YHDRA to execute the functions that the state is no longer able to perform.

Local Officials

In the LSP-targeted areas where YHDRA needed to collaborate with the local government, the LSP was viewed differently, in large part because of the different way local actors understand and position the risk of maternal mortality. First of all, at the regional level, officials regard local economic development as the top priority, even above maternal mortality. At the main entrance to Tachengzhen, one of the townships in Weixi County, where most residents are Tibetans, Naxi, and Lisu, a large banner reads: "Ecology is our foundation, culture is our strength, and industry is our prosperity. Based on these things, we can build a united, harmonious, civilized, and prosperous Tacheng." Local officials thus were reluctant to embrace the LSP in the ways that YHDRA expected.

Moreover, the local officials complained that their ability to implement the LSP was hampered by the county's poor financial status. In 2005 the gross income of Weixi County was 249,940,000 yuan (roughly US$30,113,000).[6] In a county with a population of 144,551, per capita income was US$208 a year. The LSP was part of the New Cooperative Medicine, under which a hospital would receive reimbursement from the government for each woman who gave birth in its facility. In addition, each woman would receive a 400–550 yuan subsidy from the state as an incentive to encourage hospital birth. As a result, under the LSP, hospital births should be almost free for pregnant women and their families. The central government would provide 200,000 yuan for the LSP in Weixi County each year, with the remainder of the state subsidy coming from local financing.

In one of the meetings between the experts from YHDRA and Weixi County government officials in the summer of 2008, the head of the County Treasury Bureau complained that the state financial support for the LSP was not enough; local financing was similarly insufficient. As a small-scale agricultural-based county with a formerly timber-based revenue source, recent policies prohibiting deforestation had devastated the local economy, and the local government had minimal income to spare for the LSP. Additionally, tourism is not as well developed in Weixi County as in neighboring counties. The absence of a well-established industry and poor transportation also contribute to the poor state of the local treasury. This lack increased the local officials' reluctance to implement the project.

Finally, when YHDRA interacted at the local level, it was viewed more as an NGO than as a state agency. Because of the project's cross-sectorial nature and YHDRA's self-representation as an NGO, local officials perceived the LSP neither as official nor as mandatory as other state projects. A former deputy head of Weixi County in charge of public health explained that the local health officials did not welcome YHDRA because "we did not think of it as a governmental agency." This perceived lack of legitimacy as well as authority, bordering on outright illegality, tainted the local officials' view of the project.[7]

In a report to the central government, the director of YHDRA wrote that some leaders in Weixi County did not pay enough attention to maternal health issues, which then resulted in the highest maternal and infant mortality rates in the region. After the former deputy head refused outright to recognize YHDRA's position and authority, the LSP was almost suspended in Weixi County; then a new deputy county head was elected in the spring of 2008. At a meeting with the new deputy county head, YHDRA representatives had to emphasize their relationship with the government by naming government officials who worked within YHDRA, in order to gain legitimacy and authority with local officials.

Local Health Care Providers

Another group at the local level that held its own view of risk comprised the local health care providers who participated in the LSP, including obstetricians in the Weixi County Hospital, obstetricians and pediatricians in the Weixi Mothers' and Children's Hospital, village doctors, and personnel in the County Population and Family Planning Commission. Compared to the public health experts, the local health care providers are assumed by policy makers to have less biomedical knowledge and less technical skills, as county workers generally have less professional training. Nonetheless, most of them did graduate from health schools, one form of secondary professional education of nursing and public health in the People's Republic of China; village doctors were the least skilled, having usually only a high school education with limited formal medical training. However, the position of the local health care providers was quite important within the community, since many had grown up in the area and were therefore more familiar with local cultural and religious practices. They also shared some similarities with the "barefoot doctors" of the Maoist period (White 1998), although they operated differently in the newer market economy. More significantly, many of the village doctors were multilingual in Mandarin and the local Tibetan, Naxi, and Lisu dialects and could communicate directly with the residents of Weixi County. Given the local health care workers' extramedical importance, the LSP proposed to remedy their educational shortcomings with training sessions in obstetric knowledge, including how to deal with emergencies and how to use new obstetrical equipment.

Whereas the goal of the County Population and Family Planning Commission was to control the number of unplanned births, the goal of the LSP was to lower the mortality rate regardless of whether the births were planned or not.[8] In other words, the obstetricians in the county hospital and the county Mothers' and Children's Hospital saw their mission as to save as many lives as possible—planned births or not. In my conversation with the president of Weixi Mothers' and Children's Hospital in 2008, she told me that if they did not save a pregnant woman, even though they knew she was having an unplanned birth, there would be one more name on the maternal death roll, increasing the mortality rate in Weixi County. Consequently, county leaders, the public health experts, and upper-level hospital personnel would blame them for not doing a good job. In this way, risk for local health providers lies primarily in its effect on mortality statistics. This view led to a conflict between the obstetricians and the cadres of the Population and Family Planning Commission. Although they shared the common goal of lowering the rates of maternal mortality and unplanned births—thereby making Weixi County appear more "developed" and "updated" in the state projects—the internal contradiction in birth-planning policy and the construction of a "harmonious society" that requires empowerment of the local people and more human rights inevitably led to disagreement between the two groups. As the state-mandated directing agency, YHDRA suggested enhancing the collaboration and information sharing between the obstetricians and the family planning groups to solve the puzzle, a solution too simple to be effective.

Local Residents

The local residents, the direct target of the LSP and those identified as being at risk for maternal death, articulated a still different view about risk. The local residents in Weixi County are over 66 percent ethnic Lisu, with the remainder consisting of Tibetans, Naxi, and Han, living sparsely in various locations. Most Han live in towns, whereas Naxi and Tibetans live closer to the river valley where it is relatively flat and conducive to rice cultivation. Han, Naxi, and Tibetans live within easy access to vehicle transportation and public services such as hospitals and schools. Lisu, however, often live in the mountains; the homes of close to 60 percent are above 12,000 feet, without drivable roads. For the Lisu, walking and horseback are the dominant modes of transportation (Tao et al. 1999). The great distance to hospitals and clinics and the difficult transportation limit Lisu access to the hospital and to town-based medical care. According to YHDRA's data, most of the maternal deaths in Weixi County occur among the ethnic Lisu.

In the past, home-based birth with an elder woman in the family serving as the midwife was the norm for most Lisu women living in the mountainous villages, which meant minimum prenatal care and no back-up medical services. Similar to Morsy's (1995) findings in Egypt, postpartum hemorrhage is the leading cause of death, followed by infection and heart failure. However, even under the LSP, home birth remained the norm for a number of reasons, mainly because it is more affordable than hospital birth. Although the LSP entitled women to give birth in the hospital for free, it did not cover the transportation and other expenses of family members accompanying the pregnant woman. For example, the doctor at the county Mothers' and Children's Hospital told me one woman in Tachengzhen had been hospitalized for one month before she delivered, resulting in exorbitant expense for the family members who accompanied and kept watch over her. Cases like this further impede local people's willingness to give birth in the hospital.

Moreover, many women explained, they did not want prenatal care. In my conversations with some of the local women, I was told that they are afraid of obstetric technologies like the ultrasound machine and other prenatal check-up procedures like taking a Pap smear and drawing blood for genetic screening. They also worry about the expenses associated with prenatal care that are not covered by the LSP, such as transportation to and from the health center, food, and travel incidentals. Because they are not receiving prenatal care, it is hard for the women to project their exact due date. Consequently it is hard for them to know when they should go to hospital.

For the local residents living in the mountainous regions, the village doctors are the medical care providers most readily available to provide primary care services, including obstetrics. Yet women are reluctant to see the village doctors in

Weixi County for reasons of gender: they don't want to see male doctors about maternity care, which is a female issue. Because only a few women from the villages of Weixi County graduate from high school—the prerequisite to becoming a village doctor—only twelve of the seventy village doctors in Weixi County are female. The lack of female village-based doctors puts the burden of maternity care on the county-level hospitals. The hospitals, however, are inaccessible for the people such as Lisu who live high up in the mountains, for reasons of transportation and cost, as we have seen.

Another concern the local residents expressed concerning a hospital birth was based in a desire for privacy: they did not want people outside their immediate family to know that they are going to give birth. Some local people explained that pregnancy is a very private affair. However, more were concerned about their unplanned births and the state involvement that results from this occurrence. To conceal pregnancy, home birth is a favorable choice, despite the associated risks. For some people, maternal death has been normalized as a part of one's destiny. As one middle-aged male villager explained to me: "If you die at home, you will die in hospital too."

Conclusion

Population policy has a long-standing history in the People's Republic of China, with the recent Larger Shangri-la Project being the latest manifestation in the era of a postsocialist market economy. The LSP, as a continued form of fertility regulation and supplement to family planning, was situated within the New Cooperative Medicine, a program of state health care reform intended to provide affordable health care for a large rural population. The state assumed that YHDRA, as somewhat independent from the government, would be able to bridge the different government sectors. The organization's governmental nature legitimized its existence under state socialism; its multifaceted nature increased its ability to fulfill tasks in varied situations.

The variety of discourses of risk as exemplified in the LSP indicates the idiosyncratic acceptance of state policy, depending on a group's access to power and knowledge. In other words, even though the Chinese state implemented the LSP through its official mouthpiece, not all groups viewed the policy in the same way. Current reproductive practices in Weixi County hence remain the product of ongoing negotiation among the policy makers, public health experts, local officials, local health providers, and local residents.

Notes

1. This research was funded by a Graduate Student Travel and Research Award from Temple University and the Sixteenth World Congress of the International Union of Anthropological and Ethnological Sciences.

2.   In 2010, ten yuan was equal to US$1.47, a hefty sum for a population where the gross per capita income is less than US$1.00 per day.
3.   I put these terms in quotation marks because they are used as state categories that have been naturalized through its discourse.
4.   Rose and Novas (2005) elaborate the concept of "biological citizenship" to describe the citizenship projects originating from government authorities that aim to incorporate individuals into the formation of the nation-state by emphasizing their biological existence.
5.   YHDRA also undertakes projects on behalf of international NGOs, such as the Ford and Rockefeller Foundations, and receives funding from them.
6.   The exchange rate between the U.S. dollar and the yuan was 1:8.3 in 2005.
7.   Because NGOs have only recently emerged in China, their legitimacy may not always be recognized by the government.
8.   Planned births are those that fall within the guidelines of up to two children per household. Childbirths that exceed this limit are regarded as unplanned and are officially prohibited.

References

Anagnost, Ann
   1995   A Surfeit of Bodies: Population and the Rationality of the State in Post-Mao China. *In* Conceiving the New World Order: The Global Politics of Reproduction. Faye Ginsburg and Rayna Rapp, eds. Pp. 22–41. Berkeley: University of California Press.
Anderson, Benedict
   1983   Imagined Communities: Reflections on the Origin and Spread of Nationalism. London: Verso.
Bourdieu, Pierre
   1992   The Logic of Practice. Trans. Richard Nice. Stanford, CA: Stanford University Press.
Chen, Junjie
   2009   Charting the Public/Intimate Dynamic: Fieldwork on Reproductive Politics in Rural China. Anthropology News 50(3):26.
Foucault, Michel
   1978   History of Sexuality, Volume 1: An Introduction. New York: Vintage.
   1991   Governmentality. *In* The Foucault Effect: Studies in Governmentality. Graham Burchell, Colin Gordon, and Peter Miller, eds. Pp. 87–104. Chicago: University of Chicago Press.
   1994   The Birth of the Clinic: An Archaeology of Medical Perception. New York: Vintage.
Fraser, Gertrude
   1995   Modern Bodies, Modern Minds: Midwifery and Reproductive Change in an African American Community. *In* Conceiving the New World Order: The Global Politics of Reproduction. Faye Ginsburg and Rayna Rapp, eds. Pp. 42–58. Berkeley: University of California Press.

Greenhalgh, Susan
  2003   Planned Births, Unplanned Persons: "Population" in the Making of Chinese
          Modernity. American Ethnologist 30(2):196–215.
  2008   Just One Child: Science and Policy in Deng's China. Berkeley: University of
          California Press.
Greenhalgh, Susan, and Edwin Winckler
  2005   Governing China's Population: From Leninist to Neoliberal Biopolitics. Stanford,
          CA: Stanford University Press.
Harrell, Stevan
  1995   Introduction. *In* Cultural Encounters as China's Ethnic Frontiers. Stevan Harrell,
          ed. Pp. 3–36. Seattle: University of Washington Press.
Hyde, Sandra
  2007   Eating Spring Rice: The Cultural Politics of AIDS in Southwest China. Berkeley:
          University of California Press.
Kaufert, Patricia, and John O'Neil
  1993   Analysis of a Dialogue on Risks in Childbirth: Clinicians, Epidemiologies, and
          Inuit Women. *In* Knowledge, Power and Practice: The Anthropology of Medicine
          and Everyday Life. Shirley Lindenbaum and Margaret Lock, eds. Pp. 32–54.
          Berkeley: University of California Press.
  1995   *Irniktakpunga!* Sex Determination and the Inuit Struggle for Birthing Rights in
          Northern Canada. *In* Conceiving the New World Order: The Global Politics
          of Reproduction. Faye Ginsburg and Rayna Rapp, eds. Pp. 59–73. Berkeley:
          University of California Press.
Leys, Colin
  2005   The Rise and Fall of Development Theory. *In* The Anthropology of Development
          and Globalization: From Classical Political Economy to Contemporary
          Neoliberalism. Marc Edelman and Angelique Haugerud, eds. Pp. 109–25.
          Malden, MA: Blackwell.
Morsy, Soheir
  1995   Deadly Reproduction among Egyptian Women: Maternal Mortality and the
          Medicalization of Population Control. *In* Conceiving the New World Order:
          The Global Politics of Reproduction. Faye Ginsburg and Rayna Rapp, eds. Pp.
          162–76. Berkeley: University of California Press.
Murphy-Lawless, Jo
  1999   Reading Birth and Death: A History of Obstetric Thinking. Bloomington:
          Indiana University Press.
Pinto, Sarah
  2008   Where There Is No Midwife: Birth and Loss in Rural India. New York: Berghahn
          Books.
Potter, Jack, and Sulamith Potter
  1990   China's Peasants: The Anthropology of a Revolution. Cambridge: Cambridge
          University Press.
Rose, Nikolas, and Carlos Novas
  2005   Biological Citizenship. *In* Global Assemblages: Technology, Politics, and Ethics
          as Anthropological Problems. Aihwa Ong and Stephen Collier, eds. Pp. 439–63.
          Malden, MA: Blackwell.

Scheper-Hughes, Nancy
   1993   Death without Weeping: The Violence of Everyday Life in Brazil. Berkeley:
           University of California Press.
Scheper-Hughes, Nancy, and Margaret Lock
   1987   The Mindful Body: A Prolegomenon to Future Work in Medical Anthropology.
           Medical Anthropology Quarterly 1(1):6–41.
Shore, Cris, and Susan Wright
   1997   Anthropology of Policy: Critical Perspectives on Governance and Power. New
           York: Routledge.
Tao, Yuan, Li Ruchun, Zhao Genchuan, Yin Zhitang, Li Zhongxiu, He Junqin, Chen
Yuwen, and Wu Chenghu
   1999   The County Annuals of Weixi Lisu Autonomous County. Kunming, China:
           Yunnan Nationalities Press (in Chinese).
White, Sydney
   1997   Fame and Sacrifice: The Gendered Construction of Naxi Identities. Modern
           China 23(3):298–327.
   1998   From "Barefoot Doctor" to "Village Doctor" in Tiger Springs Village: A Case
           Study of Rural Health Care Transformations in Socialist China. Human
           Organization 57(4):1–9.
Zhang, Kaining, and Xiangyuan Liu
   2007   New Countryside New Family: The Population Health Promotion Program in the
           Larger Shangri-la Area Newsletter. Yunnan Health and Development Research
           Association (YHDRA) 7(53) (in Chinese).

PART III

Struggles over the Embodiment of Reproductive Risk

CHAPTER 8

Negotiating Risk and the Politics of Responsibility

Mothers and Young Child Health among Datoga Pastoralists in Northern Tanzania

Alyson G. Young

The strategies that mothers use to prevent and negotiate infant illness are a useful interface for understanding the complex relationship between risk and reproduction on both an individual and a societal level. This chapter gives a brief background to the construction of risk and harm reduction among Datoga women and uses research on diarrheal illness in north-central Tanzania as a case study to illustrate the complexities of trying to disentangle the interrelationship between risk, responsibility, and the practice of child care and reproduction.

Diarrhea is a preventable health issue. Nonetheless, the high global mortality from diarrheal diseases is well known, especially in young children in developing areas (Black, Morris, and Bryce 2003; Bryce et al. 2005; Mara 2003). These enteric infections have profound effects on intestinal absorption, nutrition, and child development. With oral rehydration therapy (ORT), this rate has fallen to less than 2.5 million per year over the last decade. However, reviews by Kosek, Bern, and Guerrant (2003), as well as more recent work from Petri et al. (2008), show that morbidity from diarrheal diseases is continuing to increase.

The prevention of diarrhea in infants and young children depends heavily on caretaker health behavior and child-care practices. Thus, much of the public health and clinical research on diarrhea in infants and young children has focused on maternal knowledge about diarrhea, the role of maternal care and feeding in diarrhea prevention, and the use of ORT (Boschi-Pinto, Lanata, and Black 2009; CDC 1992; Holliday 1982). However, it is now widely recognized that differences in child nutritional status and mortality are embedded in larger social, economic, and political contexts. For example, Millard (1994) argued that many deleterious child-care practices are not the result of ignorance or "culture" but the by-product of poverty and other structural constraints on parental decisions (see also Gittelsohn, Thapa, and Ladman 1997; Hampshire et al. 2009; Young and Jaspars 2006).

In situations of extreme resource scarcity, the priorities of local communities and clinical health workers often differ, despite their common aim—improving child health. Health workers and clinicians may also have different perceptions of risk and vulnerability than have local parents. What outsiders perceive to be risky or neglectful caretaker behavior may seem for many Datoga women to be appropriate, adaptive, and beneficial, especially in challenging environments (Engle, Castle, and Menon 1996; Pennings and Grossman 2008). Lupton echoes this point: "The difference that is commonly observed between 'expert' and 'lay' judgments of risk is founded not on the fact that lay people cannot think in terms of probabilities, but rather that other concerns are brought to bear in the ways they judge risk" (1999:37). Nonetheless, these differences in perspectives on appropriate child care can create frustration for the health worker as well as the caretaker. These misunderstandings also feed into a discourse about reproductive risk and the politics of responsibility for child care—much of which is directed at mothers.

Ethnographic Context

The material for this chapter is based on data collected continuously from 2004 through 2006 and more recent discussions with mothers between June and August 2009. Data collection was conducted in a rural community in the Yaeda basin, located in Mbulu District near Lake Eyasi in northern Tanzania. The material presented is part of a larger project that examines the structural causes of inequality and the mechanisms linking socioeconomic marginalization and resource security to health and nutrition disparities among Datoga children (Young 2008).

The sample includes forty mother-infant dyads, with children between two and twenty-four months of age. Data were collected using a variety of methods, including participant-observation, narrative interviews, group discussions, and interviews with health workers. In this instance, the data are used as a case study to illustrate the complexities and codependency of biomedical and maternal constructions of risk, and the effect of the household context of the negotiation of these concepts on maternal decisions about child care. This chapter focuses specifically on diarrheal illness because it as an important nexus for understanding biomedical and individual constructions of risk and harm reduction and the tensions associated with making child-care decisions in resource-poor environments.

The Yaeda depression is arid, with unpredictable seasonal rainfall, limited water, and high midday temperatures. Annual rainfall is 300–500 mm. and occurs bimodally, with the short rains in November and December and the long rains from April to June (Borgerhoff Mulder 1992; Sellen 1995; Sieff 1995). Water is scarce, and most of the year it is obtained only from deep wells dug into dry riverbeds. Local vegetation consists of seasonal marshlands, salt flats, savannah grasslands, and the acacia thicket in the surrounding hills. Cultivation is difficult, and the only viable crop options are maize, millet, and squash. There is one functional road running from Haydom down to Yaeda and some of the surrounding villages, but most travel is by cattle and foot trails. Health services lie at a considerable distance: the village I focus on in this chapter is located fifteen miles from the rudimentary medical services at the government dispensary and several hours by car from the hospital. Although mobile clinics are available in some villages, few carry medical supplies, and most operate only on a monthly basis during the dry season and less frequently during the rains, when mud makes the airstrip and roads impassable.

Datoga villages in Yaeda Valley are important as a case study, because Datoga in this area represent a marginalized population who are suffering from a number of political, economic, and environmental stressors with important impacts on their health and nutrition. Datoga pastoralists have a long history of socio-economic marginalization, from the colonial era to today's postindependence period in Tanzania (Lane 1996; Ndagala 1991). Eyasi Datoga in particular are located in a marginal ecological environment, the effects of which are exacerbated by historic and political forces such as the privatization of land and health care, which amplify resource insecurity while constraining the strategies available for mitigating vulnerability (Blystad 2000; Lane 1996; Ndagala 1991).

Health Disparities between Datoga and Other Populations in Northern Tanzania

Datoga in general show higher rates of infectious disease, psychosocial stress, and malnutrition than do other ethnic groups living in the local area. Research on health disparities in the region indicates that being Datoga is a risk marker for many problems, including anemia, maternal mortality, and tuberculosis (Hinde-raker et al. 2001; Mfinanga et al. 2003; Olsen et al. 2002). Infant mortality is high among Datoga (20 percent, compared to the 2010 Tanzanian national average of roughly 7 percent), while fertility is lower than in neighboring groups (Borgerhoff Mulder 1992). Child growth is compromised by food insecurity, early weaning and supplementation, and the high prevalence of infectious disease. Sellen (1995, 1999, 2003) found that pastoral Datoga children show early growth faltering and little catch-up growth when compared to neighboring groups. My research in the area in 2008 indicated that infant and young child growth and nutrition patterns among Eyasi Datoga had not improved in the ten years since Sellen's work, despite improvements in child health for Tanzania as a whole (Young 2008).

Beyond physical distress and impacts on demographic indicators such as infant mortality, child growth, and reproduction, Datoga marginalization has taken a toll on individual emotional health and feelings of security. Informants increasingly report concerns about the unpredictability of resources, including reduced access to adequate water, food, and medical care (for both humans and animals), as well as concerns about the intrusion of other groups onto Datoga land (Blystad 2000; Hadley and Patil 2006, 2008; Ndagala 1991; Pike and Patil 2006; Rekdal and Blystad 2000; Young 2008). This combination of data on distress and health inequalities between Datoga and other communities indicates that they are psychologically and biologically incorporating the effects of sociopolitical marginalization, as well as the effects of settlement and recent socioeconomic change.

Diarrheal Illness among Datoga Children

Data from 2004–2006 show that diarrheal illness made up a significant proportion of the illnesses found among children younger than two years of age (Young 2008). Overall, gastroenteritis is the third leading cause for hospital admission among children under five in the Haydom catchment area (including the Yaeda region) (HLH 2009). Fecal samples collected from participants during this time indicated that a number of these incidences correlated with the presence of giardia, amoebas, or both in infant stool.[1] Out of 160 samples collected, 14 percent were associated with gastroenteritis, 45 percent of which tested positive for amoebas and 13 percent of which tested positive for giardia. While giardia can be self-limiting and is fairly innocuous (albeit unpleasant) in adults, it can pose significant health risks for young children. Amoebiasis is a concern for both infant and adult health depending on the type, duration, and severity of infection (Stanley 2003). Nutritional data from Datoga children that were identified as having giardia or amoebiasis showed significantly lower height for age, weight for age, and weight for height scores—especially those children that showed both amoebas and giardia at the same time and those who repeatedly tested positive for either parasite (Young 2008). The difference in these measures is important, because they indicate variations in both short-term nutritional status (weight for age) and chronic nutritional strain (height for age and weight for height).

Infant Vulnerability and Protecting Infants from Illness

Ethnographic research among Eyasi Datoga indicates that women are keenly sensitive to the cultural and environmental factors that create vulnerability in fertility and infant health outcomes (Blystad 1999; Blystad, Rekdal, and Malleyeck 2007; Sellen 1995). Datoga constructions of infant vulnerability to illness are continuous and dynamic, reflecting not just the state of the child at a particular moment but the accumulation of biosocial maternal and child experience that coalesce to create a unique individual in a particular space and time. Datoga women use a suite of behavioral, physical, and developmental cues to identify "vulnerable" children, including patterns of illness, changes in behavior/physical state (such as becoming more tired/pale, and "going backward"), and certain stages of development that are considered more risky (Young 2008).

These concepts of risk are drawn from multiple sources, including personal (both individual and group) experience and health messages (both lay and biomedical). It is important to note the individual agency in this situation: Datoga risk roles are constructed from the dynamic between individual and society and the imagery and values that flow between the two. Each mother creates her own construction of knowledge about risk and vulnerability from these plural sources and applies it (both consciously and unconsciously) to her choices in behavior, given her sociopolitical and economic locality.

Even before children are born, mothers take steps to protect them from spiritual and physical harm (Blystad 2000; Blystad and Rekdal 2003; Blystad, Rekdal, and Malleyeck 2007; Rekdal 1999). The long-term health of the child and the interaction between mother and infant are closely related to the health and well-being of the mother during pregnancy and the early neonatal period. Women have a conflicted relationship with the fetus, however. Although the growing fetus is considered vulnerable, during pregnancy women say that a tiny "strong-willed" human inhabits the woman's body (Blystad 2000). Thus, women often "close the womb with the leather skirt" or bind their leather skirts (*hanang'wenda*) tightly around their waist to prevent too much commotion from the fetus (Blystad 2000).

The fetus also has some control over the woman's diet and social behavior during pregnancy. Mothers often ask people to get the specific foods that they crave and spend more time with people they like during pregnancy because they are considered to "go well with the child" (Blystad 2000). The type of person with whom the woman shares food also comes under particular scrutiny, because eating with the wrong person can endanger the child. People with missing limbs or disfigurement are significant threats, as it is believed that the shape of the fetus can be influenced by maternal contact with physical and spiritual abnormalities or pollution (*meeta*) (Blystad, Rekdal, and Malleyeck 2007; cf. Laderman 1983; see Gálvez, this volume, and Howes-Mischel, this volume).

Labor is also considered a vulnerable time for both the mother and child, with important implications for the long-term health and well-being of the child. Datoga often identify infants and pregnant women as more susceptible to *uchawi* (witchcraft) because of their vulnerable nature (Blystad 2000). Women consistently commented about the threat of *uchawi* from strangers and people from other groups like the Iramba and Sumburu. For example, Udamaghed, a young mother with two children, described an experience that occurred with a visitor when Udamaghed was delivering her first child: "She was staring at me when I was in labor. I didn't want her there—she didn't have children. She always had troubles with children. I knew she was causing me problems."[2] The person was a guest at the house when Udamaghed was pregnant and had inadvertently come into the room while she was giving birth. Although the woman was ushered out, and appropriate actions were taken to reduce the potential spiritual ramifications of the event, Udamaghed said that she always considered this child to be "weaker" than her other children because of the intrusion.

Postnatal convalescence is also seen as a vulnerable time for women and their newborns. At this point the infant is considered a visitor, not a permanent resident of the household (Blystad 2000). Datoga culture requires that women and their newborn children be secluded for the first two to three months of the postnatal period (usually two months for boys and three months for girls). The period of seclusion for boys is shorter to encourage the male child to "grow up" more quickly. However, many women reported that they stayed in seclusion only for a month (independent of the sex of the child), generally because they needed to do household labor. The birth attendant stays on with the mother for the first couple of weeks, after which an older girl is chosen to stay with the mother and care for her and the newborn when their seclusion has ended. Normally, the midwife stays on until a male goat has been selected and ritually slaughtered, and the "song of the child" (*dumda jeapta*) has been initiated (Blystad 1999, 2000).

Cultural practices to protect older children from harm include isolating them from harmful circumstances or people (as during the early neonatal period), feeding them fatty soups and clarified butter (*ghee*) to strengthen the body, and using charms (*harmishta*) and scarification to protect the child and rid the body of toxins. Datoga mothers seek treatment and protection for children from a wide range of providers, including local herbalists, individuals renowned for their knowledge of particular ailments (such as bonesetters and healers from other local groups), as well as clinics and local hospitals (Blystad 2000). Datoga tend to see these various types of medicine as complementary and use a range of different providers according to the nature of the ailment and other practical factors.

The pattern of much preventive biomedical care by Datoga women can be categorized by what one study identifies as "social demand" (Streefland, Chowdhury, and Ramos-Jimenez 1999). There is a high demand for vaccination and other forms of treatment based on maternal understandings of the general value of immunization, biomedicine, and clinic attendance. Furthermore, biomedical uptake among Datoga does not appear to be associated with a decline of traditional practices—on the contrary, the latter continue to be used in ways that complement and sometimes support clinic attendance. This practice provides little evidence for what Nichter (1995) defines as "active demand," or an informed public that perceives the need for specific care. Parents do actively seek preventive care such as vaccinations, but they do so based on cultural understandings of what medicines do rather than on disease-specific knowledge.

The attention that Datoga women pay to diet during pregnancy, postnatal convalescence, and early child development shows an obvious concern with young child health and well-being. Nonetheless, socioeconomic and household changes are creating challenges to a balance of household demands and child care. This is especially clear from the decrease in postnatal convalescence time for mothers and the lower ages for supplementation and weaning of children.

Maternal Knowledge about Risk and Management of Diarrheal Illness

Differences in beliefs about the etiology and management of diarrheal disease have an important impact on the association of personal actions with risk for poor health outcomes among Datoga children. The most commonly cited cause of diarrheal illness by Datoga women was bugs (*wadudu*) in contaminated food and water. However, there was variability in the concept of *wadudu* and little specific knowledge about pathogenic organisms. Importantly, unlike the static biomedical model of diarrheal illness, where diseases are caused by pathogenic microorganisms directly transmitted when contaminated items are consumed, Datoga models of diarrheal illness include not just *wadudu* but also the social life of food/water, including the origin of an item, where it has been since its origination, how it has been prepared, and how it has been used. Women often explain their choices about the source of water and their strategies for treating "unsafe resources" by describing the social context of resource acquisition and the vulnerabilities associated with particular spaces. In the case of water, Datoga women mesh concerns about parasite infestation with concerns about how the social context may exacerbate the dangers associated with poor water quality.

Another challenge to the biomedical model of risk for diarrheal illness springs from Datoga women's beliefs about infant feeding and its role in infant vulnerability. The biomedical argument is "breast is best" (exclusive breastfeeding until six months), especially for infants and young children in resource-scare environments and places with high prevalence of infectious disease (Stanway and Stanway 1978; WHO 2010). Several studies have also indicated that the immunoglobulins and probiotic lactobacilli in breast milk reduce the negative impact of diarrheal illness on child health (Abrahamsson et al. 2009; Chirico et al. 2008). Thus, the insistence that breastfeeding confers unique and significant benefits upon infants underpins both government policy and health professionals' practice in Tanzania, while shaping ideas of infant risk and vulnerability to diarrheal illness. It also leaves Datoga women open to the charge of being poor mothers. In a biomedical context, deviating from global standards for infant nutrition undermines Datoga women's claims of "being a good mother," or being selfless, wise, and responsible about child care.

While Datoga women agree that breastfeeding is important for helping strengthen and nourish infants and young children, they also believe that there are some risks to the exclusive consumption of breast milk (Blystad 2000; Sellen 1995, 2003; Young 2008). In particular, women are concerned that any illness they may be harboring could be passed to the infant through the breast milk. Thus, women will actually stop breastfeeding children with chronic diarrhea because they are concerned that their milk is exacerbating the problem. In this case, women argue that although normally breast milk is a better source of nutrition and it would be preferable to continue to exclusively breastfeed, they are concerned that the long-term health implications of subjecting the child to potentially dangerous milk are far riskier than a change in the child's diet.

One example of this came from a woman, Udabaiskeli, whom I visited a number of times during the study. At the beginning of the project, I asked Udabaiskeli about her feeding plans for her then two-month-old infant. She replied that she intended to exclusively breastfeed for six months and then continue nursing until the child was a "big child." Several months later I was visiting her again when I saw her spooning gruel into the infant's mouth and actively preventing the child from breastfeeding. When I asked about the change in her feeding plans, she responded that the child had been ill, and she was concerned that her breast milk had been contributing to the problem, because she herself had been ill for a few days. When I asked whether the cessation of breastfeeding had improved the child's health, she replied that it had not. However, the reason that it had not was that she had not given the child cow's milk when very young. Since the child had not acclimated to cow's milk, it was of no help and she would have to take the child to the hospital. The mother did not want to go to the hospital, however, because she knew that the nurse would be upset that she had stopped breastfeeding. Furthermore, Uda-baiskeli was concerned that the hospital would refuse to give her ORT and just tell her to continue breastfeeding at home—a direct contradiction to Datoga beliefs about illness transmission.

This example illustrates that the construction and management of risk for diarrheal illness among Datoga mothers includes a number of social and cultural beliefs in addition to the internalization of biomedical messages. Most strategies represented by women are a balance of personal beliefs about mediating illness and harm reduction and the interpretation of community health messages about child care. However, this also illustrates the tensions that arise when women try to reconcile multiple and sometimes-contradictory messages about proper care for their children. Women lament that they often want to follow both culturally prescribed rules for care and clinical suggestions for treatment—but it is often difficult to do so effectively because of contradictions between biomedical and lay models of health.

Constraints on Infant Care

While the combination of lay and biomedical beliefs about disease etiology have an impact on the strategies that mothers use to care for and feed infants and young children, my earlier research shows that Datoga concepts of infant vulnerability actually map quite closely to biomedical indicators of child health and vulnerability. For example, 79 percent of the specific vulnerability events reported by mothers in 2005 mapped on to biomedical risk indicators for poor health (including low growth scores, low hemoglobin scores, and febrile events). However, while mothers are aware of and dedicated to treating vulnerable children, they are often constrained by structural forces working at the community and household levels. Women were able to seek treatment in only 65 percent of the cases where maternal perceptions of vulnerability synchronized with biomedical indicators of poor health (Young 2008).

In fact, these constraints were what women primarily identified as issues in seeking care. Whether it was lack of help in the household, lack of access to care in the area, or the social relationships at clinic, women consistently observed that it was not that they wanted to put other needs before child care, but that they felt they had little choice. Frequently, women reported having to make the best of a range of poor choices. Udamagisana, a young mother with two children, spoke about the way structural and household constraints interfered with child care and the perception of Datoga mothers among hospital staff. "They think we don't care for our children—of course we care [about our children]! But you start from nothing and tell me what you can do. They just don't understand what it is like here."

Household Constraints

In Yaeda, as in many other parts of the world, women bear the brunt of buffering children from resource scarcity. Everyday activities for mothers include collecting water and firewood, grinding maize, cooking, milking cattle, and child care. During the dry season, women travel long distances to collect water and firewood and to herd small stock and calves for water and grass. Rainy season workloads are lower, but women are still found planting, guarding, and harvesting household fields and working on repairing roads in exchange for maize from a local food-for-work program. Recent increases in male labor outmigration in the area and seasonal changes in household structure that are the result of the pastoral economy increase the overall number of de facto female-headed households and force Datoga women to deal with greater household production demands, as well as a need for cash income to buy food and pay medical bills (Creighton and Omari 1995). This puts female caretakers in a tense negotiation between successful tactics for coping with the household at large and strategies for maintaining the well-being of individual children.

The strongest threats to caretaking in terms of household constraints for Datoga women are less cash income, which means decreased frequency of both biomedical and traditional treatments for illness; increased labor demands, which mean more hours Datoga women must spend apart from their infant; and increased herd production ratios, which are associated with earlier ages for the cessation of exclusive breastfeeding and weaning. There is also a trend toward a higher prevalence of biomedical and traditional treatment events in households with more cattle and higher herd production ratios, even though women in households with higher labor demands were also more likely to say that they chose not to seek treatment because "no one was available to get it," meaning there were no household members that could go to the hospital, clinic, local healer, or pharmacy for medicine (Young 2008). With the closest health dispensary located fifteen miles away, women have to leave their household work for almost a full day in order to seek treatment. Therefore, women are more likely to seek treatment at periods when labor demands are low and more people are available to help in the household.

Social Constraints

There are more than just socioeconomic and educational constraints on decisions about child health, risk, and reproduction among Datoga women. Beyond the geographic and time limitations associated with travel to the clinic, there is a social aspect to clinic attendance that helps shape women's decisions to seek care. Women's narratives suggested that once they arrived, certain mothers felt excluded and worried about criticism from either mothers waiting for care or the staff at the clinic. Mothers who were more marginalized in the community, were poorer, and lacked clothing for the children, or who thought their children were "too thin," felt especially concerned about provoking disapproval from the staff and other mothers at the clinic. While I did not witness women being reproached at the clinic for the nutritional status of their children, I did witness staff members verbally harass several women for "inadequate clothing" and "waiting too long" to seek treatment for their children" (see Maraesa, this volume, for a similar reaction in Belize).

Observations at the mobile clinic and the narratives of mothers also revealed a strong perception that social connections with clinic staff and strong integration with other women would lead to privileged treatment, while lacking such connections could hamper women's social acceptance. Many women from the village would bring gifts of eggs or milk to the clinic in hopes of currying favor with the staff. This meant that poorer households were further isolated from service, because they rarely had extra eggs or dairy products that could be traded.

One example of this scenario comes from Udamekwa, a mother I visited with in 2005. Her youngest child had been suffering from a fever and diarrhea for several days, and she had not been able to get away from household work long enough to take the child to the clinic. While I was in her home, we heard the plane from the mobile clinic fly overhead. Since she lived only a short distance from the landing strip, I suggested that we take her youngest child to the visiting health workers for evaluation. Her response was: "I cannot take my child to that clinic. When we go, the women glare at me. The nurses ignore me, or worse. The only way to get care from that clinic is if the head wife takes our children. She has good relations with the nurses and they will at least speak to her." This passage illustrates that there is clearly more affecting the use of clinic services than simple distance and time constraints for Datoga women. Thus, analyses of medical resource use need to consider the impact of social trade-offs on decisions to seek care and treatment.

Structural Constraints

State-level health restructuring policies and budget cuts have had a distinct impact on the community and household levels, especially in relation to maternal strategies for child treatment and care. The role of state funding in health is of particular concern now, as Tanzania (like many other African countries) faces severe budget cuts associated with the ongoing global economic crisis. Tanzania has an annual health budget that works out to approximately four dollars per person; however, the per capita spending is even lower (Smith et al. 2008). While Tanzanian officials have worked hard to use limited resources efficiently, there are still significant gaps in the system that affect household health.

The effects of restructuring and budget modification filter down to a local level and are evident in the lack of resources available for care. For example, the government clinic located in Yaeda is often closed because it is short staffed, and when open it rarely has medical resources available. The mobile clinic run by Haydom hospital often has resources for care; however, it is located several hours by foot from the village. This poses a challenge for most women, because the clinic is available only in the mornings, when they are involved with household activities. These issues are exacerbated by the somewhat unpredictable nature of clinic services. While the hospital maintains a set monthly schedule for arrival to villages, the amount of time spent in each village varies with the number of women who arrive for the clinic. Therefore, many women say that the clinic is simply inaccessible because of the unpredictable nature of services coupled with the time/distance requirements.

Communication and the Politics of Responsibility for Child Health

There are several ways that conflicts in belief about disease etiology and structural constraints on care negatively impact the dialogue about risk and reproduction between Datoga women and clinical staff. Staff see Datoga women as "unhygienic subjects"—noncompliant and ignorant because they do not use free clinic services or follow prescribed caretaking procedures to protect infants from disease (Briggs and Briggs 2003; Briggs and Nichter 2009). Datoga women argue that free services are far from free, and biomedically prescribed strategies do not always deal with the true issue at hand.

One challenge to communication is that community health messages often focus on strategies (such as boiling water) for preventing diarrheal illness that women cannot carry out under all circumstances. Women often express their frustration about the conflict between understanding what they are supposed to do and not being able to do it because of household constraints. For example, of the forty women interviewed, 75 percent stated that they knew about boiling as a technique for treating water. However, only around 8 percent said that they consistently tried to boil water. Most said that boiling was a low priority because the types of illness that boiling water could solve were not as severe as other types (such as brucellosis, malaria, etc.). Perhaps more importantly, they argued that boiling water used up precious resources (wood and time) that were needed for other activities.

This situation is complicated by tensions between the appropriate time to seek care for ill infants and the ability of mothers to bring children to the hospital in a timely manner. While mothers and clinic staff agree that rapid treatment is the best way to ensure a positive health outcome, household constraints often extend the amount of time women have to wait to bring their infants for treatment. As time until treatment is extended, the chances of a positive health outcome decrease—to the point that women may bring children who are severely ill and dehydrated to the clinic, with limited chances of survival. Hospital staff's failure to resuscitate these children reinforces maternal concerns about the effectiveness of clinic resources, and clinical staff beliefs about maternal incompetence in infant care.

Conclusion: What Can Be Done?

The ethnographic data presented in this chapter help show how patterns of low compliance with hospital strategies for reducing risk for poor child health outcomes, conventionally assumed to be associated with lack of knowledge, are much more complicated. These patterns indicate that we need to consider a multilevel analysis of child health that includes the social life of resources, structural constraints, and household limitations on time and care when examining issues of risk and reproduction. Additionally, it is important to note that this discussion is fundamentally different from the biomedical "culture as a barrier to health," or victim-blaming argument (Crawford 1998[1977]), which penalizes individuals for their illness and proposes that, instead of relying on costly and inefficient medical services, they should take more responsibility for their health. This chapter is about how larger structural forces constrain women's ability to seek care, exacerbate tensions between clinical staff and mothers, and reinforce misapprehensions and stereotypes about the politics of responsibility on both sides of the clinical bench. There is little evidence that choices in harm reduction strategies for children are primarily associated with mothers' refusal or resistance to community health messages about diarrheal illness and child care (Young 2008). Instead, the construction of these patterns involves issues of workload, autonomy in the household, and trust in the health care provider, as well as knowledge and perceptions of young child vulnerability to illness.

Implications for Public Health Practitioners

While these challenges paint a bleak picture of communication about risk and reproduction between Datoga women and biomedical practitioners, there are ways to mediate this negative feedback loop.

One way to improve service delivery and communication is by improving relations between staff and patients, a problem the literature commonly addresses. In fact, several other African studies have identified staff rudeness and attitudes as a problem (see Helman and Yogeswaran 2004; Streefland, Chowdhury, and Ramos-Jimenez 1999). Often these staff behaviors are linked to low pay and poor incentives, staff training, and self-definition as bearers and transmitters of "superior" Western biomedicine. A similar problem exists with the mobile clinics in Mbulu District. Health staff often treats Datoga mothers as "backward" because they are poor and maintain a pastoral lifestyle. If these mothers' experiences are to be addressed, health service policy makers need to work with clinic staff to help them understand the social and relational reasons for clinic nonattendance—Datoga mothers' poverty, social exclusion, and feelings of discomfort or marginalization at the clinic.

A second way to improve services is by ensuring predictable health resources at times that the community can access them. In this case, a simple solution would be to restructure the timetable for clinic visits and schedule the clinic later in the day when women's household responsibilities are less. This would increase community participation with almost no increase in health care spending.

Finally, caution should be taken to promote local investment when designing education programs. In this setting, there is a risk that one-way or top-down approaches that promote biomedical, disease-specific views will prove counterproductive, undermining mothers' confidence in lay discourse and traditional practices that underlie the social demand for certain accepted biomedical practices such as vaccination. Instead, communication should build on existing social demand and culturally grounded active demand through dialogue-based approaches that appreciate mothers' existing views and work with them to build a better understanding of the variables that impact child health and nutrition.

Acknowledgments

Research funded by a Fulbright Hays Doctoral Dissertation Research Fellowship, NSF BCS (DDIG-No. 0451049), and a Humanities Research Enhancement Fund award from the University of Florida. I'd like to give a warm thanks to Lauren and Amíkolé for pulling this volume together. I'd also like to thank the participants and community elders of Eshkesh, the Tanzanian authorities, Haydom Hospital, J. Gwalgwa, P. Gasheka, J. Samo, A. Musa, and S. Malleyeck for their assistance with the research.

Notes

1. Giardia or giardiasis is an infection of the small intestine caused by the protozoa *Giardia lamblia*.
2. Place names are accurate, but I use pseudonyms to protect the identity of the individuals involved with this research.

References

Abrahamsson, T., G. Sinkiewicz, T. Jakobssen, M. Fredrikson, and B. Bjorkstén
    2009   Probiotic Lactobacilli in Breast Milk and Infant Stool in Relation to Oral Intake during the First Year of Life. Journal of Pediatric Gastroenterology and Nutrition 49(3):349–54.

Black R., S. Morris, and J. Bryce
    2003   Where and Why Are 10 Million Children Dying Every Year? The Lancet 361:2226–34.

Blystad, Astrid
    1999   Dealing with Men's Spears: Datoga Pastoralists Combating Male Intrusion on Female Fertility. *In* Those Who Play with Fire: Gender, Fertility, and Transformation in East and Southern Africa. H. Moore, T. Sanders, and B. Kaare, eds. Pp. 187–223. London: Athlone Press.
    2000   Precarious Procreation: Datoga Pastoralists in the Late 20th Century. Ph.D. dissertation, University of Bergen.

Blystad, Astrid, and Ole Rekdal
    2003   Datoga. *In* Encyclopedia of Medical Anthropology: Health and Illness in the World's Cultures, Vol. 2. C. Ember and M. Ember, eds. Pp. 629–38. New York: Kluwer Academic Publishers.

Blystad, Astrid, Ole Rekdal, and Herman Malleyeck
    2007   Seclusion, Protection, and Avoidance: Exploring the Metida Complex among the Datoga of Northern Tanzania. Africa 77:331–50.

Borgerhoff Mulder, Monique
    1992   Demography of Pastoralists: Preliminary Data on the Datoga of Tanzania. Human Ecology 20(4):383–405.

Boschi-Pinto, C., C. Lanata, and R. Black
    2009   The Global Burden of Childhood Diarrhea. *In* Maternal and Child Health: Global Challenges, Programs, and Policies. J. Ehiri, ed. Pp. 225–43. New York: Springer.

Briggs, Charles, and Clara Mantini-Briggs
2003   Stories in the Time of Cholera. Berkeley: University of California Press.
Briggs, Charles, and Mark Nichter
2009   Biocommunicability and the Biopolitics of Pandemic Threats. Medical
        Anthropology 28(3):189–98.
Bryce, J., C. Boschi-Pinto, K. Shibuya, and R. Black
2005   WHO Estimates of the Causes of Death in Children. The Lancet 365:1147–52.
Centers for Disease Control and Prevention (CDC)
1992   The Management of Acute Diarrhea in Children: Oral Rehydration,
        Maintenance, and Nutritional Therapy. CDC Recommendations and Reports
        41(RR-16):001.
Chirico, G., R. Marzollo, S. Cortinovis, C. Fonte, and A. Gasparoni
2008   Anti-infective Properties of Human Milk. American Society for Nutrition
        138(9):1801S.
Crawford, Robert
1998[1977] You Are Dangerous to Your Health: The Ideology and Politics of Victim
        Blaming. *In* Classic Texts in Health Care. Lesley Mackay, Keith Soothill, and
        Kath Melia, eds. Pp. 84–89. New York: Reed Publishing.
Creighton, Colin, and C. Omari
1995   Gender, Family, and Household in Tanzania. Brookfield, VT: Avebury.
Engle, Patricia, Sarah Castle, and Patricia Menon
1996   Child Development: Vulnerability and Resilience. Social Science and Medicine
        43(5):621–35.
Gittelsohn, J., M. Thapa, and L. Ladman
1997   Cultural Factors, Caloric Intake and Micronutrient Deficiency in Rural Nepali
        Households. Social Science and Medicine 44(11):1739–49.
Hadley, Craig, and Crystal Patil
2006   Food Insecurity in Rural Tanzania Is Associated with Maternal Anxiety and
        Depression. American Journal of Human Biology 18(3):359–68.
2008   Seasonal Changes in Household Food Insecurity and Symptoms of Anxiety and
        Depression. American Journal of Physical Anthropology 135(2):225–32.
Hampshire, Katherine, Catherine Panter-Brick, Kate Kilpatrick, and Rachel Casiday
2009   Saving Lives, Preserving Livelihoods: Understanding Risk, Decision-Making and
        Child Health in a Food Crisis. Social Science and Medicine 68(4):758–65.
Harkness, Sarah, and Carol Super
1994   The Developmental Niche: A Theoretical Framework for Analyzing the
        Household Production of Health. Social Science and Medicine 38(2):217–26.
Haydom Lutheran Hospital Annual Report (HLH)
2008   www.haydom.no/facts_and_map.aspx, accessed June 4, 2011.
Helman, C., and P. Yogeswaran
2004   Perceptions of Childhood Immunisations in Rural Transkei—a Qualitative Study.
        South African Medical Journal 94(10):835–38.
Hinderaker, Sven, Bjorg Olsen, Rolv Lie, Per Bergslo, Peter Gasheka, and Gunnar Kvale
2001   Anemia in Pregnancy in the Highlands of Tanzania. Acta Obstetrica et
        Gynecologica Scandinavica 80(1):18–26.

Holliday, M.
  1982   The Evolution of Therapy for Dehydration: Should Deficit Theory Still Be
         Taught? Pediatrics 98(2):171–77.
Kosek M., C. Bern, and R. Guerrant
  2003   The Global Burden of Diarrhoeal Disease, as Estimated from Studies
         Published between 1992 and 2000. Bulletin of the World Health Organization
         81(3):197–204.
Laderman, Carol
  1983   Wives and Midwives: Childbirth and Nutrition in Rural Malaysia. Berkeley:
         University of California Press.
Lane, Charles
  1996   Pastures Lost: Barabaig Economy, Resource Tenure, and the Alienation of Their
         Land in Tanzania. Nairobi: Initiatives Publishers.
Lupton, Deborah
  1999   Risk. New York: Routledge.
Mara, D.
  2003   Water, Sanitation and Hygiene for the Health of Developing Nations. Public
         Health 117(6):452–56.
Mfinanga S., O. Morkve, R. Kazwala, S. Cleaveland, J. Sharp,
G. Shirima, and R. Nilsen
  2003   The Role of Livestock Keeping in Tuberculosis Trends in Arusha, Tanzania.
         International Journal of Tuberculosis and Lung Disease 7(7):695–704.
Millard, Ann
  1994   A Causal Model of High Rates of Child Mortality. Social Science and Medicine
         38(2):253–68.
Ndagala, Daniel
  1991   The Unmaking of the Datoga: Decreasing Resources and Increasing Conflict in
         Rural Tanzania. Nomadic Peoples 28:71–82.
Nichter, Mark
  1995   Vaccinations in the Third World: A Consideration of Community Demand.
         Social Science and Medicine 41(5):649–63.
  2003   Harm Reduction: A Core Concern for Medical Anthropology. In Risk, Culture,
         and Health Inequality: Shifting Perceptions of Danger and Blame. Barbara Herr
         Harthorn and Laury Oaks, eds. Pp. 15–33. Westport, CT: Praeger.
Olsen, B., S. Hinderaker, P. Bergsjo, R. Lie, O. Halgrim, E. Olsen, P. Gasheka,
and G. Kvale
  2002   Causes and Characteristics of Maternal Deaths in Rural Northern Tanzania. Acta
         Obstetrica et Gynecologica Scandinavica 81(12):1101–9.
Pennings, Joost, and Daniel Grossman
  2008   Responding to Crises and Disasters: The Role of Risk Attitudes and Perceptions.
         Disasters 32:432–48.
Petri, William, Mark Miller, Henry Binder, Myron Levine, Rebecca Dillingham,
and Richard Guerrant
  2008   Enteric Infections, Diarrhea, and Their Impact on Function and Development.
         Journal of Clinical Investigation 118:1270–90.

Pike, Ivy, and Crystal Patil
    2006   Understanding Women's Burdens: Preliminary Findings on Psychosocial Health
        among Datoga and Iraqw Women of Northern Tanzania. Culture Medicine and
        Psychiatry 30(3):299–330.
Rekdal, Ole
    1999   Cross-Cultural Healing in East African Ethnography. Medical Anthropology
        Quarterly 13(4):458–82.
Rekdal, Ole, and Astrid Blystad
    2000   "We Are as Sheep and Goats: Iraqw and Datooga Discourses on Fortune, Failure,
        and the Future." *In* The Poor Are Not Us: Poverty and Pastoralism in Eastern
        Africa. David Anderson and Vigdis Broch-Due, eds. Pp. 125–46. Athens: Ohio
        University Press.
Sellen, Daniel
    1995   The Socioecology of Young Child Growth among the Datoga Pastoralists of
        Northern Tanzania. Ph.D. dissertation, University of California, Davis.
    1999   Growth Patterns among Semi-nomadic Pastoralists (Datoga) of Tanzania.
        American Journal of Physical Anthropology 109(2):187–209.
    2003   Nutritional Consequences of Wealth Differentials in East African Pastoralists: The
        Case of the Datoga of Northern Tanzania. Human Ecology 31(4):529–70.
Sieff, Daniella
    1995   The Effects of Resource Availability on the Subsistence Strategies of Datoga
        Pastoralists of Northwest Tanzania. Ph.D. dissertation, University of Oxford.
Smith, M., S. Madon, A. Anifalije, M. Larazzo-Malecela, and E. Michael
    2008   Integrated Health Information Systems in Tanzania: Experience and Challenges.
        Electronic Journal on Information Systems in Developing Countries (EJSCD)
        33:1–21.
Stanley, S.
    2003   Amoebiasis. The Lancet 361:1025–34.
Stanway, Penny, and Andrew Stanway
    1978   Breast Is Best: A Commonsense Approach to Breast Feeding. London: Pan.
Streefland, P., A. Chowdhury, and P. Ramos-Jimenez
    1999   Patterns of Vaccination Acceptance. Social Science and Medicine
        49(12):1705–16.
World Health Organization (WHO)
    2010   Breast Is Always Best, Even for HIV-Positive Mothers. Bulletin of the World
        Health Organization 88(1):1–80.
Young, Alyson
    2008   Young Child Health among Eyasi Datoga: Socioeconomic Marginalization,
        Local Biology, and Infant Resilience within the Mother-Infant Dyad. Ph.D.
        dissertation, University of Arizona.
Young, H., and S. Jaspars
    2006   Meaning and Measurement of Acute Malnutrition: A Primer for Decision-
        Makers. Humanitarian Practice Network Paper no. 56. Overseas Development
        Institute.

CHAPTER 9

Shifting Maternal Responsibilities and the Trajectory of Blame in Northern Ghana

Aaron R. Denham

One afternoon early in my fieldwork in the Upper East Region of Ghana, I accompanied a local NGO worker and a community health nurse to visit a sick three-year-old girl named Azuma, her mother, Abiiro, and their extended family.[1] The NGO worker had concerns not only about Azuma's poor health, but also about circulating rumors that the family suspected her of being a "spirit child"— a malicious spirit from the bush with a grave intention of destroying the family. From the NGO worker's perspective, Azuma was at risk because of her medical condition and the chance that family members would administer to her a deadly poisonous concoction. From the family's perspective, Azuma represented a risk to her mother, the family's livelihood, and its continued existence in this and in the ancestral world.

Upon arriving at the family's compound we sat in the shade of a baobab tree with eight slight children under the watchful eye of the family elder and waited for Abiiro. She soon emerged from her near-collapsing mud home, limping from a filariasis infection and carrying Azuma, to sit on a bench across from us with Azuma on her lap.[2] Azuma, arms around her mother, regarded us with concern from an askew right eye as she breathed uneasily, mouth open. After we exchanged customary greetings with the family, the nurse examined Azuma and talked with Abiiro.

As we spoke about her condition, Azuma made repeated attempts to breastfeed. Abiiro pushed Azuma away, mentioning that she had stopped producing milk several months earlier. Azuma's medical card, issued by the Ministry of Health at its free postnatal care clinic, indicated that the three-year-old was consistently underweight, never exceeding eleven pounds. The nurse tried, to no avail, to get Azuma to stand unaided. Her lean legs bowed outward with each unsuccessful attempt.

Abiiro estimated that she was around thirty-four years old, although she appeared much older. She had given birth four times and had three surviving children, including Azuma, the youngest. Abiiro's most significant complaint was that Azuma cried day and night, rarely slept, and insisted on being carried in her arms, which interfered with her work. At subsequent visits with the family, it became apparent that she was greatly concerned about the disruption and impact of Azuma's condition on the larger family. Also, the family described an increase in interpersonal family conflict that coincided with Azuma's birth. These complaints were indicative of potential spiritual danger and ancestral displeasure. Other than her frailty, Azuma's most noticeable feature was a strabismus in her right eye. This "look" troubled family members. Wandering eyes are perceived as evidence that a child or adult is up to something spiritual and cannot be trusted.

I was surprised that the nurse, after a brief examination, quickly pronounced Azuma fine and said Abiiro simply needed to provide her with "proper nutrition" and vitamins to stimulate her appetite. She prescribed vitamins, antibiotics for Azuma's respiratory infection, and medication for a suspected malaria infection. "That wandering eye is caused by the child failing to get the proper eyedrops during birth," the nurse explained. "The mother must have had gonorrhea when she gave birth. If she would have gone to the hospital to deliver, none of this would have happened." The nurse questioned Abiiro about Azuma's birth, stressing that all women should give birth in hospital. "Why didn't you call the midwife or go to the hospital to give birth?" the nurse asked. "You even had complications and still did not go." Abiiro said she was unable to send for the local midwife because she went into labor at night and lived a five-hour minibus ride away from the nearest hospital.

While hospital and clinic births represent the Ministry of Health's official position aimed at reducing maternal risk, my subsequent visits with Abiiro and other community members revealed a complex set of unofficial risks that overshadowed sanctioned safe-motherhood messages. First, Abiiro had gone into labor after sunset. Although midwives employed by the Ministry of Health encourage families to contact them at all hours, Abiiro later revealed that she did not want to bother the midwife at night. Community members, particularly expectant mothers, rarely travel along paths at night because of the increased presence of dangers such as witchcraft, sorcery, and various spiritual beings. Giving birth in the family compound is often preferred, since babies born along a road or path—a liminal, ambiguous, and potentially dangerous place—may never fully integrate into the social/earthly world (see Smith-Oka, this volume, for similar beliefs among Mexican women). Moreover, the local interventions for difficult delivery require the woman to be in the family compound connected to the uterine or agnatic kin, rather than in a depersonalized clinic (see Cassiman 2006:234). Several women also equated home birth with a valued ethic of endurance and strength. Finally, rumors of birth experiences in hospitals or clinics warned of nurses beating women who labor too slowly, and of medical staff mishandling or dropping and thus injuring or killing infants.

Abiiro's notion of responsibility for Azuma's condition was understood within an epistemology that emphasized the local social, ancestral, and spiritually based perceptions of risk. The nurse redirected and focused on Abiiro's individual responsibilities as a mother disconnected from the social and economic realities of the kin system, a biomedical risk discourse that emphasized the importance of regular antenatal clinic attendance, family planning and birth spacing, and improved nutrition. In this and other encounters I observed, it was apparent that biomedical health providers regarded mothers as individual agents who are responsible to make the choices, as communicated by health professionals and educators, that are in their best interests (cf. Pinto 2008).

During my research among the Nankani, the local ethnic group, I became interested in the disjuncture between and integration of traditional ways of knowing in relation to the transnational models incorporated in Safe Motherhood campaigns and biomedical programs. Cases like Azuma's spurred my interest in local subjective understandings of maternal risk and blame. Based on my early impressions, mothers appeared subject to a double burden of blame ensuing from both the biomedical and the traditional models. However, upon viewing blame from a processual framework—resulting from long-term relationships and ongoing case studies—a difference between biomedical and traditional models of blame emerged.

This chapter uses Nankani perceptions of the spirit child phenomenon to explore notions of maternal and infant risk, responsibility and blame. In this descriptive and critical analysis, I identify a trajectory of blame associated with risk at the intersection of the local and the biomedical. That is, I present a diachronic, temporal perspective of (1) how agents perceive risk and attribute blame accordingly, (2) how agents resolve or sustain ongoing blame, and (3) in a dialectical manner, how blame influences future perceptions of risk. A close examination of the spirit child phenomenon grounds maternal risk perception within the broader social system and illustrates both traditional and biomedical perceptions of maternal and infant risk and the shifting trajectories of blame.

Context

This chapter is based on ethnographic research in several rural Nankani communities in the Kassena-Nankana District (KND) of Ghana in 2006–2007, followed by three shorter trips between 2008 and 2010.[3] Nankani families are patrilineal, virilocal, and organized according to a segmentary lineage pattern. Polygyny is practiced, although it is less common than in the past and is dependent on a man's financial resources. The family head, usually the eldest male in the extended family compound, is responsible for decision making. Gatekeeping by the family head is common, particularly when significant decisions affecting the family are considered, such as those involving finances or health. Elders' decisions consider and often prioritize the interests of the larger family and community, including deceased ancestors, over individual needs. When faced with maternal health decisions, a woman often follows a hierarchical protocol, for example, to seek permission and money from her husband and father-in-law to attend a clinic, pay for transportation, and purchase medicine.

Traditionally, fertility rates have been high, and families attribute their pronatalist beliefs to a history of high infant mortality. Religious and kinship expectations, particularly those that center on ensuring intergenerational continuity, are also important, as is the prestige of having a large family. Despite these imperatives, the district's fertility rate has fallen in conjunction with community health and family-planning projects and other regional demographic changes (Debpuur et al. 2002:141). Between 1995 and 1999, the total fertility rate in the KND declined from 5.1 to 4.1 (Baiden et al. 2006). In 2004, the Navrongo Health Research Center indicated that the total fertility rate was 3.9.

The KND is a rural, semi-arid Guinea savannah with one annual rainy season. Because of the dependence on a single growing season, food insecurity, periods of famine, and seasonal malnutrition are persistent threats. Thus, the challenges facing mothers begin long before birth. The public health literature and professionals identify mothers as being at high risk as a result of significant disease burden, care-seeking delays resulting from geographic or economic constraints, and limited access to health facilities equipped to handle serious obstetric cases (Ngom et al. 1999:142). Community members recognize the dangers of the perinatal period and infancy in terms both of serious biomedical health risks such as infectious diseases and of the presence of spiritual dangers.

Data from the Navrongo Health Research Center indicate that in 2003 a skilled birth attendant was present at 20 percent of births in the KND (Navrongo Health Research Center 2004). After the Ministry of Health and Navrongo Health Research Center launched targeted health campaigns in the mid-1990s, maternal mortality in the KND was reduced from 636 deaths per 100,000 in 1995–1996 to 373 in 2002–2004 (Mills et al. 2008). Infant and child mortality rates, while still excessive, also fell. Before the health campaigns, it was estimated that one in nine children did not make it to age five (Binka et al. 1999). However, the most recent statistics indicate that infant mortality (0–<1 year) was 84.6 deaths per 1,000 births and postinfant child mortality (1–<5 years) was 82.9 deaths per 1,000 births (Binka et al. 2007). The primary causes of infant and child mortality in the KND include malaria, diarrheal diseases, acute respiratory infections, and meningitis (Baiden et al. 2006).

Medicalization, Risk, and Blame

It is incorrect to assume that people living in areas where biomedical treatment options are limited lack health knowledge, await biomedical enlightenment, or will readily replace local ethnomedical beliefs. In Northern Ghana, government and internationally funded community health clinics and maternal health education programs have expanded families' knowledge of maternal and infant risk factors, and these programs have had a tremendous impact on community health. Despite these programs, such models have not necessarily supplanted local notions of risk. Rather, families frequently incorporate public health messages into their understanding of reproductive vulnerabilities (cf. Cassiman 2006:250).

The social science literature has discussed the globalization of biomedicine and its related impacts at length (Conrad 1992; Finkler 2000). Critical perspectives have noted how biomedical systems obscure the root causes of illness, such as poverty, inequality, and power relationships. Biomedicine has been critiqued as assuming moral neutrality and freedom from culture (Mishler 1981), as casting social experiences in medical terms (Kleinman and Kleinman 1991), and as treating sufferers as agents independent of social context (Mogensen 2005:238). Within the intervention discourse present in Safe Motherhood programs specifically, Pinto describes a "neoliberal logic in which health is a private good and responsibility largely that of individuals," enacted with the goal of making women informed and efficient consumers of health care resources (2008:191). Even my own experiences receiving biomedical treatment in Ghana demanded culpability, a Foucauldian-like surveillance and controlling discourse, and assigned blame.

Biomedical programs primarily address what are described as the "official risks" that are seen as harmful to women during pregnancy and childbirth. "Unofficial risks," such as concerns about witchcraft, receive less attention by those in the public health system, although they might be of greater concern to the community (Allen 2004:9). Consequently, official risks may not accurately reflect the realities of women's experiences of pregnancy and childbirth, often leading to one-size-fits-all solutions for reducing maternal mortality (Allen 2004:8–9).

Nankani unofficial risks include jealousy, witchcraft, benevolent and malevolent sorcery, hidden forces or intentions, ancestral demands, spirits, destiny, and a range of behavioral taboos that govern kinship boundaries and restrict women's movement. These play a role in identifying deviants and assigning blame. For example, some families may attribute prolonged labor to possible adultery and demand that the mother confess to speed childbirth.

In an analysis of Arab and African Muslim women's perspectives on maternal risk, Allen found that women were responding to two aspects: risks *of* motherhood (as articulated by the government's Safe Motherhood strategy) and risks *to* motherhood (as articulated by the healing strategies adopted by women in the community) (2004:10). Throop's (2010) thoughts on experience, perceptions, and experiences of risk that resist categorization or dwell on the fringes of interpretation and articulation are also important domains of investigation. Finally, while these perspectives contribute a pluralistic understanding of specific risks, a consideration of risk's temporal dimensions reduces the potential for static or incomplete representations. In this way, we consider the variability of individual and social perceptions of risk and resultant blame, which are subject to factors such as the degree of perceived control (Foege 1988:335).

People's risk interpretations and blaming processes are rarely far from their local moral worlds and attempts at meaning making. Individuals have used blame throughout history to understand events, for example, to "make mysterious and devastating diseases comprehensible and therefore possibly controllable" (Nelkin and Gilman 1988:362). In this way, blaming is part of a larger post-misfortune existential inquiry, part of a process that results from what Zizek and other scholars have described, in one form or another, as "the temptation of meaning" (2009:157). Or in terms more familiar to anthropologists, blaming is a way to answer the questions, Why me? Why now?

For a community, the process of assigning blame identifies the source of misfortune so that members can take steps to control and order the risks, resolve the anxiety, and fix or reduce vulnerability in the future (Nelkin and Gilman 1988:362–63). While blame contributes to local definitions of normality and healthy behavior, it also establishes psychological and sociopolitical boundaries within and between groups. These boundaries reinforce community ideals, working as an othering process a community can attach to ideological concerns (Douglas 1994:63; Nelkin and Gilman 1988:363). In this way, communities can identify scapegoats, and blame becomes a means to control deviant or threatening individuals and groups, thereby teaching accepted beliefs and behaviors.

Trajectories of Blame

The assessment and assignment of blame is a key dimension of understanding what is at stake in the negotiation of maternal and infant risk (Mogensen 2005:235). Considering the trajectory of that blame, moreover, enhances our understandings of risk experiences and how they shape behavior. Specifically, the trajectory of blame is a model that emphasizes a diachronic, temporal consideration that encompasses the shifting movement from the initial perceptions, explanations, meanings, and notions of risk for a particular circumstance, diagnosis, or misfortune, to the way responsibility is assessed, how blame is attributed and resolved, and how this process dialectically influences future perceptions of risk and preventive actions. I do not wish to conflate this notion of a trajectory with a unidirectional, deterministic perspective that lacks human agency. Rather, I find insightful a praxis orientation or, as Devisch (1985) describes, a praxecological perspective that focuses on the purposeful articulation of how human action alters or creates meaning.

Illness narratives are an important element in the process of gathering accounts of and analyzing trajectories blame. A trajectory of blame can emerge, in part, within the temporal process of narrative emplotment, exemplified in the role that narrative plays "in shaping the ways an individual is able to reflect on past experience, give meaning to ongoing interaction while also setting a course for future action" (Throop 2010:259). Finally, taking stock of the role of multiple factors, actions, and meanings that influence blame over time provides a more holistic account of the notions and experiences of risk and blame. This approach is more likely to include important contextual domains—social and power relations, beliefs, history, and culture—and how these forces shape the experience of blame over time.

The Spirit Child

I choose the spirit child as a focal point for this discussion because it represents an extreme yet infrequently occurring risk that has significant power to shape families' behaviors. Last (1992) recognizes that focusing on extremes of experience, rather than on the normative or mundane, proves more significant for understanding a community's response to misfortune. Jackson (2005) also remarks that a focus on the mundane may miss what he describes, in Kleinman's terms, as "what's at stake" (1995:98) for individuals and their community and the significant events that people strive to achieve or to avoid. Using Durkheim's argument in *Suicide* (1951), Bledsoe remarks that "apparent aberrations should not necessarily be regarded as separate from the rest of the population. Rather, they may be extreme manifestations of the entire shape of normality in a particular society" (2002:3). In regard to health interventions or policy determinations, research that seeks to establish the average or focuses on common risks is liable to miss what is significant for people; "thus health campaigns based on such interpretations are likely to be seriously flawed" (Last 1992:799). Even simple descriptions of a particular phenomenon such as the birth of a disabled infant are overshadowed by the fears provoked by the birth and the associated risks and consequences the infant brings into the world. It is these beliefs and fears that people respond to that might disproportionately skew actions and ideas away from the norm (ibid.).

Nankani community members believe that some children are born into the family not as human beings, but as spirits in the guise of a child. These spirit children come from the "bush" (undomesticated forest spaces) to cause misfortune and destroy the family. After an extensive identification process to confirm their suspicions, families conduct a ceremony that involves the intentional administration of a poisonous concoction to the child with the goal of returning the spirit to the bush and reestablishing normality within the family.

From a biological perspective, all the spirit children I observed had suffered damage from an infection, had a congenital disability, or had experienced trauma during the birthing process. I also encountered seemingly healthy children suspected to be spirit children because their mothers died during childbirth. The majority of spirit child cases fit within the common anthropological explanations of infanticide practices: fitness-oriented explanations, parental investment strategies, ecologically based perspectives, local and global political economies, and structural violence (Farmer 2005). While these theoretical perspectives offer detailed etic insights into why infanticide occurs, much like the official maternal health risks they do not capture parental experiences and sentiments, decision-making processes, perceptions of maternal risk, and the blaming that shapes practice.

In addition to identifying spirit children through their physical status, families also detect spirit children through the various misfortunes they are believed to cause, such as loss of livestock, family conflict, sickness, death, infertility, and maternal complications. When asked to describe a spirit child, a Nankani mother remarked: "A spirit child comes from a woman who gives birth, continuously falls sick, and doesn't appear to get well." A member of a local women's group said: "It is a child that has been born and the mother dies immediately." Many men in the community described unfortunate encounters with spirit children. An elder recalled: "Years ago my wife gave birth and would not stop bleeding. The child died soon after it was born. I went to get herbs to treat my wife, but she too died. After that, I went to the diviner and found that my wife had given birth to a spirit child."

Another man said: "I have witnessed my own wife give birth to a spirit child. She was very sick and just lying around. The child would cry all the time, day and night, even if it had breastfed already."

Although the community discourse on spirit children is prevalent through vocalized suspicions, myths, stories, and rumors, infanticide does not occur in all cases. Many spirit children die from common diseases or congenital conditions (Denham et al. 2010). While infanticide of nonviable infants does occur, families commonly use the spirit child diagnosis as a postmortem explanation for the ultimate cause of death or misfortune, such as why a child died from malaria or why a mother became ill or died during childbirth. The spirit child diagnosis is a way for families to signify, as one community member indicated, a child "not meant for this world" and to explain the ultimate risks and reasons for maternal and infant misfortune. Despite its infrequency, the birth of a spirit child is a concerning risk that families are conscious of avoiding. The following sections describe the traditional notions of risk associated with spirit children—a necessary first step in outlining a trajectory of blame.

The Spirit Child and the Unofficial Risks of Maternal and Infant Misfortune

How does a family come to have a spirit child, and what unofficial risks attract spirit children? The violation of traditional taboos, social norms, kinship structure boundaries, and geographic boundaries are the most commonly identified maternal risks for having a spirit child. Spirit child discourse indicates that families are vigilant about potential destructive activities, such as conflict, illicit sexual relations, illegitimate children, and sickness. In turn, they are attuned to the physical and social boundaries that prevent spirits, or these antisocial acts, from entering the family. In the following descriptions of spirit child risk and causation, each violation must occur before the mother becomes pregnant. In other words, a fetus or infant cannot "catch" a spirit; most families believe it is a spirit child from or near the time of conception.

First, taboos stipulate that a woman must sit down inside of the home to eat. Eating while walking is the most common behavior by which a woman can attract a spirit. If a woman walks anywhere outside the home while eating, pieces of food may fall to the ground. Spirits crave human food and are always looking for opportunities to eat. If spirits are nearby, they will follow her and enter her womb. A woman described the danger in this way:

> If you are fond of eating while walking, those spirit children will follow you and pick up the food as you drop it. They will say, "This woman is good, she likes me. That's why she's dropping all this food." The spirit will follow the woman all the way to her house. If the ancestors are not strong, the spirit will be able to enter the house and find a way to enter the woman. Before you realize it, you give birth to a spirit child.

Second, spirits, sex, and sexual taboos are common themes. Male spirits are described as desirous of women. "Anytime the spirit is just standing there and a woman passes by, it can follow her," a male informant said. "For the woman, maybe she cannot see it, but it sees her. The spirit will follow her and have intercourse with her and she'll not know." A woman risks catching a spirit child if she has "illegal sex," that is, intercourse outside the home or in the bush. A man explained: "If a spirit is passing by while you are having sex, [it can enter you] immediately when you finish, or just before you start; it can move so fast. That is why it's advisable for men not to have intercourse with a woman outside the house."

Third, women are discouraged from urinating in various prohibited locations, especially those considered spiritually dangerous, liminal, or ambiguous. The most important are places where spirit children are buried. A woman told me: "The place where they bury the spirit children—there are so many spirit children there—if a woman goes there to urinate, the spirit can easily have intercourse with her." Failing to squat or to properly conceal oneself while urinating can also attract a spirit. "Some women don't want to squat, sometimes they want to stand as men do," a male informant said. "So when they do that, the spirit, because they are always roaming about, can easily enter the woman and make her give birth to a spirit child."

Men may also attract a spirit child, albeit less frequently. Most commonly, a man's failure to take the necessary precautions around an adulterous relationship may catch a spirit. Informants explained that after having sex with someone other than his wife, a man must not rush home immediately. Rather, he should wait for some period of time and bathe before entering his room. Spirit children are attracted to sex and would follow the "unclean" man, enter the home, and possibly enter his wife. As one woman explained: "Coming home from the outside [after sex] may mean that you are importing the evil spirits into the house."

Additionally, the intentional killing of a totem animal can cause misfortunes for a family and anger the ancestors, particularly if a woman eats it. "Human beings and animals have a spirit," a male informant said. "When you kill a spirit animal, we believe that the spirit in that animal will jump into a human being." This spirit can move itself into a woman and bear a spirit child. Other risks that attract spirits include using unapproved entrances and exits to a house, washing another woman's calabashes at the riverside, and bathing at night.

An analysis of these themes reveals the need for family members to attend to and to maintain the distinction between the "house" and the "bush"—the domesticated and ancestrally protected versus the undomesticated space where spirits dwell and malevolent or antisocial events occur. Family members must be aware of the boundaries of the family system and the risks and behaviors that can weaken these and create an opportunity for spirits, as sources of misfortune or impurity, to literally enter the woman and disrupt the family system. In this case, the meanings of sicknesses, maternal misfortunes, and the bodily states of spirit children threaten the balance of social and domestic relations, since the body is a profound historical and moral site (Livingston 2005; Rapp and Ginsburg 2001).

While it is apparent that the woman bears a burden of blame for the causation of a spirit child, blame is divested away from the mother in a variety of ways. First, through interpretive divination, the family elder divines in order to understand the misfortune, establish its ultimate cause, and determine further actions, such as ancestral sacrifices. Sociopolitically, divination redirects or diffuses blame to individuals or groups and from individuals to the ancestors or to a spiritual or nonhuman scapegoat (see Mendonsa 1982). During a divinatory session, while the mother may be identified as attracting a spirit, the ultimate cause of the misfortune, such as a desirous spirit, is often targeted.

Second, the family identifies the offending spirit as a scapegoat and blames it for the ultimate reasons why misfortune occurred. The spirit comes to embody the antisocial or destructive causes that result in sickness, maternal misfortune, or conflict. Consequently, attributing responsibility and blame to the spirit through ceremonial means redirects and expunges the blame for the misfortune from the mother to the untamed and antisocial forces of the bush.

Third, if the family identifies the child as a spirit, they perform several purification, appeasement, and preventive rituals. While there is considerable variation, the basic ceremony involves animal sacrifices, pouring of libations, appeals to the ancestors for protection and to spirits to remain in the bush, sharing of food with the extended family, and purification of the mother and father through ritual bathing, cutting of the hair, and disposal of clothing. The sacrifices and related rituals ensure that the dangerous spirit does not return and engages the wider family and ancestral world in the protection of the mother and, ultimately, the larger family. In essence, the family and larger social network transforms the responsibility and blame.

Finally, because mothers and fathers understand the spirit child as not human, most reported that their suffering and despair were less with the death of a believed spirit child than with the death of a normal child. Future research will explore this important area of parental sentiments.

Changing Perceptions: Integrating Public Health Knowledge

Community members indicated that improvements in access to maternal health services over the past fifteen years have significantly reduced the number of spirit child deaths. Some maintained that the spirit child no longer exists, because of medical treatment. According to one woman: "Just in the olden days of the ancestors, if the child grows sick or lean then they say that such a child is a spirit child. . . . But now, if a child is sick, they can send for treatment." A male elder noted:

> I live near the hill where they abandoned the spirit children. When I was a child, we would follow the animals as they grazed, watching over them. In those days, there were so many spirit children abandoned there. . . . These days it's no longer so, because of the medical treatment we have for them . . .

and because the women attend antenatal care, these days when you go to the hill you rarely see any spirit children.

Women who attend maternal health clinics and those with some formal public education are increasingly integrating biomedical notions of causation into local spirit child frameworks. The mother of a three-year-old boy with cerebral palsy, a suspected spirit child, easily shifted between traditional and biomedically related causes for his condition by equally attributing two risks: a difficult, prolonged labor and cesarean section, and eating beneath a baobab tree where spirits dwell.

Traditional stipulations regarding taboo foods now include contemporary taboos, such as use of alcohol and drugs and misuse of pharmaceuticals. Other risk factors identified as causing spirit children include lack of prenatal checkups, premature births, severe malaria, prolonged labor, and a heavy workload during pregnancy. One woman explained the role of prenatal nutrition: "In the old days there were not as many nutrients, they were not eating the way we do today. That's why in the old days there were more spirit children. Today we learn what to eat. If you don't get the proper nutrients, your baby will not develop well and you can easily give birth to a spirit child."

While biomedicine is increasingly recognized as reducing risk, families explicitly identified poverty and the cost of many biomedical services as a cause of spirit children and a barrier to accessing prenatal and antenatal care. "If you are poor and give birth to a child, you can't go to the hospital," a mother said. "If the child is sick, you can't care for the child, you can't buy drugs, you can't do anything. It's because of all these things that it's a spirit child." Another woman added: "You have to buy this thing, that thing, get eggs, and eat more so the child will form well. But when you come home and tell your husband, he will tell you he has nothing, that he has no money. If you have some money it helps, but if not, you will not be able to help the child, so it will be abnormal—a spirit child."

Finally, several men and women identified weak or poor-quality sperm as a risk. A young man explained: "Men who are up to sixty or seventy years and are still having children. At that time, their sperm are weak. They still have intercourse with woman but they give birth to children who are not properly formed." This is the only risk that is the sole domain of the male.

Azampana: A Biomedical Trajectory of Blame

Mogensen describes how families use biomedical frameworks to access alternative notions of blame, responsibility, and ways to interpret sickness. These alternatives open other ways of linking events such as misfortunes and connect people to what are perceived as "modern" practices (Mogensen 2005:242). Biomedical models place responsibility on the health care system, genetics, or impersonal factors or causes that result in no one being blamed, according to Mogensen (238). On the contrary, my research indicates that blame and the biomedical are connected. Beyond the benefits of biomedicine acknowledged by community members, the expanding reliance on biomedical explanations for maternal health and risk in the KND has incredible potential to cast unofficial risks as outdated and, consequently, to focus blame upon individual women.

Early one morning, Joe, a local NGO worker, rushed me to the compound of a family that had recently given birth to a possible spirit child. He refused to provide details, saying that no words could explain what he had seen. In the compound, Apoka emerged from the traditional women's room with her eight-day-old son, Azampana, completely covered and protected from dangers carried by the strong wind. The elders softly urged Apoka and Azampana to move forward. Upon removing his cloth, Apoka revealed Azampana's bilateral cleft palate and infected spina bifida. We all looked on in silence.

After Apoka and Azampana retreated, I asked the other family members what caused his condition. I was expecting them to describe Azampana as a spirit child, since the families I had worked with previously indicated that such characteristics are surely those of spirit children. However, not one person recognized him as such. "Actually, I cannot tell what is wrong," replied the family head. "It's the first time I've seen something like this." The child's father remarked: "I think it could be the mother's sickness. Maybe she had an infection when she was pregnant and through [the sickness] the child has those deformities." Her brother and sister-in-law added that she might not have followed all the antenatal care visit recommendations. In a later conversation, Apoka agreed, saying she was unsure of the cause but might be responsible for not following all the maternal health recommendations. That afternoon, Joe and I took Apoka and Azampana to the regional hospital, where the hospital staff speculated about vitamin supplements and maternal responsibilities. Azampana was admitted but died two days later. The evening of his death, the family buried him in a brief ceremony in an empty field next to the compound. The family elder did not perform the traditional divination to examine the causes of Azampana's death, since it was "probably just some illness." In this biomedically framed case, the ultimate responsibility for Azampana's condition, whether lack of nutrients, defective genes, or failure to closely follow health recommendations, rests with his mother.

Families throughout KND widely agreed that a child with spina bifida or a cleft palate would be identified as a spirit child, both historically and in significant numbers today. After Azampana's brief funeral, I thought about the circumstances and considered how they would have differed if the family had attributed his death to spiritual causes. If the family understood his condition from a traditional perspective, the purification and spirit child rituals previously described would have been performed. Were Azampana a spirit "not meant for this world," the family would not have attributed the ultimate responsibility and blame for his condition and death to any one individual; rather, it would rest with malevolent spirits and the broader social system.

Azampana's case illustrates an increasing trend toward interpreting instances of maternal or infant misfortune through a biomedical public health model rather than a traditional framework. This shift, which results in part from public health campaigns and improved access to community health resources, is changing community members' understanding of maternal and infant misfortune and is resulting in a trajectory of blame that differs from those of traditional models. When families accept a situation as solely a biomedical problem caused by individual behaviors the woman should have performed or avoided, the trajectory of blame fixes upon the mother throughout the course and resolution of the misfortune. This notion of individual responsibility and trajectory of blame does not address or diffuse responsibility throughout her larger kin and social system. Rather, the rhetoric of responsibility and burden of blame is directed at the mother for making "incorrect choices" or for making no choice at all (Pinto 2008:228). When misfortune occurred, the resulting maternally directed blame is a disciplining discourse that (re)emphasized biomedical risk reduction and frequently set off wide speculation, with questionable accuracy or basis, as to why the mother, as an individual agent, failed. The health provider's intention behind this discourse—as illustrated in Azuma's case—appeared to be positive and in good faith; however, the burden and other effects it placed on mothers were less so.

Traditional healing and care practices in this region are "molded by kinship" and social responsibilities (Bierlich 2007:146; Fortes 1949). Similar to Bierlich's observations among the Dagomba, a neighboring group in the Northern Region of Ghana, the epistemological foundations central to biomedical education and services are incompatible with and frequently in opposition to Nankani social and kin-based healing epistemologies and practices. Traditional practices engage and affirm existing social relationships and obligations, whereas biomedical care is individual or "person-centered." Consequently, community members frequently do not understand the reasoning behind biomedical practices (Bierlich 2007:144–46). Serious maternal and infant health concerns, such as spirit children, involve the entire Nankani family system in diagnosis, confirmation, and resolution. The biomedical model, however, can short-circuit this trajectory and kin involvement, shifting blame and notions of responsibility from the broader kin system and antisocial spirits onto the individual mother.

Families frequently employ biomedical and traditional treatments and preventive methods simultaneously, such as the use of pharmaceuticals alongside herbal preparations. While treatments are concurrent or integrated, the fundamental models or frameworks used to interpret and understand illness and misfortune often remain distinct because of their epistemological incompatibility. Attribution of responsibility and the trajectory of blame are connected to the epistemological model family members use to determine causation. Thus, if sickness is identified as having a spiritual origin, even if family members treat it with pharmaceuticals, it remains framed as traditional and retains the corresponding trajectory of blame. Finally, what families practice in public or when subject to a biomedical gaze can differ from what occurs in private. For example, when NGO field-workers and a community health nurse offered assistance to a family who attributed their infant son's illness and disability to spiritual causation, the family readily accepted the nurse's biomedical explanations for their infant's condition. Community members remarked, however, that the family temporarily eschewed their traditional beliefs only to appease the powerful community figures and gain access to valuable resources. The field-workers were not surprised. They openly acknowledged the power differential and accepted the duplicity. Weeks later, when the child died from its illness, the family invited them to the brief ceremony where they buried the child as "a normal human being." Later, a field-worker offhandedly remarked that the burial was a show for the NGO. The family likely still believed he was a spirit child and would rebury him as a spirit and conduct the necessary ceremonies.

Concluding Thoughts

The increasing availability of community health clinics in the KND is having an overwhelmingly positive effect on maternal health outcomes and has been instrumental in reducing the risks of motherhood. It is not the intention of this chapter to discredit these efforts. Rather, I want to direct consideration to externalities and changes associated with this growth and, specifically, how it is shifting local understandings of risk, responsibility, and blame. As biomedical understandings are becoming more prominent in the region, I question if families will cease to use traditional frameworks of risk and related trajectories of blame for maternal and infant misfortune. I suppose that much of the answer depends on how public health campaigns and services are packaged and implemented.

Biomedical forms of knowledge and risk might not always be incompatible with local healing frameworks. Ideally, providers can tailor public health interventions and services to fit within existing local frameworks, giving primacy to local belief systems. However, difficulty in resolving epistemological differences, notions of authority, and hegemonic power differentials embedded within biomedical models might complicate such integration.

A social work–oriented model that gives primacy to traditional models while integrating public health messages and practices appears to work well. In Azuma's case, the local NGO, acting as a mediary or buffer between the family and public health services, was able to connect the family with needed biomedical care and resources, which, as depicted earlier, initially placed Azuma's condition upon Abiiro's shoulders. In conjunction with the medicine and food provided, the community-based field-worker engaged the family on its terms within its cultural model for understanding risk. Working from a position that gave primacy to traditional and kin-based ways of knowing, the field-worker encouraged the *family* to take responsibility for Azuma and Abiiro's condition, emphasizing the kin-based system of care while also explaining how biomedical treatments could help. Rather than discounting the "unofficial" risks, he recognized how they play a significant role in shaping the family's experience, power dynamics, and decision making.

Soon after her initial encounter with the nurse, Azuma and Abiiro entered a three-month residential feeding program in the regional capital. Upon returning home, Azuma began speaking and could walk without assistance. On my most recent visit with Azuma, now almost seven years old, she was healthy, laughing, and running and playing with the other children. Although Azuma's language development is delayed and it takes longer for her to complete some tasks, her family no longer believes she is a spirit child. What made the difference in Azuma's case was that while the family recognized biomedical treatment and notions of causation, with the help of the NGO they integrated these within the traditional social frameworks for managing sickness, responsibility, and blame. Abiiro, the family elders, and in-laws readily dispersed a significant portion of the responsibility and blame for Azuma's condition and related misfortunes to the obligations of the father and elders as well as the family's economic state. Rather than remaining singled out and saddled with the brunt of blame for Azuma's condition, Abiiro and her family were later empowered to consider Azuma's condition in biomedical terms while also framing it within the social, economic, and spiritual context of the family system.

In summary, I propose that investigations into experiences of risk and blame consider an integrative approach that accounts for not only official and unofficial risks, but also how people attribute and resolve blame over time. I have illustrated how biomedical and traditional risks associated with the spirit child play an important role in shaping maternal perceptions of risk and demonstrated how these different models espoused divergent trajectories of blame. Finally, I suggest that if health services and Safe Motherhood programs are tailored to the cultural contexts; acknowledge the role that unofficial risks play in shaping experience, choice, and trajectories of blame; and are integrated within local social frameworks and models for maternal risk, it will be less likely—at least within the context of the KND— that mothers will bear a fixed burden of blame for misfortune.

Notes

1. I use pseudonyms throughout this chapter.
2. Lymphatic filariasis is a parasitic disease caused by filariae, or worms, that are transmitted by mosquitoes. A common symptom is elephantiasis in the lower extremities, which is a result of the worms living in the lymphatic system. Filariasis can result in long-term disability.
3. This research was supported by the University of Alberta Fund Supporting International Development Activities (FSIDA), the University of Alberta Department of Anthropology, Northern Arizona University Faculty Grants Program, and Northern Arizona University Department of Anthropology.

References

Allen, Denise
    2004   Managing Motherhood, Managing Risk: Fertility and Danger in West Central Tanzania. Ann Arbor: University of Michigan Press.
Baiden, Frank, Abraham Hodgson, Martin Adjuik, Philip Adongo, Bawah Ayaga, and Fred Binka
    2006   Trend and Causes of Neonatal Mortality in the Kassena-Nankana District in Northern Ghana, 1995–2002. Tropical Medicine and International Health 11:532–39.

Bierlich, Bernhard
    2007   The Problem of Money: African Agency and Western Medicine in Northern
            Ghana. Oxford: Berghahn Books.
Binka, Fred, Bawah Ayaga, James Phillips, Abraham Hodgson, Martin Adjuik,
and Bruce MacLeod
    2007   Rapid Achievement of the Child Survival Millennium Development Goal:
            Evidence from the Navrongo Experiment in Northern Ghana. Tropical Medicine
            and International Health 12(5):578–83.
Binka, Fred, Pierre Ngom, James Phillips, Kubaje Adazu, and Bruce MacLeod
    1999   Assessing Population Dynamics in a Rural African Society: The Navrongo
            Demographic Surveillance System. Journal of Biosocial Science 31:375–91.
Bledsoe, Caroline
    2002   Contingent Lives: Fertility, Time, and Aging in West Africa. Chicago: University
            of Chicago Press.
Cassiman, Ann
    2006   Stirring Life: Women's Paths and Places among the Kasena of Northern Ghana.
            Uppsala: Uppsala University.
Conrad, Peter
    1992   Medicalization and Social Control. Annual Review of Sociology 18:209–32.
Debpuur, Cornelius, James Phillips, Elizabeth Jackson, Alex Nazzar, Pierre Ngom,
and Fred Binka
    2002   The Impact of the Navrongo Project on Contraceptive Knowledge and Use,
            Reproductive Preferences, and Fertility. Studies in Family Planning 33(2):141–64.
Denham, Aaron, Philip Adongo, Cindy Freydberg, and Abraham Hodgson
    2010   Chasing Spirits: Clarifying the Spirit Child Phenomenon and Infanticide in
            Northern Ghana. Social Science and Medicine 71(3):608–15.
Devisch, Rene
    1985   Perspectives on Divination in Contemporary Sub-Saharan Africa. *In* Theoretical
            Explorations in African Religion. Wim van Binsbergen and Matthew Schoffeleers,
            eds. Pp. 50–83. London: KPI.
Douglas, Mary
    1994   Risk and Blame: Essays in Cultural Theory. London: Routledge.
Durkheim, Emile
    1951   Suicide: A Study in Sociology. New York: Free Press.
Farmer, Paul
    2005   Pathologies of Power: Health, Human Rights, and the New War on the Poor.
            Berkeley: University of California Press.
Finkler, Kaja
    2000   Diffusion Reconsidered: Variation and Transformation in Biomedical Practice, a
            Case Study from Mexico. Medical Anthropology 19(1):1–39.
Foege, William
    1988   Plagues: Perceptions of Risk and Social Responses. Social Research 55(3):331–42.
Fortes, Meyer
    1949   The Web of Kinship among the Tallensi. London: Oxford University Press.
Jackson, Michael
    2005   Existential Anthropology: Events, Exigencies, and Effects. New York: Berghahn
            Books.

Kleinman, Arthur
  1995 Writing at the Margin: Discourse between Anthropology and Medicine. Berkeley: University of California Press.
Kleinman, Arthur, and Joan Kleinman
  1991 Suffering and Its Professional Transformation: Toward an Ethnography of Interpersonal Experience. Culture, Medicine, and Psychiatry 15(3):275–301.
Last, Murray
  1992 The Importance of Extremes: The Social Implications of Intra-Household Variation in Child Mortality. Social Science and Medicine 35(6):799–810.
Livingston, Julie
  2005 Debility and the Moral Imagination in Botswana. Bloomington: Indiana University Press.
Mendonsa, Eugene
  1982 The Politics of Divination. Berkeley: University of California Press.
Mills, Samuel, John Williams, George Wak, and Abraham Hodgson
  2007 Maternal Mortality Decline in the Kassena-Nankana District of Northern Ghana. Journal of Maternal and Child Health 12(5):577–85.
Mishler, Elliot
  1981 Viewpoint: Critical Perspectives on the Biomedical Model. *In* The Social Contexts of Health, Illness, and Patient Care. Elliot Mishler, Lorna Amarasingham, Stuart Hauser, Ramsay Liem, and Samuel Osherson, eds. Pp. 1–23. Cambridge: Cambridge University Press.
Mogensen, Hanne
  2005 Medicalized Experience and the Active Use of Biomedicine. *In* Managing Uncertainty: Ethnographic Studies of Illness, Risk and the Struggle for Control. Vibeke Steffen, Richard Jenkins, and Hanne Jessen, eds. Pp. 225–44. Copenhagen: Museum Tusculanum Press.
Navrongo Health Research Center
  2004 Community Health and Family Planning Panel Survey Report 2003. Navrongo: Ghana Health Service.
Nelkin, Dorothy, and Sander Gilman
  1988 Placing Blame for Devastating Disease. Social Research 55(3):361–78.
Ngom, Pierre, Patricia Akweongo, Philip Adongo, Bawah Ayaga, and Fred Binka
  1999 Maternal Mortality among the Kassena-Nankana of Northern Ghana. Studies in Family Planning 30:142–47.
Pinto, Sarah
  2008 Where There Is No Midwife: Birth and Loss in Rural India. New York: Berghahn Books.
Rapp, Rayna, and Faye Ginsburg
  2001 Enabling Disability: Rewriting Kinship, Reimagining Citizenship. Public Culture 13(3):533–56.
Throop, C. Jason
  2010 Suffering and Sentiment: Exploring the Vicissitudes of Experience and Pain in Yap. Berkeley: University of California Press.
Zizek, Slavoj
  2009 Slavoj Zizek: Ecology. *In* Examined Life: Excursions with Contemporary Thinkers. Astra Taylor, ed. Pp. 155–83. New York: New Press.

CHAPTER 10

Imaging Maternal Responsibility
Prenatal Diagnosis and Ultrasound among Haitians in South Florida

Lauren Fordyce

One afternoon toward the end of my ethnographic fieldwork in South Florida, I received a call from the nurse-practitioner at Prenatal Clinic, the public clinic where I was conducting participant-observation. Portia told me that she had given my name and number to a local obstetrician.[1] She explained: "Dr. Albert is the perinatologist who runs the ultrasound clinic where I send the patients who don't have Medicaid. She has some questions and concerns about her Haitian patients, and I told her she should talk to you." Within a week, I was sitting across from Dr. Albert in her patient waiting room with my digital recorder and a list of questions.

Dr. Albert explained that she wanted to speak with me about her frustrations with prenatal counseling among her Haitian patients:

> They make it very hard to do antenatal diagnoses and counseling. [I will say to them,] "As far as I see this on the ultrasound, I think there's an increased risk that your baby might have Down syndrome" or [explain] what Down syndrome is. "This is that, and implies this and that, and you know, we want to try and give you the option of knowing before the baby is born, if the baby has this or not?" I do amnios [amniocentesis] here, but they always decline. I've never had a Haitian patient consent to an amnio.

Dr. Albert's comments echoed much of what I was finding to be most salient in my research with providers who administer prenatal care to Haitian women—that is, the ways in which narratives of risk and responsibility figure prominently within the biopolitics of contemporary pregnancy care (Fordyce 2009). Underlying the choice to use prenatal diagnosis, such as ultrasound or amniocentesis, is the notion that pregnant women have a responsibility to understand the genetic "risks" to their unborn child, as well as a responsibility to use biomedical technologies to "know" these risks (Browner and Press 1995; Hunt and Voogd 2003; Kenen 1996; Lupton 1999b; Rapp 2000; Weir 2006). Ultrasound examinations, an important component of prenatal diagnosis and a gateway to further diagnostic measures, provide a particularly important site for research into these narratives of risk and responsibility in biomedical prenatal care.

While initially used as a diagnostic tool in high-risk pregnancies, ultrasound has become a ubiquitous aspect of prenatal care in the United States, such that it is rare for a woman not to have at least one scan, if not many, during her pregnancy (Georges 2008; Mitchell 2001; Mulcahy 2004; Taylor 2008). For women who have no insurance or Medicaid coverage, ultrasounds done at County Hospital cost US$750, but Dr. Albert, the supervising physician at the private Ultrasound Clinic, worked out an arrangement with Prenatal Clinic by which these patients received an ultrasound for US$175. The majority of the Haitian women I interviewed saw ultrasound as a valuable part of the pregnancy experience and therefore a necessary expense for their families. Questions about their experiences with ultrasound exams solicited a show-and-tell of their fetal photos. Often they would interrupt our conversation to get the images to show me—from their purse or the baby album, in a frame next to their bed, or, in one case, from the glove compartment in the car. Clearly, ultrasound examinations are a highly valued aspect of pregnancy experiences among Haitian immigrant women, yet Dr. Albert's comments on prenatal diagnosis speak precisely to what makes ultrasound such an interesting case study: the ways in which ultrasound is situated as a both a diagnostic tool and a pleasurable experience.

Discourses of risk and responsibility contribute to the creation of particular kinds of subjects: "autonomous, self-regulating moral agents" who voluntarily take up government imperatives and embrace expert advice (Lupton 1999a:105). Yet far from docile bodies, Haitian women are reflexive about the narratives of risk in their everyday lives. And by situating the technologies of prenatal risk within women's experiences in pregnancy, we can begin to explore the varied and dynamic ways in which Haitian women encounter and respond to these discourses of risk and responsibility.

Biopolitics of Being Haitian in the United States

I imagined that when I moved to South Florida I would find the Haitian community bounded by a shared culture, language, and pride in Haiti's legacy as the first black republic, yet one also fractured by notions of race, class, and gender (Glick Schiller and Fouron 2001; Stepick 1997). What I did not expect was that this community was created by much more than the shared history of Haiti; being Haitian in the United States is increasingly shaped by the biopolitics of HIV/AIDS (Farmer 2006[1992]; Sangaramoorthy 2008). No longer simply defined by nation, race, or history, this is a community also shaped by the shared experience of stigma, political violence, diaspora, and notions of risk (Glick Schiller and Fouron 2001; Santana and Dancy 2000; Stepick 1997). While a number of scholars have interrogated the biopolitical links between Haitians in the United States and epidemiological risks for HIV/AIDS (Marc et al. 2010; Marcelin, McCoy, and DiClemente 2006), my own research argues that technologies of risk are also inherently gendered, and by focusing on the everyday practice of prenatal care I wish to draw attention to the proliferating technologies of risk management that inform expectations for maternal behavior. Technologies are not simply the tools and machines used in biomedicine but also the techniques of quantification, systematization, and routinization that aim to manipulate and control risk, as well as to create outcomes assumed to be beneficial to individuals and society (Escobar 1995; Lock and Kaufert 1998). Haitian women, historically linked to analyses of risk based on sexuality and nation, provide an important case study into how women experience technologies of risk in their everyday lives.

The data for this chapter were collected in South Florida over a two-year period, 2004–2006, using qualitative and ethnographic research methods. Recent census figures estimate there are over 200,000 Haitians living in South Florida, but Haitian advocates argue that this number is highly underrepresentative, as an accurate census count of this community remains difficult because of distrust of federal agencies and lack of funding to do necessary outreach in immigrant communities (Brookings Institution Metropolitan Policy Program 2005; Stepick 1997). There were over 11,000 live births to Haitian women in Broward and Miami-Dade Counties during the years 2004 through 2006 (Florida Department of Vital Statistics 2004–2006). According to recent maternal and child health data, Haitian women living in the United States are at risk for poor birth outcomes; they experience higher rates of infant mortality, preterm birth, and low-birth-weight infants than do women of other ethnicities in Miami-Dade County (Healthy Start Coalition of Miami-Dade 2005). Other research indicates a disproportionate rate of congenital anomalies among babies born to Haitian women living in Florida, including atrial septal defects, pulmonary artery anomalies, Down syndrome, and microcephalus, particularly in comparison to "White," "African-American," "Cuban," and "Mexican" women (Beckerman 2005:99).[2] These statistical portraits of risk underscore the growing attention by local health advocates and professionals to Haitian women's use of prenatal diagnosis technologies during pregnancy.

Reproduction provides an important site within contemporary analyses of risk, where fundamental connections between individuals and the collective, the technological and the political, and the legal and the ethical highlight the links between technologies of risk and the making of subjects (Rabinow and Rose 2006). Ideal subjects are expected to be responsible for managing their own risk, as well as to assume responsibility for refraining from actions that may harm themselves or others (Ruhl 1999). This behavior is expected to conform to specific expert advice, and, in the case of health care, to guidelines created by health professionals and biomedical providers. This expert knowledge is in turn informed by biomedical and epidemiological techniques that assist in the identification, treatment, and management of individuals or groups of people. Such expert discourses are particularly significant within prenatal care, where pregnant women are simultaneously cast as an authority and agent in the care of themselves and their fetus, yet also haunted by the specter of the "irresponsible pregnant woman" who threatens the health and well-being of her "unborn child" (Ruhl 1999; Tsing 1990).

Contemporary notions of responsible behavior are shaped by the biomedicalization of pregnancy, as well as structured by notions of class, race, and nation (Ginsburg and Rapp 1991, 1995; Ruhl 1999). Changing notions of fetal subjects, informed by the visualization of fetal life, have also begun to influence expectations for maternal behavior during pregnancy. Building on the legacy of feminist work on fetal images and visualization (Duden 1992, 1993; Haraway 1997; Hartouni 1998; Morgan and Michaels 1999; Stabile 1998, 1999; Taylor 1992, 1997, 2008), this chapter broadens the discussion to include experiences of women outside North American private obstetrical offices (cf. Bashour, Hafez, and Abdulsalam 2005; Gammeltoft 2007; Georges 1997, 2008; Harris et al. 2004; Rapp 2000). Haitian women's experiences with the technologies of pregnancy reflect not only their interests as individuals but also the wider sociopolitical fields of shared engagements and interests (cf. Gammeltoft 2007; Rapp 2000). As the contemporary management of pregnancy increasingly focuses on fetal health, in conjunction with and at times in opposition to maternal health, ultrasound becomes an ever more important space for investigating the links between the narratives of risk and responsibility and the making of subjects.

Staging an Ultrasound

During the past twenty years, ultrasound has become a frequent component of prenatal care because of its perceived value as a simple and noninvasive diagnostic technology. Initially used to detect fetal anomalies such as spina bifida or anencephaly, ultrasound is now used to verify viability, detect gestational age, check for multiples, detect the heartbeat and placenta location, and assist in other diagnostic techniques such as amniocentesis (Taylor 1997). I spent three days observing obstetrical ultrasounds at Dr. Albert's clinic, where I primarily shadowed Cindy, a young, Anglo-American woman who had recently completed her training to become a certified sonographer, and who was responsible for producing the majority of scans at this clinic.[3] Although my observation periods did not correspond with any scans of pregnant Haitian women from Prenatal Clinic, I attained a general understanding of the typical experience the ultrasound scan provided.

While the importance of the inscriptions or fetal images themselves can be overestimated, it is through the staging or scene setting that this set of dramatized inscriptions becomes central. As Taylor notes in her work on ultrasound: "Nothing about the physics of high-velocity sound waves, nor the medical imaging devices constructed to exploit them, *requires* that a diagnostic ultrasound procedure be performed in just the way that it has come to be in this country" (2002:368, emphasis in original). Dr. Albert's clinic has three examination rooms: two devoted to clinical visits and one for ultrasound examinations. Appointments for an ultrasound were scheduled to last half an hour. The scans are performed by a certified technician, such as Cindy, and then reviewed by Dr. Albert. The room was large (particularly in comparison to those at Prenatal Clinic), with discreet lighting and many comfortable leather chairs set around the room for any family and friends who might have accompanied the pregnant woman to the ultrasound screening.

On my first visit to Ultrasound Clinic, I was quickly ushered into a room where a scan was in progress. To my surprise, the pregnant woman reclining next to the ultrasound machine (as the technician rubbed the transducer across her belly) was not even facing the machine's screen. I then realized that the woman and her husband were staring straight ahead, where a large flat-screen TV hung on the wall in front of them. While the technician narrated what they were seeing, the woman and her husband could look at the fetal images in a seemingly cinematic transmission.

During the exam, the sonogram technician stood facing the machine; using her left hand, she adjusted the dials and knobs to obtain various views of the fetus. With her right hand she moved the transducer over the woman's belly or positioned the transvaginal transducer for a particular angle. While I spent only a few days at Ultrasound Clinic, the comments that both Cindy and Dr. Albert expressed to me highlighted their frustration at the view of many women that the point of this experience was only to "see the baby," disregarding the ultrasound's role as an important diagnostic tool. For instance, Cindy told me of a recent patient who had received her twenty-week scan, bringing her entire family, including her five children. The woman did not speak English, so her daughter was translating Cindy's comments into Spanish for her. As they were doing the scan, the daughter started getting excited about what she thought were twins, while Cindy realized that what the young girl thought was another fetus was actually the single fetus's bowels and stomach floating outside of it. She tried to move quickly through the exam and pointed out the findings to Dr. Albert outside the room. They suspected Trisomy 18, which was confirmed by a subsequent amniocentesis.[4] Cindy expressed frustration to me a number of times during my visits when patients seemed to appropriate the technician's diagnostic skills, or when they seemed interested only in the sex of the fetus or in getting a good view.

Many who have been confronted with 2-D ultrasound images can attest to the difficulties in interpreting them without a radiologist or sonographer. Ultrasound involves the use of high-energy sound waves that bounce off internal structures and are converted into electrical signals that are displayed on a screen (Taylor 2008). When we look at an ultrasound, we are not looking at a photograph of a fetus but at a photograph of the scan—that is, the movement that produces the image is the movement of the scanner. These scans actually come from the ultrasound machine and reflect the rendering of the inside of a woman's body (Strathern 2002). These sonographic echoes require interpretation, and a requisite part of the ultrasound examination is the narration/interpretation by the sonographers, describing fetal "life" for the parents-to-be (Georges 2008; Mitchell 2001; Rapp 1997, 2000; Taylor 2008). Countless still images are taken during the course of the examination, and the technician tries to pick the best ones to send home. In some cases, Cindy spent much of the exam trying to get the fetus to roll over or turn a certain way in order to get a face shot or another highly valued shot, such as the feet or the hands (or the genitalia). Particularly in early scans, the feet or the hands are considered most humanlike, attesting to their popularity as well in the world of antiabortion images (see also Ginsburg 1998[1989]:105). Some machines allow the ultrasound technician to tag a descriptive to the scan, such as "leg" or "arm." It is not unusual to see images with the tagline "It's a boy" next to a blurry image of a penis, or "Hi Mommy!" next to a seemingly waving hand.

All the Haitian pregnant women I interviewed had received at least one ultrasound scan during their pregnancy. A portion of these women had received their ultrasound at Dr. Albert's clinic or at the hospital linked to Prenatal Clinic, while many others described for me their ultrasound examinations conducted at a private physician's office or at Jackson Memorial Hospital, the large public hospital in Miami-Dade County. As I have mentioned, most of the women added to their responses to my questions about their ultrasound by showing me their printed ultrasound images and, in some cases, sharing a series of early and later scans. Many women talked about saving their ultrasound images in an album, along with the images from previous pregnancies. Danise, who had saved the images from her pregnancy with her son, already had an album prepared for this child.

> Lauren Fordyce: Did they give you any pictures?
> Danise: Uh-huh. Yeah, it's in my bedroom. I looked, yeah, I did it yesterday.
>   I was looking at it this morning, last night—"Well, how are you?"
> Lauren: Are you going to save it?
> Danise: Yeah, I already have an album, so I am going to put it in there.

Danise assumed that the ultrasound images taken throughout her pregnancy were just more baby photos to save along with other firsts in her baby album. Many women told me that they interacted with their fetal photos, talking, singing, even tickling the image, a contemporary means of bonding with their baby-to-be.

In some cases, ultrasounds reaffirmed potential kin ties between partners. Valerie, whose current pregnancy was with a new partner, used her ultrasound image to announce this new development in their relationship. Her first ultrasound was performed at three weeks for the provider to verify her pregnancy.

> Valerie: Yes, but at three weeks, there was nothing. [Laughter]. Just a little
>   ambiance, yeah, not a big thing.
> Lauren: Do you keep the pictures?
> Valerie: Yes, yes. Because I keep the, the first one—when I was three weeks.
>   I gotta have it home, 'cause the father, he don't know. I feel the thing
>   [the pregnancy], but I don't tell him nothing. I just go on the weekend,
>   the doctor tell me you have to make a sonogram, I say okay, and I make
>   it. He say, "Now you are three weeks pregnant." I take it, and I buy a
>   little card. I put it inside and I give it to the father. When he see, he say,
>   "What's that?!" [Laughter]. I say, "That's your baby." He say, "What?!"
>   and he start to cry.

These ethnographic examples illustrate the ways in which ultrasound imaging can be experienced as pleasurable. "Seeing the baby" is a means for women to demonstrate to potential partners their new kin ties, proof of their nascent family. These sorts of multiplicities of experiences with sonogram imaging validate how tensions between pleasure and risk management become ever more complicated with reproductive technology such as ultrasound and its use in prenatal diagnosis.

Many of the women I spoke with expressed frustration when they did not experience the ultrasound exam as pleasurable, as they had expected. Rose, who was nineteen years old and pregnant with her first child, was living with her aunt and cousins in western Broward County when we spoke one afternoon. She had left Haiti two years earlier to live in Florida and was planning to raise the child herself with the help of her family, as the father of her child lived in Haiti. I met Rose through my work at Prenatal Clinic, and because she qualified for the grant—that is, her prenatal care was subsidized through the county—she had received her ultrasounds at the local hospital. She explained to me that she had four ultrasounds during her pregnancy, and I asked her to describe these experiences.

> Rose: When I went over there, they told me to drink a lot of water, and the first technician, she was good. She tried to help you and she handle [that] you need to pee. She tried to do it quickly, and when she do it she explain everything. "This your baby head, this your baby body, something happened, everything good." I was so excited. That's the only thing, because now you can't feel the baby.
>
> Lauren: And the other technicians, they weren't as helpful, they didn't tell you so much?
>
> Rose: No, no. They didn't tell you. Like the last one, I told her, "How many pounds is the baby?" She didn't say anything. I think she just get out of the university or something and she don't have much experience. I think, if she or they give me a file, a paper to fill out for her, that's going to be bad for her. I am going to complain. She didn't tell me anything.

These tensions of ultrasound as pleasure versus diagnostic technology were returned to again and again, both in my interviews with Haitian women and with Cindy and Dr. Albert. And while the sonographer at Dr. Albert's office had expressed frustration that many of the patients who came to be scanned only wanted to see the baby or learn the sex, Cindy also felt "sorry" for the ultrasound technicians who worked in the hospital. She explained: "At the hospital, they are not allowed to tell the patient anything because of liability issues. Here, I don't point out any abnormalities—Dr. Albert does that. But I can show the patients the hands, the feet, the anatomy, and the sex. I can tell them if things look good. It is too bad for patients who go to the hospital and get no real interaction with the technician."

As described earlier, experiences of ultrasound as enjoyable are not unique to Haitian women. In most cases, ultrasound exams are staged to provide a pleasurable event for the pregnant woman and her family. This practice has only broadened with the move of 3-D ultrasound examinations into consumer spaces in the new industry called "keepsake imaging" (see Taylor 2008).

Keepsake imaging is the newest wave in pregnancy experiences. Located in shopping malls or in strip malls, fetal photo studios often have names like Peek-a-View, Baby Insight, Fetal Fotos, or Womb with a View. These studios advertise fetal photos solely as entertainment for the pregnant woman and her family and encourage the accompaniment of guests. Women are expected to provide documentation of prenatal care and a previous diagnostic sonogram before they can access the services, thereby affirming that this practice is exclusively for pleasure and holds no medical or diagnostic value.

Eugénie, the only woman I interviewed who had received a 3-D/4-D ultrasound, was very excited to share the images with me and describe how meaningful an experience it was. For her, seeing the 3-D/4-D ultrasound allowed her to recognize characteristics of the baby's father in the fetus and facilitated "bonding" with her future daughter. Yet what I think is most intriguing about Eugénie's experience is that it was unique among the women I interviewed. She was the only woman I spoke with who referred to "bonding" in reference to her ultrasound experiences, and the only one who argued that "seeing" the fetus made her "feel" more pregnant.

> I guess with today's modern technology and you can see the kid, it makes the bonding that much closer. At seven weeks when I first saw it, I felt immediately bonded to her. If I didn't go to that doctor appointment [where they did an ultrasound], I probably wouldn't know I was pregnant because I had no symptoms. But once I knew I was pregnant, I suddenly felt pregnant, and I became more conscious. Now I was very conscious of, Oh my God, I can't do this, I can't do that.

While Eugénie's narrative is unique among the women I interviewed, it remains instructive, as it demonstrates contemporary discourses about maternal responsibility and behavior in pregnancy. Early proponents of ultrasound posited its benefit for shaping positive maternal behavior, and innovations in ultrasound technology, particularly the 3-D/4-D keepsake imaging, has contributed to changing notions of fetal life in the contemporary United States (Dewsbury 1980; Fletcher and Evans 1983; Ginsburg 1998[1989]; Hartouni 1997; Mitchell 2001; Petchesky 1987; Taylor 1997). Yet fundamental to this experience is also the presumed value of the sonogram as a key diagnostic tool in prenatal screening. In addition, underlying notions of risk and responsibility become particularly clear in providers' expectations for women's narratives of genetic histories, collected in conjunction with prenatal testing.

Eliciting Risk

Dr. Albert was particularly vocal about her frustrations in soliciting genetic histories from her Haitian patients. In addition to describing these women as indifferent to both ultrasound and prenatal diagnosis, she expressed concern about her ability to adequately assess the risks for Haitian women because they did not recount their medical histories in much detail:

> And the other thing that I find that makes it very difficult to relate to Haitian patients is that they're not always very forthcoming with clinically very significant information. You know, it took me seven antenatal visits to find out that [a Haitian patient] had hemorrhaged at a previous C-section, that she'd had a DVT [deep vein thrombosis] after her first C-section. And, you know, when I recommended anticoagulants and the risk of transfusion, and it's like she wanted nothing of that. And she didn't even think that it was relevant that she mentions these complications to me. She didn't understand why I was upset that she kept that information from me on the initial intake.

This comment echoes Rapp's (2000) ethnographic investigation of the use of amniocentesis by a diverse sample of women in New York, in which she describes how genetic counselors portrayed recent immigrants as having little knowledge of their own heredity, resulting from a lack of awareness about either genetic risks or previous health problems in their family.

Dr. Daniel was a Haitian obstetrician who provided care at a free clinic in Little Haiti, a predominantly Haitian neighbored located in northeastern Miami-Dade County. She provided an alternative analysis as to why Haitian women were less than forthcoming about their genetic history, explaining that many of her patients also differentiate between "natural" illnesses and "spiritual" illnesses, such as deaths resulting from vodou.[5]

> A lot of their family members died from whatever illness. But because they didn't know what illness it was, therefore, it was something not natural. That's very common. "What did your mother die of?" "Somebody didn't like her. They did something [vodou] to her." Nobody in my culture seems to be dying of natural causes. So therefore I reinforce to them—because a lot of my patients are hypertensive or have diabetes—and I say to them, "Your blood pressure is 240/100, you don't have any problem or a headache or anything like that. If you drop dead, your parents are gonna say that somebody did something to you, but the fact is that it's your blood pressure that's so high it's gonna kill you." So I try to put it in perspective for them.

For many Haitian women, family members who died in Haiti may never have received biomedical care and therefore never received a biomedical diagnosis for the illness that might have ultimately led to their death. Throughout Haiti, preventive and emergency biomedical care is unaffordable for most people; furthermore, for those in the rural areas, clinics are few and far between, and for those in Haiti's large urban centers of Port-au-Prince and Cap-Haïtien, years of civil unrest and environmental disasters have exacerbated the difficulties in accessing health care. The coup d'état in Haiti in 2004 was followed by three years of civil unrest characterized by high rates of kidnapping and political violence (Fordyce 2008; Thompson 2005). More recently, the earthquake that devastated Port-au-Prince in January 2010 destroyed the fragile health infrastructure within the capital city, and also resulted in high numbers of displaced people throughout the nation (McRuer 2010).

Gender also remains a key dynamic in the narration of medical histories during prenatal intakes and screenings. It was not uncommon for Haitian women attending Prenatal Clinic to rely on their husbands to translate for them, as many were not completely comfortable with speaking English and not all the nurses spoke Haitian Creole. Kathia, a young Haitian American community health worker at Prenatal Clinic, described for me how many of the older Haitian women defer to their husbands during the intake process

> because husbands don't care [about pregnancy]. Especially Haitian husbands, they are, like, "Whatever, it's a woman thing." They know nothing, nothing about the whole pregnancy thing. They will come here with their wives. And during intake, [the nurse] has a series of questions that she asks them, where she says things, like, you know, "If you're dying, can we give you blood?" And 90 percent of them will turn around and look at the husband, so the husband can answer it. You have some women who have had abortions in their past life and their husbands didn't know, or if they had miscarriages and their husbands don't know. On more than one occasion they'll tell me one thing when their husband is there on their first visit, and then on their next visit they'll say, "I told you last time I had two pregnancies but it was really three." And you gotta go back to the paperwork and put three instead of two. Because the husband is very strict, Haitian husbands are very strict.

What we see in these narratives are certain expectations for how a patient is supposed to behave, what communication between partners is supposed to be, and what is considered to be an autonomous decision. Pregnant women are assumed to embody individualized maternal subjects who take responsibility for knowing not just their genetic history but the sorts of risk such a history presents to their unborn child.

Knowing and Biomedical Technologies of Risk

Amniocentesis is one of the most common forms of genetic testing during pregnancy: a long syringe, guided by ultrasound, is inserted into the amniotic sac to extract a small amount of amniotic fluid. Amniocentesis is recommended for all women over thirty-five years of age, and for any woman who has received a positive maternal serum alpha-fetoprotein test or a problematic ultrasound screening

(ACOG 2002).[6] As I described in the introduction to this chapter, Dr. Albert commented to me that none of her Haitian patients had consented to an amniocentesis, even when it was recommended that they receive one. She felt that even when faced with a troubling ultrasound examination, the Haitian patients were not interested in discussing any further genetic testing, evidently believing "that their baby is going to be the way that it's going to be, you know, with two heads and three legs, and that's the way its going to be. They're not really interested in or they don't seem to grasp the whole concept of antenatal diagnosis. . . . They just take what comes, and they don't—they're on a different level of reality, you know?"

A number of anthropologists have looked at the moral issues that develop in conjunction with prenatal testing during pregnancy, particularly when families are faced with the possibility of deciding to terminate in cases of a positive diagnosis (Browner and Press 1995; Landsman 2008; Rapp 2000; Rothman 1993). But for Dr. Albert, a patient's knowing is equally as valuable, and it was problematic for her that her Haitian patients were uninterested in "knowing" whether their fetus had chromosomal anomalies and therefore uninterested in preparing and educating themselves for living with disabled children.

> Yeah, even if you're not thinking of terminating, there are advantages in
> knowing. First of all, most of the time you'll have good news and you can
> take that out of your mind for the rest of the pregnancy. And you know,
> God forbid there is something wrong with your child, then you'll be able to
> prepare yourself. And to read up on it, and contact resources in your area,
> you know, to help you take care of a child with special needs.

This choice for knowing has begun to inform our everyday notions of pregnancy in the United States, where the decision to not know becomes almost an immoral act. Some scholars have referred to providers' assumption that parents want to know as the "gift of knowing" (Kenen 1996; see also Hunt and Voogd 2003). This gift of knowing is grounded in the assumption that knowledge is intrinsically good, and that knowing the results of prenatal diagnosis would enable parents to make informed decisions. The possession of knowledge is equated with empowerment, as prenatal diagnosis is assumed to result in parents who are empowered to make rational, informed choices (Kenen 1996). Dr. Albert's frustration that Haitian women and their partners refused this gift of knowing illustrates the ethics of responsibility that underlie the contemporary biopolitics of risk management in pregnancy. It is a woman's responsibility to be informed of her fetus's predicted health status and to plan for this future, regardless of the outcome (Lupton 1999b). Yet Haitian women's narratives about prenatal diagnosis illustrate the ways in which it is important to contextualize moral decisions on life and illness within local moral worlds, where women's knowledge, relationships, and lived experiences intersect with this gift of knowing.

In some cases, it was basic ideas about risk that informed Haitian women's choices to use or not use amniocentesis. There is a slight risk of spontaneous abortion after an amniocentesis, and it is estimated that 1 percent of women experiencing this procedure after fifteen weeks' gestation will have a miscarriage (ACOG 2002). Dr. Jean, a Haitian family practitioner who practiced at a regional hospital in South Dade, shared with me her own experience with amniocentesis during her last pregnancy: "They tell you they're gonna put a needle in your stomach, and you wonder what if they hurt the baby. Then they tell you the risk that it might hurt the baby. After the amnio, I lost some fluid, and I had to stay in bed for two days."

And although she understood the risk of the procedure, for her the benefits outweighed this risk. Other Haitian biomedical providers also characterized patients' refusal of prenatal diagnosis as reflecting the simple fact that most Haitian women would not "understand the concept." As Dr. Daniel commented: "Another aspect also with amnio referral, I'm not sure that in the end even if the amnio revealed that there was something wrong with the baby, I'm not sure that they would be able to comprehend what it means. And two, what to do with it? That you have to put a needle in their belly to figure if the baby has a problem with the brain?"

Very few of the women I interviewed had been offered amniocentesis, mainly because the majority of the women I spoke with were under the age of thirty-five or had not been flagged for further genetic testing through ultrasounds or blood tests. Only two acknowledged being offered amniocentesis during the current pregnancy. Marie, a thirty-six-year-old who was pregnant with her third child, explained to me that she was asked to do special tests because of her age: "Uh, they ask me, for a special test, to take some water—that's what I heard. Yeah, so, I told them I don't want the test. Because I heard some people say when you do that, you maybe lose the baby. That's why I told them no, I don't want to do it." Notions of scientific literacy inform the practice of prenatal diagnosis; that women comprehend the risk of miscarriage versus the benefits of knowing is understood to be clear for all women (Rapp 2000).

Haitian providers also pointed out that for many Haitian women, by the time it is recommended that they receive prenatal testing, they have already committed to the pregnancy and therefore would not choose to terminate even if there were a problem. For instance, Dr. Daniels evoked the common belief among Haitian families that humans are unable to interfere with what God determines is meant to be: "Because God gives children, once they have accepted to carry the pregnancy, they will accept it no matter what the consequences." This disinterest in late-term abortion is not evidence that Haitian culture is highly forgiving of disabled individuals. In fact, disabilities are often stigmatized and many families attribute them to interaction between the natural and supernatural world, rather than to genetic or medical origins. For some families, a baby born with a physical or mental disability is paying the price for a family member's spiritual transgression or misdeed (Jacobson 2003). Therefore, this notion that you can know about a disability before birth is not culturally acceptable for many families.

For Marie-Lucie, a thirty-five-year-old who was offered amniocentesis because of her advanced maternal age, this act of knowing would not change the way she felt about her pregnancy or her child-to-be:

I have to say, when they do the amniocentesis, they going to found the baby has a Trisomy 18 or Down's syndrome, or spina bifida, everything. I just ask them, "What am I going to do after that?" So after I get the results I have to either decide to keep it or not. But I already decide to keep it, so I just keep praying. Not that I am, like, not pro-technology or stuff. I just don't see why I am going to do this. If it was something just draw my blood or something, but I don't like invasive procedures. All this for nothing. For some people they may want to terminate the pregnancy or the baby is not well, but I am not gonna do that.

Finally, Haitian biomedical providers question whether telling a woman that she is going to have a disabled child actually helps her in any way. As Dr. Daniel commented to me: "So therefore, if I'm not helping her in any other way but just telling her that she's gonna have an abnormal child, then I haven't done anything for the patient. So let her have her baby and let her see for herself that as he grows or she grows this isn't a normal child."

In other words, cultural understandings about disability and family also influence Haitian women's acceptance of the responsibility to know genetic risks during pregnancy.

Conclusion

In the introduction to this chapter, I described one perinatologist's frustration with providing prenatal care and diagnosis to her Haitian patients. She was interested in speaking with me in order to gain an understanding of what she felt was their indifference to the value of prenatal diagnosis, and particularly, her frustrations in soliciting reproductive and genetic histories and promoting risk management among her Haitian clients. Much of this frustration illustrates the tensions that exist with the use of ultrasound in contemporary pregnancy care: it is a technology that has come to be situated as both pleasurable and diagnostic. Central to these tensions are specific narratives of risk and responsibility. Underlying the choice to use prenatal diagnosis is the notion that pregnant women must be aware of the genetic risks for their unborn child and take advantage of biomedical technologies to know these risks (Rapp 2000).

In this chapter, I used an ethnographic investigation of ultrasound and prenatal diagnosis in pregnancy among Haitian women living in South Florida to critically examine the links between the technologies of risk and the making of subjects. Building on the work of contemporary scholars of reproduction who focus on pregnancy to draw attention to the proliferating technologies of risk management, this chapter demonstrates the plurality of experiences that influence Haitian women's use of ultrasound and prenatal diagnosis. Notions of risk are embodied and understood in dynamic ways, where ideas about family, genetics, disability, and gender shape these experiences (Browner and Press 1995; Landsman 2000; Rapp

1998, 2000). While ultrasound examinations were highly valued for the chance to see the baby, opportunities for knowing prenatal risks for disability and chromosomal problems were problematic both ethically and culturally.

While my ethnographic work with providers in South Florida sensitizes me to the difficulties and frustrations in working within a diverse and impoverished community with little resources, it is also relevant for providers to become aware of the realities and ideologies that inform Haitian families' decisions to engage with profiles of risk. For instance, Dr. Daniel, a Haitian obstetrician who practices at both the large public hospital in Miami and a small satellite clinic in Miami's Little Haiti neighborhood, explained how her "cultural competency" played an important role in making decisions about what constitutes the best care for her "high-risk" patients: "I want to do what's best for the mother. But I also know that sending them to Jackson [Memorial Hospital] is not necessarily the best thing for them. So, therefore, I would rather follow a high-risk pregnancy with my cultural competency and a very close one-on-one relationship than have her sent to the big Jackson where she's gonna be a number and not understand what's going on." I am not suggesting that pregnant Haitian women will receive the best care only from Haitian obstetricians, but I wish to illustrate the varied and dynamic ways in which Haitian women respond to and experience these discourses of risk and responsibility. Providers must become mindful of discourses of scientific literacy, which are assumed within recommendations for prenatal diagnosis and some of which do not conform to lived experiences of pregnancy, disability, and notions of risk for poor birth outcomes (see Rapp 2000). In addition, this work reveals how changing notions of fetal subjects, particularly the contemporary emphasis on knowing the intimacies of fetal life, have come to be intricately linked to ideas about maternal responsibility, as well as how these ideas have come to shape the biomedical management of maternal bodies.

Acknowledgments

This research was funded by a National Science Foundation—Science, Technology and Society Dissertation Improvement Grant. This chapter has benefited greatly from the revisions and suggestions of Florence Babb, Traci Yoder, Michael Ames, and Amínata Maraesa, as well as from the helpful comments of two anonymous reviewers.

Notes

1. All names in this chapter are pseudonyms. This research was approved by the University of Florida Institutional Review Board and the Ethics Board, North Broward Hospital District.
2. While no research has evaluated the high rates of these anomalies among Haitian women, in my own discussions with Haitian providers they emphasize that these data reflect high rates of birth defects among infants "born" to Haitian women. They argue that because of the rejection of late-term abortion by Haitian women, most likely the high rates of "birth defects" in comparison to those in other racial/ethnic com-

munities in Florida result from continuing pregnancies that most likely would have been terminated among other groups (see also Fordyce 2008).

3.   Cindy was known only by her first name to patients at the ultrasound clinic, which may reflect her lower-status job as a health professional with little authority. For more discussion on obstetric ultrasonography as "women's" work, see Taylor (2002).

4.   Trisomy 18 is a genetic disorder related to the eighteenth chromosome. There is a very low rate of survival among infants born with Trisomy 18, often because of heart abnormalities, kidney problems, and other internal organ disorders (ACOG 2002).

5.   Vodou is a form of religious practice and ideology prevalent in Haiti. Although practitioners of vodou emphasize its healing modalities, popular and sensationalized depictions of vodou practices emphasize its malevolent expression.

6.   The maternal serum alpha-fetoprotein test is given to pregnant women to measure alpha-fetoprotein as a means to screen for a number of developmental abnormalities, such as neural tube defects and Down syndrome. The test itself does not signal that these problems definitively exist but results in a referral for more high-level testing, such as ultrasounds and amniocentesis (ACOG 2002; Browner and Press 1995).

References

American College of Obstetrics and Gynecology [ACOG]
   2002   Guidelines for Perinatal Care. Fifth Edition. Elk Grove Village, IL: American Academy of Pediatrics; Washington, DC: American College of Obstetricians and Gynecologists.

Bashour, Hyam, Raghda Hafez, and Asmaa Abdulsalam
   2005   Syrian Women's Perceptions and Experiences of Ultrasound Screening in Pregnancy: Implications for Antenatal Policy. Reproductive Health Matters 13(25):147–54.

Beckerman, Adela
   2005   Birth Defects as an Indicator of the Health Status of Haitian Women and Their Children. Journal of Health and Social Policy 22(1):93–109.

Brookings Institution Metropolitan Policy Program
   2005   The Haitian Community in Miami-Dade: A Growing the Middle-Class Supplement. www.brookings.edu/reports/2005/09cities_sohmer.aspx, accessed June 4, 2007.

Browner, Carole, and Nancy Ann Press
   1995   The Normalization of Prenatal Diagnostic Screening. *In* Conceiving the New World Order: The Global Politics of Reproduction. Faye Ginsburg and Rayna Rapp, eds. Pp. 307–22. Berkeley: University of California Press.

Dewsbury, Anton
   1980   What the Fetus Feels [letter]. British Medical Journal (16 February):481.

Duden, Barbara
   1992   Visualizing "Life." Science as Culture 3(4):562–600.
   1993   Disembodying Women: Perspectives on Pregnancy and the Unborn. Cambridge, MA: Harvard University Press.

Escobar, Arturo
   1995   Encountering Development: The Making and the Unmaking of the Third World. Princeton, NJ: Princeton University Press.

Farmer, Paul
  2006[1992]   Aids and Accusation: Haiti and the Geography of Blame. Berkeley:
     University of California Press.
Fletcher, John, and Mark Evans
  1983   Maternal Bonding in Early Fetal Ultrasound Examinations. New England Journal
     of Medicine 308(7):392–93.
Florida Department of Vital Statistics
  2004, 2005, 2006   Annual Report 2004–2006. Tallahassee, Florida. www.flpublichealth
     .com/VSBOOK/VSBOOK.aspx, accessed November 14, 2007.
Fordyce, Lauren
  2008   Birthing the Diaspora: Technologies of Risk among Haitians in South Florida.
     Ph.D. dissertation, University of Florida.
  2009   Social and Clinical Risk Assessment among Pregnant Haitian Women in South
     Florida. Journal of Midwifery and Women's Health 54(6):477–82.
Gammeltoft, Tine
  2007   Sonography and Sociality: Obstetrical Ultrasound Imaging in Urban Vietnam.
     Medical Anthropology Quarterly 21(2):133–53.
Georges, Eugenia
  1997   Fetal Ultrasound Imaging and the Production of Authoritative Knowledge in
     Greece. In Childbirth and Authoritative Knowledge: Cross-Cultural Perspectives.
     Robbie Davis-Floyd and Carolyn Sargent, eds. Pp. 91–112. Berkeley: University
     of California Press.
  2008   Bodies of Knowledge: The Medicalization of Reproduction in Greece. Nashville:
     Vanderbilt University Press.
Ginsburg, Faye
  1998[1989]   Contested Lives: The Abortion Debate in an American Community.
     Berkeley: University of California Press.
Ginsburg, Faye, and Rayna Rapp
  1991   Politics of Reproduction. Annual Review of Anthropology 20:311–43.
  1995   Introduction: Conceiving the New World Order. In Conceiving the New World
     Order. Faye Ginsburg and Rayna Rapp, eds. Pp. 1–18. Berkeley: University of
     California Press.
Glick Schiller, Nina, and Georges Fouron
  2001   Georges Woke Up Laughing: Long-Distance Nationalism and the Search for
     Home. Durham, NC: Duke University Press.
Haraway, Donna
  1997   Modest_Witness@Second_Millenium.FemaleMan©_Meets_OncoMouse™. New
     York: Routledge.
Harris, Gillian, Linda Connor, Andrew Bisits, and Nick Higginbottam
  2004   "Seeing the Baby": Pleasures and Dilemmas of Ultrasound Technologies for
     Primiparous Australian Women. Medical Anthropology Quarterly 18(1):23–47.
Hartouni, Valerie
  1997   Cultural Conceptions: On Reproductive Technologies and the Remaking of Life.
     Minneapolis: University of Minnesota Press.
  1998   Fetal Exposures: Abortion Politics and the Optics of Allusion. In The Visible

Woman: Imaging Technologies, Gender and Science. Paula Treicheler, Lisa Cartwright, and Constance Penley, eds. Pp. 198–216. New York: New York University Press.

Healthy Start Coalition of Miami-Dade
    2005   Healthy Start Needs Assessment. www.hscmd.org/NeedsAssessment.asp, accessed October 5, 2006.

Hunt, Linda, and Katherine de Voogd
    2003   Autonomy, Danger, and Choice: The Moral Imperative of an "At Risk" Pregnancy for a Group of Low-Income Latinas in Texas. *In* Risk, Culture, and Health Inequality: Shifting Perceptions of Danger and Blame. Barbara Herr Harthorn and Laury Oaks, eds. Pp. 37–56. Westport, CT: Praeger.

Jacobson, Eric
    2003   An Introduction to Haitian Culture for Rehabilitation Service Providers. CIRRIE: Center for International Rehabilitation Research Information and Exchange. Buffalo: State University of New York.

Kenen, Regina
    1996   The At-Risk Health Status and Technology: A Diagnostic Invitation and the "Gift" of Knowing. Social Science and Medicine 42(11):1545–53.

Landsman, Gail
    2008   Reconstructing Motherhood and Disability in the Age of "Perfect" Babies. New York: Routledge Press.

Lock, Margaret, and Patricia Kaufert
    1998   Introduction. *In* Pragmatic Women and Body Politics. Margaret Lock and Patricia Kaufert, eds. Pp. 1–27. Cambridge: Cambridge University Press.

Lupton, Deborah
    1999a   Risk. London: Routledge Press.
    1999b   Risk and the Ontology of Pregnant Embodiment. *In* Risk and Sociocultural Theory: New Directions and Perspectives. Deborah Lupton, ed. Pp. 59–85. Cambridge: Cambridge University Press.

Marc, Linda, Alpa Patel-Larson, H. Irene Hall, Denise Hughes, Margarita Alegría, Georgette Jeanty, Yanick Sanon Eveillard, Eustache Jean-Louis, and National Haitian-American Health Alliance
    2010   HIV among Haitian-born Persons in the United States, 1985–2007. AIDS: Official Journal of the International AIDS Society 24(13):2089–97.

Marcelin, Louis Herns, H. Virginia McCoy, and Ralph DiClemente
    2006   HIV/AIDS Knowledge and Beliefs among Haitian Adolescents in Miami-Dade County, Florida. Journal of HIV/AIDS Prevention in Children and Youth 7(1):121–38.

McRuer, Robert
    2010   Reflections on Disability in Haiti. Journal of Literary and Cultural Disability Studies 4(3):327–32.

Mitchell, Lisa
    2001   Baby's First Picture: Ultrasound and the Politics of Fetal Subjects. Toronto: University of Toronto Press.

Morgan, Lynn, and Meredith Michaels, eds.
    1999   Fetal Subjects, Feminist Positions. Philadelphia: University of Pennsylvania Press.

Mulcahy, Nicholas
  2004   Obstetric Ultrasound More Common Than Previously Reported. Ob.Gyn. News
          39(12):5.
Oaks, Laury
  2000   Smoking and Pregnancy: The Politics of Fetal Protection. New Brunswick, NJ:
          Rutgers University Press.
Petchesky, Rosalind Pollock
  1987   Fetal Images: The Power of Visual Culture in the Politics of Reproduction.
          Feminist Studies 13(2):263–92.
Rabinow, Paul, and Nikolas Rose
  2006   Biopower Today. BioSocieties 1(2):195–217.
Rapp, Rayna
  1997   Real-Time Fetus: The Role of Sonogram in the Age of Monitored Reproduction.
          In Cyborgs and Citadels: Anthropological Interventions in Emerging Sciences and
          Technologies. Gary Lee Downey and Joseph Dumit, eds. Pp. 31–48. Sante Fe:
          School of American Research Press.
  2000   Testing the Woman, Testing the Fetus: The Social Impact of Amniocentesis in
          America. New York: Routledge.
Rothman, Barbara Katz
  1993   The Tentative Pregnancy: How Amniocentesis Changes the Experience of
          Motherhood. New York: W. W. Norton.
Ruhl, Lealle
  1999   Liberal Governance and Prenatal Care: Risk and Regulation in Pregnancy.
          Economy and Society 28(1):95–117.
Sangaramoorthy, Thurka
  2008   Invisible Americans: Immigrants, Transnationalism, and the Politics of Difference
          in HIV/AIDS Research. Studies in Ethnicity and Nationalism 8(2):248–66.
Santana, Marie-Anne, and Barbara Dancy
  2000   The Stigma of Being Named "Aids Carriers" on Haitian-American Women.
          Health Care for Women International 21(3):161–71.
Stabile, Carol
  1998   Shooting the Mother: Fetal Photography and the Politics of Disappearance. *In*
          The Visible Woman: Imaging Technologies, Gender and Science. Paula Treicheler,
          Lisa Cartwright, and Constance Penley, eds. Pp. 171–98. New York: New York
          University Press.
  1999   The Traffic in Fetuses. *In* Fetal Subjects, Feminist Positions. Lynn Morgan and
          Meredith Michaels, eds. Pp. 133–58. Philadelphia: University of Pennsylvania
          Press.
Stepick, Alex
  1997   Pride against Prejudice: Haitians in the United States. Needham Heights, MA:
          Allyn and Bacon.
Strathern, Marilyn
  2002   On Space and Depth. *In* Complexities: Social Studies of Knowledge Practices.
          John Law and Annemarie Mol, eds. Pp. 85–115. Durham, NC: Duke University
          Press.

Taylor, Janelle
  1992   The Public Foetus and the Family Car: From Abortion Politics to a Volvo
          Advertisement. Science as Culture 3(4):601–18.
  1997   Image of Contradiction: Obstetrical Ultrasound in American Culture. *In*
          Reproducing Reproduction: Kinship, Power and Technological Innovation.
          Sarah Franklin and Heléna Ragoné, eds. Pp. 15–45. Philadelphia: University of
          Pennsylvania Press.
  2002   The Public Life of the Fetal Sonogram and the Work of the Sonographer. Journal
          of Diagnostic Medical Sonography 18:367–79.
  2008   The Public Life of the Fetal Sonogram. New Brunswick, NJ: Rutgers University
          Press.
Thompson, Ginger
  2005   A New Scourge Afflicts Haiti: Kidnappings. New York Times, June 6.
Tsing, Anna
  1990   Women Charged with Perinatal Endangerment. *In* Uncertain Terms: Negotiating
          Gender in American Culture. Faye Ginsburg and Anna Tsing, eds. Pp. 282–89.
          Boston: Beacon Press.
Weir, Lorna
  2006   Pregnancy, Risk and Biopolitics: On the Threshold of the Living Subject. New
          York: Routledge.

CHAPTER 11

A Competition over Reproductive Authority
Prenatal Risk Assessment in Southern Belize

Amínata Maraesa

By six o'clock on Wednesday mornings the market in the town of Punta Gorda is already buzzing with distant villagers and local townspeople. While there are a few Garinagu merchants selling cassava sweets and Mestizo-owned dry-goods storefronts, most of the vendors are rural-dwelling Kekchi- and Mopan-speaking Maya—primarily women—who come into town to sell a variety of harvested items such as root vegetables, beans, and culantro leaves. Meanwhile, their children are dispersed throughout town selling vegetables from plastic buckets they carry door-to-door for the townspeople who might not get to the market to shop. "You no wan' buy?" is a familiar query heard through the house windows, which at 6:30 a.m. are just beginning to open to the day's sun and the fresh breeze blowing off the Bay of Honduras that borders this anything-but-sleepy town in the Toledo District of southern Belize.

Although the rural communities of Toledo are seemingly isolated from town life—scattered throughout a mountainous and water-logged topography, separated by long stretches of dirt road where few vehicles pass—the population of this relatively small geographic region is connected within itself and to the urban center in various multistranded relationships of blood, marriage, and commerce (Williams 1973). All roads lead to town, where villagers use the early-morning shopping time to make some money, obtain goods, and catch up on the latest news and gossip from within the region and beyond. After making their initial purchases and marking larger items to be picked up by the bus driver for their return trip, many of the pregnant women who have come to town on this day head away from the market commotion in the direction of the local hospital. Swaying under the weight of their protruding bellies, the women trickle into the faded yellow public health building, which opens every Wednesday morning at eight o'clock to serve the thirty or so women who come in from the surrounding villages for prenatal care each week.

This chapter looks at the interplay between nurse-midwives and pregnant women concerning reproductive risk, as the prenatal examination room becomes an arena for competing knowledge systems where nurse-midwives and pregnant women often negotiate opposing viewpoints concerning maternal and child health. Although they represent a purportedly acultural biomedical authority, the rural and public health nurse-midwives in charge of administering the Ministry of Health prenatal care services in the Toledo District are part of the local cultural matrix, adjusting the administration of standardized protocols to try to accommodate a local reality. Nonetheless, pregnant women in this area continue to make their reproductive decisions based on their preexisting beliefs—incorporating only the advice that is feasible given the concrete realities of their daily lives (cf. Markens, Browner, and Press 1999). As nurse-midwives struggle to convey and maintain the authority of international biomedical standards and a discourse of risk that relies on a constructed objectivity to validate its superiority, pregnant women have their own perception of risk and interpret the health of their pregnancies through a reliance on an embodied understanding of their previous and current reproductive conditions as well as their social and environmental realities. Usually these contrasting perspectives result in disregard by the pregnant women for the information relayed to them by the Ministry of Health nurses during the prenatal examination. At times, these divergent understandings erupt into heated—yet respectful—competition for authority.

Some Notes on Language

Because of its unique history, Belize is the only English-speaking country in Central America. Despite the increasing influx of Spanish-speaking immigrants from neighboring Latin America, English remains the national language. More commonly heard, however, is Belize Creole, an English-based language that contains words derived from Amerindian and African languages, as well as words and phrases from Spanish and American English (Young 1995). Despite the frequency of Garifuna linguistic communication among the Garinagu residents of Toledo and the prevalence of Kekchi and Mopan as the first languages of these Maya populations, Belize Creole is the lingua franca of social life and a common communicative thread that binds the multiethnic and multilingual populations in the Toledo District.

In this chapter, I have transcribed the words of individuals speaking Belize Creole, including those speaking Belize Creole as a second language, as they were uttered to include grammatical structures that do not conform to the rules of Standard English. However, I have chosen to minimize my use of phonetic transcription to facilitate the readability of direct quotations. Although the full effect of the Belizean "voice" (accent) may not be readily perceived, I believe that the transcripts are easier to comprehend and require less translation. One common Belize Creole linguistic structure that occurs throughout the speech reported in this chapter is the copular variant *di* [pronounced "dee"] (present tense) and *mi* [pronounced "mee"] (past tense), which is used in place of the Standard English verb "to be" (Escure 1992). "I mi see it" means "I did see it" or "I saw it." "I di see it" means "I am seeing it" or "I see it." When this grammatical element of Belize Creole has been used, I have not translated transcripts unless other aspects of the speech are difficult to comprehend by a Standard English speaker.

The Influence of Demographic Particularities

Belize is located in Central America, surrounded by Mexico to the north, Guatemala to the west and south, and the Caribbean Sea to the east. Its territory includes a multitude of small islands and mangrove tangles that dot the Great Barrier Reef off its Caribbean coastline. The estimated 2009 midyear population of 333,200 individuals is almost equally divided male/female and found in near equal proportion in both urban and rural settings, with an extremely low average population density of 31.9 persons per square mile (Statistical Institute of Belize 2007, 2009). The Belizean census enumerates its population by its six predominant ethnic groups (Creole, Mestizo, Garifuna, Maya, East Indian, and Chinese), leaving room for "Other," yet statistically ignoring the many interethnic unions that characterize the country's self-proclaimed melting pot.

Indeed, research among primary school children in the town of Punta Gorda revealed that close to half the students were ethnically mixed (Haug 2002). Nonetheless, when looking at contemporary Belizean society, it is impossible to ignore the continued colonial legacy of racial/ethnic hierarchy (Bolland 1977) and Belize's current relationship with the United States and its two-tiered racial system (Shoman 2000). These racial—and racist—ideologies influence the social hierarchy to the extent that most people I spoke with in Toledo were undisturbed by interethnic relationships, yet many expressed a strong desire to lighten the complexion of their offspring by forming a relationship with a person of a lighter skin tone. For many, ethnic identity was often secondary to skin color when choosing a sexual partner and may suggest a more "dynamic" understanding of race and ethnicity (Barnett 2002; Bolland 2003[1988]:210). While race and ethnicity are crucial to understanding the cultural practices that shape women's reproductive lives, I do not take race or ethnicity prima facie. I use ethnically based statistical social indicators to frame my data and address these categories as they entered my research. The arguments I put forth in this chapter thus prioritize the lived social realities of the residents of the Toledo District, emphasizing the strong influence of geographical constraints and environmental factors unrelated to somatic categories of difference.

Moreover, the Toledo District is unique when compared to national statistical averages. The African-descended Garinagu settled the district's only urban center, the town of Punta Gorda, in 1859 (Hall 2007:23). Representing 6.2 percent of the country's total population, they are a statistical minority; however, they remain a significant presence in Toledo at 30.8 percent of the district's urban population (Central Statistical Office 2006). The overwhelming majority of Toledo's residents, however, are rural (82.2 percent) and dominated by the Kekchi- and Mopan-speaking Maya, who make up a 65.4 percent majority compared to a 10.6 percent national average (Central Statistical Office 2006; Statistical Institute of Belize 2009).[1] Although the linguistically distinct Maya populations are lumped together for purposes of census taking, each group has a distinct history of immigration and settlement, which, in the Toledo District, is characterized by a fluid border relationship with family and economic markets in neighboring Guatemala.

Indeed, in the Toledo District the distinction between urban and rural residency patterns often maps onto ethnicity. This relates to my research in that I found both ethnicity and environment to influence the type of care available to pregnant women in the Toledo District and the choices they make about their reproductive lives, as well as the choices from which they have to select. At the same time, I argue that the unique and distinct economic and geographical constraints in Toledo often serve to flatten intradistrict ethnic distinction (see Grant 1976) while still emphasizing the stratification of Toledo women's reproductive practices (Colen 1995).[2] In other words, the social categories of ethnicity and race at play in the Toledo District are linked to structural factors (like accessibility) and cultural practices (like the prevalence of home births) that tangibly affect women's reproductive lives. Yet certain attitudes and practices surrounding issues of shame and force remained consistent, with varying degrees of intensity, throughout the district's populations. Moreover, Toledo as a whole occupies an inferior social position relative to rest of the country's five districts—linked no doubt to its unique environmental circumstances, obscuring intradistrict variation vis-à-vis the Belizean totality.

The dual influences of structure and culture are apparent in the prenatal care available to and sought out by Monica and Rossana, eighteen- and nineteen-year-old Kekchi-speaking women from San Lazaro village in Toledo, which is located thirty-five miles from town and within walking distance of Guatemala. They are both in the last month of their third pregnancies—both had their first babies at age fifteen—and they left their children, who range in age from two to four, in San Lazaro with their mothers-in-law. Monica and Rossana had their first prenatal examinations a few weeks ago at the mobile clinic that sets up an ad hoc facility every six weeks in the village's community center. During this visit they were advised by the nurse-midwife to go to the prenatal clinic in town for the complete physical routinely conducted on the first visit. In addition to a check of general physical condition, medical personnel take blood at this first appointment to measure hemoglobin levels and to check for sexually transmitted diseases, including HIV. Nurse-midwives check the breasts for cancerous lumps and examine the vagina for infectious secretions. None of these procedures are done at the mobile clinic for a number of reasons; most notably, the lack of hygienic and private space prohibits getting undressed, and blood vials cannot be adequately transported by the mobile health team.

When Monica and Rossana arrived at the hospital's prenatal clinic, they learned that their blood results would not be ready before their babies were born, and any medication prescribed for the yeast and urinary tract infections from which they were both suffering would have little effect, as it would be prescribed so late in their pregnancies. Based on a physical assessment of their inner eyelids and their general pallor, they were deemed anemic and given more iron pills and folic acid tablets. While they had also received iron pills from the mobile health team a week earlier, raising iron levels in the blood takes months that neither Monica nor Rossana have before they give birth. Possible complications from anemia include postpartum hemorrhaging—the leading cause of maternal mortality worldwide (USAID 2007) and in Belize (PAHO 2001).

Initiating prenatal care at such a late stage obviates the ability to correct nutritional deficiencies, which may result in babies with low birth weight or other maternal complications such as anemia. As part of the Safe Motherhood initiatives prescribed by the World and Pan American Health Organizations in the late 1990s, rural health nurses are promoting an early and increased use of prenatal care, advising pregnant women served only by the mobile clinics to come to one of the permanently stationed prenatal clinics, since the six-week mobile schedule—corresponding to vaccination booster shots—provides inadequate coverage for the monthly prenatal schedule. Because women in the Toledo District are known on average to begin prenatal care in their second trimester, the subsequent mobile visit—ever contingent upon weather and road conditions—might occur too late to avoid complications or to treat medical high risk, if present. Often it arrives in time to vaccinate the newborn, as the woman has already given birth in the interim. These standardized cycles of care make sense from the administrative perspective of national health care officials and international program advisers, but they often do not correspond to individual pregnancy cycles. As one rural health nurse lamented: "By the time we see her again, she done have the baby." Indeed, for Monica and Rossana, the next mobile clinic would arrive after their babies are due. Although the prenatal visit occurred too late to help them lower their risk of anemia-induced hemorrhaging, they took the advice of the rural health nurse and came to the clinic at the town hospital. But their reasons may well have been nonmedical. Being in town gave them a chance to do some shopping.

Engaging Risk: Belief Systems and Compliance

Active participation and collaboration is instrumental to the public health initiatives of the Belizean Ministry of Health. The prenatal clinic is no exception. Using the language of community-based public health, local health officials expect women to "join" the prenatal clinic to minimize the risk factors that might result in an unhealthy pregnancy and possible maternal or child death. The rural and public health nurses advise them to do so through active outreach, using a participatory language of encouragement to convey the need to begin prenatal care within the first trimester. However, they have also been known to use a culturally sanctioned pedagogy of scolding women in public when they are seen on the street pregnant but have yet to "join clinic" (see Young, this volume, for a similar reaction in Tanzania). This shame-inducing linguistic act often prompts women to join clinic lest they incur social disapproval. Although nurse-midwives emphasize the need to begin early prenatal care, most pregnant women come only after they have experienced the embodied confirmation of pregnancy with the sensation of fetal movement that usually occurs in the second trimester. Since many women in the Toledo District do not have the extra money to pay for a pregnancy test, once they have ceased to menstruate they verify that they are pregnant when they first start to feel fetal movement at around the fourth or fifth month of gestation. Even then, they might wait until they feel minor discomfort or intolerable pain that suggests a possible complication before seeking some form of prenatal care. Sometimes, women are too busy with their daily lives to begin the monthly clinic schedule, which, depending on the distance traveled, could take the better half of an entire day. Others are motivated only by the need for a prenatal record to facilitate the birth registry. And some seek to avoid the intake examination until they have felt the nurse's verbal "lashings."[3]

Because of the country's small population (a little over 300,000) and participatory health care strategies (including the vigilante watchfulness of individual nurses), the Belizean Ministry of Health is able to monitor its pregnant population, ensuring that every pregnant woman is accounted for at the ministry's prenatal clinics. While the official statistics of Belize boast a near 100 percent coverage for prenatal care, with the Toledo District ranking at complete coverage (Government of Belize 1997; Belize Ministry of Health 2005), pregnant women start prenatal care late into their pregnancies and may be seen by a nurse-midwife only once or twice before their baby is born. This behavior may be partly attributed to the distance traveled and time needed for rural-dwelling women to attend the prenatal appointment. However, urban women are just as likely to begin prenatal care well into the second trimester.

Another salient factor contributing to the late onset of prenatal care is the woman's marital status and the cultural stigma associated with unwed motherhood that is prevalent in this Catholic-dominated community. As with other regions in the Caribbean, common-law unions are the dominant form of heterosexual conjugational relations in the Toledo District. Nonetheless, many women having their first child are not necessarily in a long-term or stable union and may be more apt to concealing their pregnancies as long as possible. Indeed, all but one of the nine women from town who attended a class held at the hospital to educate primaparas about pregnancy and newborn care were unmarried, and only the married woman expressed her happiness at finding out that she was pregnant. Most of the women explained that they were "vexed" when they discovered the pregnancy and did not tell anyone until they could no longer deny their condition.

Other cultural edicts are likewise inhibiting. Although pregnancy is considered a normal condition for women of childbearing age and is perceived as a rite of passage into womanhood (Kerns 1997[1983]; McClusky 2001), Belizeans in the Toledo District across ethnic lines generally view anything related to female genital activity as a cause for shame. As such, pregnancy, indexical of genital intercourse, is inherently shameful. The shame is further compounded if the woman is not married. Furthermore, childbirth itself is perceived as a source of shame because the baby emerges from the woman's vagina. Any public exposure or public discussion of the genitals is likewise shame inducing. Most women therefore remark that they dread the first prenatal examination "when they naked you" to check for infectious vaginal secretions and potentially cancerous breast lumps. A twenty-three-year-old Kekchi-speaking Maya woman from a village relatively close to town questioned: "Why the nurse have to naked you the first time you go to clinic? The Indian no got AIDS!" And women who live in town are just as likely to begin the prenatal clinic at this late stage because of the shame involved in the first examination. At a discussion between a nurse-midwife and a group of first-time mothers from town, a twenty-one-year-old Garifuna woman exclaimed: "Mek I strip naked de worst part!" to which the nurse-midwife—also Garifuna—rhetorically asked: "How uno mek de baby if uno shame to take off uno clothes?" [How did you (plural) make the baby if you (plural) are so ashamed to take off your clothes?]. This disdainful comment elicited gales of laughter from the women at the table, but it probably did nothing to ease the restrictive cultural beliefs surrounding women's reproductive bodies and activities. For the nurse-midwives who are trying to locally situate the objective prenatal care recommendations of the Safe Motherhood campaign, shame emerges as a prevalent and gendered risk factor that, compounded with environmental constraints and women's busy quotidian lives, effectively inhibits the ability of the nurse-midwives to attain its goals of providing early and consistent prenatal care. Nonetheless, nurse-midwives are active in their pursuit of pregnant bodies to provide regular and individualized forms of culturally relevant and culturally informed prenatal care whenever—and wherever—possible.

Risk as a Category of Differential Understanding: Assessment, Interpretation, and Agency

Nurse Ical is a Mopan speaker and the only male nurse-midwife in the entire country. He conducts prenatal examinations at the town hospital and on mobile clinics to remote villages. These examinations last roughly ten to fifteen minutes and cover a range of standardized diagnostic questions in addition to a physical examination of the fetus, for which Nurse Ical palpates the uterus and listens to the fetal heartbeat, discerning gestation by measuring the height of the fundus with a tape measure.[4] Often he would laugh and say, "They didn't teach us this in nursing school," as he verified the tape measurement with a technique learned from the now deceased home-birth nanny midwives who practiced in Toledo well into the 1990s: from the pubis to navel measured twenty-four weeks; then each finger, held tightly against the adjacent fingers, represented an additional week to the top of the uterus. "But my fingers are thick, so I have to cup them like this," he explained, as he squeezed his fingers together even tighter to embody what he perceived to be a more accurate measurement of the fundal height. Some women expressed to me their shame at having a man touch their bellies. However, many also cited Nurse Ical's mix of traditional practices with more modern ones as a form of superior midwifery knowledge that outweighed his gender shortcoming. Based on the information gathered during the examination, Nurse Ical offers advice concerning diet and nutrition interspersed with limited psychological counseling.

Pursuant to a survey conducted in 1988, which found that 40.2 percent of pregnant women attending the prenatal clinic were anemic, the Belizean Ministry of Health launched an iron-supplement campaign (Hof 1989). Notwithstanding supplementation, the ministry found that eight years later the rates of anemia had gone up to 51.7 percent (Belize Ministry of Health 1996). In Toledo, the percent of anemic women was even higher at 58.9 percent (ibid. 1996). While there have been no subsequent studies for comparative purposes, at the time of my fieldwork in 2006, nurse-midwives in Toledo saw numerous cases of anemia. Similar to the findings also discussed in the 1996 study, iron supplements were often unavailable for distribution. Nurse-midwives routinely advised women to eat locally obtainable green leafy vegetables like callaloo and chaya that are rich in iron but know that few will do so. On two occasions I observed a public health nurse interacting with a large group of pregnant women and asking them: "Who knows how to make callaloo? Who eats callaloo?" Both questions were answered by silence. Echoing research conducted by Wilk (2006) on the trends in Belizean food preparation and consumption, the rural health nurse-midwives also explained to me that the diets of pregnant women have changed with increased access to canned meats and other fast foods that are high in salt and poor in nutrition. They reasoned that these processed foods might be contributing to the continued and increasingly high instances of anemia that they encounter.

During their prenatal examinations, nurse-midwives are met with varied responses from the pregnant women, who are not cued into international discussions of maternal health and pick and choose which pieces of advice to follow based on their own frames of reference. Ilana, a twenty-three-year-old Kekchi-speaking Maya woman living in a rural village, was attending her third prenatal visit for her current pregnancy. She was classified as high risk because this was her fifth pregnancy. Ilana did not know the date of her last menstrual period but, at the time of the prenatal examination that I observed, Nurse Ical measured her to be around thirty-seven weeks' gestation. Ilana began attending the prenatal clinic at around twenty-five weeks (well into her sixth month of pregnancy), because "I mi too busy with me pickney [children] for join." Her blood results had not returned from the lab, but she continued to have the physical signs of anemia Nurse Ical observed at her first prenatal examination three months ago—pale lining of the eyelids and craving the consumption of clay. Nurse Ical gave her indirect commands to eat callaloo ("callaloo has plenty iron") and to stay away from caffeine ("no coffee for pregnant ladies"). Like most of the pregnant women attending the prenatal clinic, Ilana disregarded the callaloo suggestion and strongly objected to the thought of giving up coffee by asking: "What for drink then?" Nurse Ical suggested lime juice. While he admitted that it is usually prepared with equal amounts of sugar, he believed it is beneficial for "building blood" [increasing blood iron levels], and it does not contain iron-inhibiting caffeine. However, Ilana complained that lime juice takes longer to prepare than the instant coffee she enjoys with her meals. When Nurse Ical asked if she was taking the ferrous sulfate tablets that he gave her at her last prenatal examination, she admitted that she was not, because she thought that they were making her feel sick. Ilana also said that she has pain when she lies down and sits. Nurse Ical then conducted a physical examination during which he palpated her abdomen, measured fundal height to determine gestation and fetal growth, and listened to the fetal heartbeat—all of which were within a standardized normal range. However, he referred her to one of the general practitioners located in the adjacent main hospital building for a Tylenol prescription to help relieve her pain.

Ilana has been pregnant every one to two years since she was sixteen and has a very pragmatic attitude surrounding her pregnancy. All four of Ilana's prior deliveries were conducted in the hospital without complication, and she has no reservations about having a hospital delivery for her fifth baby. When I asked her why she delivered in the hospital and not in her village, she replied: "'Cause no one di there to pick the baby [up from the floor when it is born], so that's why I come."[5] Ilana's village is without a trained home-birth attendant, her mother lives in another village, she is not comfortable around her mother-in-law, who tends to be verbally abusive about her housekeeping abilities, and her husband is often in the field tending his crops. Without someone "to pick the baby up from the floor when it is born," she felt the need to come to the hospital for her deliveries. Ilana's decision was not based on fear of complications due to a high-risk classification. Instead, her worries were directed toward the immediate care of the newborn. This known risk influenced Ilana's behavior more than did the invisible risk of postpartum hemorrhaging caused by her anemia or of a prolapsed uterus from giving birth for the fifth time in seven years. Furthermore, her pragmatic rationale is not uncommon, as many women without family assistance find comfort in the hospital—a relatively soft bed, nurses to help wash and tend to the baby, and quiet time away from household chores.

Ilana addressed her diet with the same sensible reasoning. If she cannot drink coffee, what else is there? Since caffeine inhibits iron absorption, Nurse Ical suggested lime juice. Ascorbic acid (the Vitamin C contained in citrus fruits) enhances the absorption of iron into the blood. However, lime juice Belizean-style is made with more sugar than is any other fruit juice, and sugar intake is related to gestational diabetes. Nurse Ical reasoned that since Ilana's urinalysis did not show high levels of blood sugar and she did not have swollen extremities (edema), she did not appear at risk for diabetes—yet. Orange juice, which also aids in the absorption of iron, is made with less sugar. However, there is a strong belief across ethnic groups that consumption of orange juice during pregnancy will turn the white parts of the fetus's eyes yellow. Moreover, limes are the cheapest and most abundant citrus fruit obtainable in Toledo. Nonetheless, Ilana objected, because making lime juice entails more time than does making instant coffee. As a woman who is often alone with her four children, she may not have the time to make lime juice, which she would need to make fresh each time since she has no refrigerator to keep a ready supply on hand.

Finally, Ilana chose not to take the iron pills given to her at the prenatal clinic because they upset her stomach. This is a common result of taking nonchelated iron supplements, which are cheaper, and thus more easily obtainable by government health care services in poor countries such as Belize. Moreover, iron supplements are best absorbed on an empty stomach, which is also when they can cause the greatest discomfort. Many pregnant women I observed during their prenatal examinations complained to the nurse-midwives about an upset stomach because of "de li' red pills" and chose not to take them because of this. All these examples suggest that pregnant women often chose to prioritize their embodied daily experiences over a distant risk analysis. Indeed, Ilana has yet to experience the potential risks associated with anemia, whereas the painful stomachaches are a reality that she deals with right now.

Communicating Risk: The Intensification of Conflict

A blood pressure reading is always taken at the onset of each prenatal examination conducted under the auspices of the Ministry of Health. However, the professional experiences the nurse-midwives in the Toledo District have with unreliable or aging equipment, as well as variations in ethnic diagnostic measurement, mean that the science of medicine and objective data are open to subjective interpretation—and dissent (Rapp 1999). Moreover, when laboratory results go missing and iron pills make women feel sick, the authority of medicine—its classification forms, definitions of high risk, and standardized protocols—becomes suspect. In the absence of laboratory evidence, Nurse Ical diagnosed Ilana's anemia based on his interpretation of physical signs, and he encountered resistance when he suggested preventive measures that opposed Ilana's embodied understanding of health or that she assessed as difficult for her to implement. Since she had already determined that a hospital birth was practically conducive to her lifestyle, Nurse Ical did not have to persuade Ilana to deliver her baby in the hospital. However, if Ilana had faced realities such as those lived by many other women in the Toledo District—cultural inhibitions, male-dominated heads of household, or socioenvironmental factors like distance from the hospital and transportation costs—Nurse Ical might have been put in a more difficult position to persuade her otherwise.

Likewise, Nurse Caal—a woman of mixed Mopan-speaking and Creole descent, who conducted a weekly prenatal clinic in one of the permanently stationed rural health centers, struggles to maintain medical authority while acknowledging the cultural belief systems of her pregnant constituency. Although Nurse Caal tries to overcome the disembodied language of biomedicine by blending traditional beliefs with medical knowledge, in the following truncated transcript of Miss Prudencia's prenatal examination, the thirty-year-old Mopan-speaking Maya woman who was in the last weeks of her ninth pregnancy often contested Nurse Caal's medical authority with her embodied experiences, cultural beliefs, and socioeconomic realities. The exchange with Miss Prudencia indicates the struggle Nurse Caal faces to retain her medical authority. Often she must share it. At times, she yields completely.

Miss Prudencia: On Tuesday I feel sick. I feel like it [the fetus] no want let
me to walk too much, just a little. But I get tired. I no want to rest too
much. I get tired and my back have too much pain.

Nurse Caal: So you have pain and you're not resting good. How about in the
night? Are you sleeping good?

Miss Prudencia: Li' bit, but not too good.

Nurse Caal: You know the last time you were here, we gave you pills to
control your pressure 'cause your pressure was high. And today your
pressure is still high. Actually, it gone up. The last time you came, your
pressure was 120 over 80. Today it is 120 over 90. Your pills, how many
times a day are you taking your pills?

Miss Prudencia: Three times.

Nurse Caal: Three times. You don't miss it?

Miss Prudencia: No.

There followed a long discussion of the foods Miss Prudencia had eaten over
the past week, the types of liquid she had drunk, and the need to avoid salt and to
drink "plenty water." This was Miss Prudencia's ninth pregnancy, and her first pregnancy to be considered high risk for reasons other than parity. Her urinalysis on the
morning of this prenatal exam indicated trace amounts of protein (proteinuria).
Her blood pressure was high, and she complained of a burning sensation when she
urinated.

Nurse Caal: So how about your pills? We'll give you a little bit more. . . .
So you will be taking four pills. Doctor say you have to cut down on
your fatty food, your starchy food—like your sweet yam and the yampi,
so not too much of that, okay? Potato. And the neck and back [of the
chicken], remember that you told me about? Remember that the neck
and back have a lotta fat. You have to take off the skin if you are going
to eat that. That have a lotta fat, okay? The lard is not too good to cook
with. . . . And then your pressure is high, and you are passing the protein. Remember I told you the only time you pass the protein is when
your pressure is high. The thing is, yes, you are on pills, but then if you
are not sleeping and you are not watching what you're eating and you
are worrying too much, your pressure will not go down, okay? . . . You
will have to increase the amount of times you take the pills . . . and then
you will have to do your part by watching what you are eating, okay?
Because if you don't, no matter how many pills you take, the pressure
will go up. Do you worry about it? Do you feel like you worry about it
a lot?

Miss Prudencia: I don't know. Sometimes I don't worry. Sometimes maybe I
worry.

In the unabbreviated transcript of the prenatal examination, Miss Prudencia explained that she did not have swollen ankles or headaches. Even though she had traces of protein in her urine and high blood pressure, she indicated that she does not add salt to her food, she does not eat a lot of fatty foods, nor does she drink coffee. Nonetheless, Nurse Caal addressed Miss Prudencia from an internationally scripted risk management template that Nurse Caal culturally modified to fit the foods of Belize (chicken neck and back, lard, and yampi [a starchy root vegetable]) that may contribute to high blood pressure. Her "narrative containment of risk" universalizes Miss Prudencia's individual pregnancy, placing it in the category of statistical possibility (Skinner 2000).

After Nurse Caal palpated Miss Prudencia's abdomen and listened to the fetal heart, she discerned that the fetus was in a head-down position, low in the pelvis, and due to be born in about a week's time. Miss Prudencia's first five births were delivered without complication at home with her husband; her sixth pregnancy ended in a miscarriage. Her subsequent two pregnancies were successfully delivered with the assistance of the village-based birth attendant trained by the Ministry of Health; however, this attendant had since moved from the village. Miss Prudencia was apprehensive about going to the hospital for the first time, but she did not feel that she had any alternatives.

Nurse Caal: Because of your high pressure, you for have this baby in hospi-
   tal. Did you talk to Ricardo [Miss Prudencia's husband] about this?[6]
Miss Prudencia: Yes.
Nurse Caal: And what did he tell you?
Miss Prudencia: He told me that I have to go to the hospital.
Nurse Caal: And how you feel about that? Do you want to go?
Miss Prudencia: Well, nobody could see me at home. Nobody could make
   . . .
Nurse Caal: Help you?
Miss Prudencia: . . . could help me with the baby. 'Cause last time we have
   this lady, Miss Teodora [the village-based birth attendant], see me, but
   nobody could see me or could told me something.
Nurse Caal: The thing is, Miss Prudencia, because of your pressure, even if
   Teodora was here, I would not advise you to have your baby at home
   because your pressure is high, okay? So if Teodora was here and you decided that you would go to deliver with her, you know that sometimes,
   if your pressure goes too high, she will not be able to help you, okay?
   That is why we are telling you, you have to go to hospital with this one,
   because your pressure is not good, okay? And if you stay at home and
   you try to deliver, and the pressure go too high, you will have fits, and if
   you have fits, your baby will die. And sometimes you can die from this
   as well, okay? So we advise you to go to town to have this baby. Should
   in case your pressure go too high, they can give you medicine to bring
   your pressure down. That is not the medicine that we are giving you

to drink. That's the medicine in the drips [intravenous fluids usually
administered at the town hospital to keep the laboring woman hydrated
and energized during prolonged labor; these fluids are also beneficial for
women suffering from eclampsia during childbirth].

Miss Prudencia: Oh, the drips, uh-huh.

Nurse Caal: Uh-huh, to help you to bring your pressure down, okay? That
is why we are saying you have to deliver in hospital, because of the pressure, okay? So you wouldn't stay at home. So you must explain to Ricardo that any questions, tell him to come, and I will talk to him about
it if he doesn't understand, okay? Why we say hospital is not because we
just want you to go. It's because of your pressure, okay? Your pressure.

Gestational hypertension and pre-eclampsia are conditions that carry the risk
of complications during pregnancy and childbirth ranging from low birth weight,
premature birth, or stillbirth to eclampsia (seizures during delivery). Eclampsia is
the second leading cause of maternal death in the United States. According to the
statistics of the Pan American Health Organization, eclampsia is also a leading
cause of maternal mortality in Belize (PAHO 2001). The international standardization of routine preventive measures and education about perinatal risk conditions relies on a myth of "transpositional objectivity" that validates its knowledge
system as superior to the subjective knowledge of the bodies it seeks to regulate
(Kleinman 1995:87). However, the power of the international health sector's claim
to objective reality is comprehensible only if it is adapted and accepted into local practice. Although eclampsia does adversely affect maternal mortality rates in
Belize, women in the Toledo District do not have an embodied recognition of
the fatalities emphasized in much of the international risk discourse. Of the eight
maternal deaths that have occurred in the Toledo District since 2000, none were
caused by eclamptic conditions. National maternal mortality rates doubled between 2004 and 2005, when the 61.9 maternal deaths per 100,000 live births (five
actual deaths) jumped to 119.1 maternal deaths per 100,000 live births (ten actual
deaths). Two of these 2005 fatalities occurred in the urban Toledo area with ready
access to a medical facility. However, both deaths were statistical anomalies in that
one occurred six months after delivery because of a preexisting cardiac condition,
while the other was an ectopic pregnancy that resulted in a ruptured fallopian tube.
The only maternal death in the Toledo District while I conducted my fieldwork in
2006 occurred in a remote village located some distance from medical care. Only
the woman's husband was attending to her labor and delivery, and she died of postpartum hemorrhage caused by a retained placenta.

While this last death was widely cited by the village-based birth attendants as
a reason why they should have access to injectable medication to stop postpartum
bleeding, the fear of bleeding to death at home rarely entered the risk discourse
of the pregnant women I spoke to. Instead, they claimed that if they went to the
hospital and heard the other laboring women in the shared maternity ward "bawl,"
they would be too scared to deliver: "I mi frightened when I hear them ladies

bawl with them pickney [giving birth to their child]." One woman explained how the nurses "like cuss and beat the ladies, because some ladies like bawl and cry when they have pain." Another corroborated: "They scold you if you make noise." Pregnant women also believed that the nurses in the maternity ward "forced" the baby to be born "before time" by applying external pressure to the fundus. Since epidural anesthesia is not available to women delivering at the local hospital, this pressure undoubtedly causes discomfort. However, it is an approved obstetrical technique that is often used to hasten delivery, and it does not cause the irreparable physical harm cited by the women who believe the risks involved in this proce-dure outweigh the risks of delivering at home.[7] Moreover, their primary concern was the possibility of "getting cut" (a cesarean section)—a procedure they believed would cause certain death. Indeed, the recent village fatality did not alter women's perceptions of risk, and the hospital continued to appear far riskier to the many women who cited numerous reasons to stay away from the hospital during labor and delivery.

Many of the risks Nurse Caal tried to convey to Miss Prudencia were incom-prehensible to her. They did not even reside in the realm of the imaginable because of the distance from the self as referent. Since women in Toledo tend to process information through experience, hypothetical risk situations do not generate the same fear that will motivate women to action. Because Miss Prudencia answered vaguely, "Sometimes I don't worry. Sometimes maybe I worry," Nurse Caal in-creased the emphasis on her high blood pressure and gave her a concrete cause and effect by affirming that she "will have fits [seizures]. And if you have fits, your baby will die. And sometimes you can die from this as well, okay?" ending with a col-laborative linguistic signal, "okay?" that permeated the interaction, thereby keeping Miss Prudencia engaged in the conversation as well as responsible for understand-ing and complying with Nurse Caal's recommendations. Indeed, public health ini-tiatives require the active participation of the population; thus Nurse Caal used a language of encouragement for Miss Prudencia "to do your part by watching what you are eating, okay? Because if you don't, no matter how many pills you take, the pressure will go up."

Nurse Caal must emphasize the dangers of high blood pressure in compliance with Safe Motherhood initiatives, which the Belizean Ministry of Health has insti-tuted in its efforts to minimize the risk of maternal death. However, the potential risks from a pre-eclamptic condition are difficult to convey because the symptoms usually disappear within six weeks of the birth. Since many women with symptoms of pre-eclampsia have healthy babies without complications, high blood pressure, swollen ankles, and headaches are easily normalized by women in Toledo as com-mon pregnancy-related conditions, like back pain and abdominal cramping, that likewise will disappear after the birth.

The risk of intangible probabilities pales in comparison to experiential reali-ties (Rapp 1999). Pregnant women in Toledo do worry about death, but their fears stem from hearing stories of actual women who died—the majority of whom die in the hospital setting. Indeed, most of the maternal deaths countrywide do not occur in the villages but in urban hospital settings—confirming experiential perceptions of risk (Belize Ministry of Health 2006). As recently as 1999, the national referral hospital in Belize City, the Karl Heusner Memorial Hospital [KHMH], was dubbed "Kill Him. Murder Her" after the death of two babies and public outcry regarding the shortage of staff, medical supplies, and equipment (KHMHA 2007:10). Inadequate medical care, prematurity, low birth weight, and the relatively high instances of stillbirths and miscarriages (which are not statistically compiled but are duly noted as high-risk factors on women's prenatal cards) are the concrete risks associated with poverty and arduous living conditions that Farmer framed as the "structural violence" over which individuals have little control (2005).

A Final Competition for Authority

It can be argued that nurse-midwives and pregnant women in the Toledo District are not in direct opposition. Both seek to minimize the risks associated with pregnancy and birth; however, their experience with and construction of reproductive risk are not the same. Moreover, the authority of pregnant women is often questionable when it comes into conflict with the ministry's health care mandates. The concern and personalized education offered by the rural and public health nurses during the prenatal examination is a process of medical socialization, which serves to reinforce the power of an international discourse of standardized medical and obstetric knowledge while minimizing the embodied experiential knowledge of pregnant women. Contrastingly, it is this embodiment of their current and past pregnancies as well as their socioeconomic realities that justify the decisions made by pregnant women, which often clash with the recommendations of nurse-midwives.

Like health care providers in other countries who deal with disprivileged clients, nurse-midwives often code-switch, or move between languages of biomedically defined risk, culturally defined gender roles, familial responsibility, and economic and environmental realities when trying to convey information regarding risk factors and the ways to decrease the chances of a poor birth outcome (Rapp 1999). It soon became apparent through my observations of prenatal examinations that the nurses employed by the Belizean Ministry of Health have a clear understanding of the pregnant women for whom they are providing prenatal services—tailoring their recommendations and adjusting protocols to accommodate their realities. Biomedical discourse assumes an acultural medium of delivery, as if the practitioner disseminating the information is devoid of cultural bias. However, the nurse-midwives in the Toledo District often come from the constituencies for whom they provide services. While distinguishable from other types of community health workers by degree and depth of training, they remain steeped in many of the same culturally held beliefs as the pregnant women for whom they care. Nonetheless, their medically authoritative training is often confronted with competing empirical and cultural authorities, which have a far greater impact on pregnant women like Monica, Rossana, and Ilana who base their reproductive decisions on a variety of factors having little to do with the international mandates the Ministry of Health would like to see put into practice. Indeed, women's empirical realities color their perception of risk, such that the information conveyed during their prenatal examinations—regardless of how it is delivered—often does little to influence their perinatal decisions.

Sometimes, however, the nurse-midwife succeeds in conveying the biomedical and authoritative understanding of risk, and the advice given in the prenatal examination room is followed. However, the high rate of fertility ensures that the exchange between nurse-midwife and pregnant woman will be repeated—this time with more experienced actors. Indeed, two years after recording the heated discussion between Nurse Caal and Miss Prudencia, I followed up on her risks of seizure and death and found that the birth of Miss Prudencia's then two-year-old daughter at the local hospital went without complication. When I met her on the street one day, Miss Prudencia pointed to the infant being carried by an older accompanying child and defiantly stated that for the birth of the subsequent child, number ten: "That's why I mi stay at home for this one."

Acknowledgments

Research for this chapter was made possible by generous funding from Wenner Gren Foundation for Anthropological Research, International Women's Anthropology Caucus, and New York University. This chapter owes its existence to the people of southern Belize who allowed me to "peep" into their reproductive worlds. I thank my writing partner, Lauren Fordyce, for her invaluable support and laughter. And I am forever thankful for the involvement of Rayna Rapp throughout my life as an anthropologist and beyond.

Notes

1. The Belizean Census category "Maya" includes Mopan, Kekchi, and Yucatec speakers, the latter of which are virtually absent from the Toledo District.
2. In Palacio's study of the socioeconomic status of the Garinagu people, he laments: "Unfortunately, there are no studies of economic indicators among ethnic groups in the country" (2005:113).
3. A legacy of colonial enslavement, "lashing" refers to the use of physical abuse to coerce behavior.
4. The fundus is the top of the uterus. Before the routine use of ultrasound, and in places like Belize where ultrasound is not customary, the standard medical practice for determining gestation is by measuring the height of the fundus in centimeters from the top of the pubic bone to the top of the uterus. The number of centimeters usually corresponds to the number of weeks of gestation.
5. Women birthing at home often use a squatting position and explain that the baby is then born onto the floor.

6. Even if they are married, women are often called "Miss" as a linguistic marker of respect.
7. Also known (and referred to by Belizean nurse-midwives) as the "Kristeller maneuver," external pressure is often applied to the fundus when the laboring woman has a decreased ability to expel the fetus with her own force (Parvin 1895:443). Samuel Kristeller (1820–1900) was a German obstetrician known for his obstetric research and innovative forceps technology (Hibbard 2001; O'Dowd and Philipp 1994).

References

Barnett, Carla
    2002   Defining Ethnicity in Belize: Understanding Our History. www.cavehill.uwi.edu/BNCCde/belize/conference/papers/Barnett.html, accessed June 8, 2011.
Belize Ministry of Health
    1996   Study of Iron Deficiency Anaemia among Pregnant Women in Belize. MOH, INCAP, PAHO/WHO, and UNICEF: data collected by Anne Luke, UCLA, and Ellen MacDonald, State University of New York, Cortland.
    2005   Belize Basic Health Indicators 2004. Belmopan: Office of the Director of Health Services, Epidemiology Unit.
    2006   Personal communications with the Safe Motherhood Committee in Belmopan.
Bolland, O. Nigel
    1977   The Formation of a Colonial Society: Belize, from Conquest to Crown Colony. Baltimore: Johns Hopkins University Press.
    2003[1988]   Colonialism and Resistance in Belize: Essays in Historical Sociology. Belize: Cubola Books.
Central Statistical Office
    2006   Abstract of Statistics for Belize: 2006. Ministry of National Development, Investment and Culture. Belmopan, Belize.
Colen, Shellee
    1995   "Like a Mother to Them": Stratified Reproduction and West Indian Childcare Workers and Employers in New York. In Conceiving the New World Order: The Global Politics of Reproduction. Faye Ginsburg and Rayna Rapp, eds. Pp. 78–102. Berkeley: University of California Press.
Escure, Genevieve
    1992   Gender and Linguistic Change in the Belizean Creole Community. In Locating Power: Proceedings of the Second Berkeley Women and Languages Conference. Kira Hall, Mary Bucholtz, and Birch Moonwomon, eds. Pp. 118–31. Berkeley: University of California Press.
Farmer, Paul
    2005   Pathologies of Power: Health, Human Rights, and the New War on the Poor. Berkeley: University of California Press.
Government of Belize
    1997   From Girls to Women: Growing up Healthy in Belize. Belize: Cubola Productions.
Grant, Cedric Hilburn
    1976   The Making of Modern Belize: Politics, Society, and British Colonialism in Central America. London: Cambridge University Press.

Hall, Norris
    2007   Places in Belize: Punta Gorda. Belize Today 20(3):19–25.
Haug, Sarah Woodbury
    2002   Ethnicity and Multi-ethnicity in the Lives of Belizean Rural Youth. Journal of
            Rural Studies 18:219–23.
Hibbard, Bryan
    2001   The Obstetrician's Armamentarium: Historic Obstetric Instruments and Their
            Inventors. San Anselmo, CA: Norman Publishing.
Hof, Annagret
    1989   Survey on Anaemia in Pregnant Women Attending Prenatal Clinics in Belize in
            1988. Unpublished manuscript.
Karl Heusner Memorial Hospital Authority (KHMHA)
    2007   Public Sector Modernization, Belize, a Country Case Study: A Chronicle of the
            Evolution of the Karl Heusner Memorial Hospital (KHMH), the Journey from
            "Kill Him, Murder Her" to "The People's Hospital." Unpublished manuscript.
Kerns, Virginia
    1997[1983]   Women and the Ancestors: Black Carib Kinship and Ritual. Chicago:
            University of Chicago Press.
Kleinman, Arthur
    1995   Writing at the Margin: Discourse between Anthropology and Medicine. Berkeley:
            University of California Press.
Markens, Susan, Carole Browner, and Nancy Press
    1999   "Because of the Risks": How U.S. Pregnant Women Account for Refusing
            Prenatal Screening. Social Science and Medicine 49(3):359–69.
McClusky, Laura
    2001   "Here, Our Culture Is Hard": Stories of Domestic Violence from a Mayan
            Community in Belize. Austin: University of Texas Press.
O'Dowd, Michael, and Elliot Philipp
    1994   The History of Obstetrics and Gynecology. New York: Parthenon Publishing
            Group.
Palacio, Joseph
    2005   The Multifaceted Garifuna: Juggling Cultural Spaces in the 21st Century. *In*
            The Garifuna: A Nation across Borders. Joseph Palacio, ed. Pp. 105–22. Belize:
            Cubola Books.
Pan American Health Organization (PAHO)
    2001   Country Health Profile. www.paho.org/english/sha/prflbel.htm, accessed June 8,
            2011.
Parvin, Theophilus
    1895   The Science and Art of Obstetrics. Philadelphia: Lea Brothers.
Rapp, Rayna
    1999   Testing Women, Testing the Fetus: The Social Impact of Amniocentesis in
            America. New York: Routledge.
Shoman, Assad
    2000   Thirteen Chapters of a History of Belize. Belize City: Angelus Press.
Skinner, Jonathan
    2000   The Eruption of Chances Peak, Montserrat, and the Narrative Containment of
            Risk. *In* Risk Revisited. Pat Caplan, ed. London: Pluto Press.

Statistical Institute of Belize
  2007   Abstract of Statistics. Belmopan: Central Statistical Office, Ministry of National
          Development.
  2009   Mid-Year Population Estimates. www.statisticsbelize.org.bz/dms20uc/
          dynamicdata/docs/20100112164405_2.pdf, accessed June 8, 2011.
U.S. Agency for International Development (USAID)
  2007   Postpartum Hemorrhage Prevention. www.pphprevention.org/pph.php, accessed
          June 8, 2011.
Wilk, Richard
  2006   Home Cooking in the Global Village: Caribbean Food from Buccaneers to
          Ecotourists. Oxford: Berg Publishers.
Williams, Raymond
  1973   The Country and the City. New York: Oxford University Press.
Young, Colville
  1995   Language and Education in Belize. Belize City: National Printers.

Afterword

Rayna Rapp

The chapters of *Risk, Reproduction, and Narratives of Experience* that you have just read all operate in an existential gap: in this gap, each woman's pregnancy is in deep, abstract conversation with every woman's pregnancy as experts aggregate and analyze them, whether in urban Los Angeles and Puebla, Mexico, or rural Belize, Ghana, and China. In this existential gap, the twinned concepts of risk and responsibility compress each woman's pregnancy story into the statistics by which experts come to know and intervene in what they consider high-risk pregnancy and birth practices. Expert discourse then shapes, bullies, or disciplines against such risky business.

Some of our authors invoke the contemporary Foucauldian concept of "responsibilization" as an optical technology of the neoliberal state, suggesting how individual maternal citizens are made to dutifully care for themselves and their growing fetuses in the terms of governmentality that they have ostensibly internalized. Yet in the existential gap, these very notions of responsibility/responsibilization may be quite experience-far, as the anthropological accounts collected in this book tell us. Experts rarely recognize the gap, as they consolidate their powerful, authoritative knowledge by articulating local variants of its universal dictates. Thus, physicians in Puebla, Mexico, tell their resident anthropologist that midwives are "very good . . . at attending the birth," while cautioning that midwives don't have "actual knowledge." The gap is present when obstetricians express frustration as Haitian patients in Florida refuse "the gift of knowledge" that a recommended amniocentesis might bring, without inquiring about the women's reasoned refusals; or when they label Guatemalan midwives the biggest risk to Guatemalan pregnant women's birthing experiences. The gap is widened and manipulated as health planners, policy makers, and government statisticians aggregate maternal/child morbidity and mortality knowledge at a distance. Classically, they peer over the gap, pondering birth outcomes by region, claiming that "ignorant Indians" (Guatemala) or "dirty tribal practices" (Tanzania) or "backward ethnicities" (China) are responsible for birthing under conditions they denounce. Rarely do they traverse the gap to investigate the washed-out mountainous or tropical roads of rural Belize or Oaxaca or the Shangri-la northwest Yunnan region of China, where money and transport to bring a laboring woman to clinic is sorely lacking, and barriers are physical and sometimes punitive as well as social-structural. In the gap, there is a logic used by many experts who blame pregnant women themselves for the structural violence which shadows poor women's reproduction. Sometimes, even the well-meaning addition of standardized risk discourse serves only to increase risky practices, as Alicia Gálvez's analysis of Mexican women giving birth as new immigrants in the United States shows us.

Policy strategies and debates have long circulated across international gaps. Sometimes, policy experts dictate that, for example, local empirical birth attendants be trained and empowered outside their hometowns and villages, while at other times that they be left in place but provisioned with discrete tools and hierarchies of command and oversight. For more than half a century, WHO and UNICEF have conversed with ministries of health in poor countries, sometimes approving, sometimes disapproving local midwives, always already agglomerated into TBAs, traditional birth attendants, a concept which may itself increase the gap between what local female curers, *parteras*, and *iyom* know in situ, and what their standardization is intended to produce. This ping-pong game of labeling birth attendants as competent/incompetent without attending to the specifics of their gender and training itself too often produces costly abstractions rather than teamwork in the interest of medical service, as these multiple Mexican and Guatemalan examples show us. And Qingyan Ma's analysis of shifting policy aimed to reduce maternal mortality in one mountainous, multiethnic region of the countryside illustrates the irrationality of rational governmental and NGO changes as they systematically ignore the effects of the existing market socialism in China.

Pregnant women, of course, often have their own local and deep-seated understandings of the dangers of their liminal, birthing state and the real possibilities of miscarriage, stillbirth, and infant death, which shadow their lives. For them, risk can operate in the existential gap, as well: these essays show us how drug-addicted Los Angeles women feel acutely the risk of being without their illegal highs, unable to imagine the risks that intravenous drug use might bring to their blood-tethered fetuses; and Guatemalan pregnant women and their attendants speak of "angel pacts" by which empirical midwives have been called to their dangerous profession. In rural northern Ghana, parents, kinsfolk, and neighbors may blame "spirit children" for reproductive misfortune, while in small-town and urban Mexico, Oaxacan women speak about "doing just what the doctor told me" while dismissing the very "creencias" of diet, dress, and demeanor that continue to be part of their strategic and successful health pluralism. Local beliefs, expertise, and practices may well be denigrated by the too-often overworked and frustrated medical/health professionals who dwell on the other side of the gap.

But we readers have been lucky: the hard work of our authors has made *Risk, Reproduction, and Narratives of Experience* available to us. Their abundance of field-based knowledge takes the perspectives of birthing women, their local supports and constraints, and available health care providers and puts these into a conversation with the abstractions and standardization concerning risk by which an existential gap is necessarily created. While policy, statistics, and best-evidence practices can, in principle, reduce what Matthew Dudgeon here labels the "dense cloud of risk" in which women of reproductive age too often live, they will rarely succeed without reasoned understanding of the real threats that each pregnancy faces in its complex context. The authors whose work appears in *Risk, Reproduction, and Narratives of Experience* excavate that gap, making the possibilities for its transcendence more experience-near.

Contributors

Carole H. Browner is a professor in the Department of Anthropology, Department of Women's Studies, and the Center for Culture and Health in the Semel Institute for Neuroscience and Human Behavior at the University of California, Los Angeles. She is also the chair of the Department of Anthropology. Her recent books include the coauthored book with H. Mabel Preloran, *Neurogenetic Diagnoses: The Power of Hope and the Limits of Today's Medicine* (Routledge, 2010), and *Reproduction, Globalization, and the State: New Theoretical and Ethnographic Perspectives,* coedited with Carolyn Sargent (Duke University Press, 2011).

Sheila Cosminsky is an associate professor in the Department of Sociology, Anthropology, and Criminal Justice at Rutgers University, Camden. She is the coauthor, with Ira E. Harrison, of the two-volume bibliography *Traditional Medicine: Implications for Ethnomedicine, Ethnopharmacology, Maternal and Child Health, Mental Health, and Public Health* (Garland Press, 1983).

Aaron R. Denham is an assistant professor in the Department of Anthropology at Macquarie University, Sydney, Australia.

Matthew R. Dudgeon is a doctoral candidate in medical anthropology at Emory University, where he is also completing an MD. He is a resident at Stanford Hospital and Clinics in obstetrics and gynecology.

Lauren Fordyce is a visiting assistant professor in the Department of Sociology and Anthropology at Bucknell University.

Alyshia Gálvez is an assistant professor in the Department of Latin American and Puerto Rican Studies at Lehman College of the City University of New York. She is the author of *Guadalupe in New York: Devotion and the Struggle for Citizenship Rights among Mexican Immigrants* (New York University Press, 2009). Her second book, *Patient Citizens, Immigrant Mothers: Mexican Women, Public Prenatal Care and the Birth Weight Paradox,* is forthcoming in the Critical Issues in Health and Medicine series (Rutgers University Press). She edited *Performing Religion in the Americas: Media, Politics, and Devotion in the 21st Century* (Berg/Seagull, 2007).

Alison B. Hamilton is an associate research anthropologist in the Integrated Substance Abuse Programs at University of California, Los Angeles.

Rebecca Howes-Mischel is a doctoral candidate in the Department of Anthropology at New York University.

Qingyan Ma is a doctoral candidate in the Department of Anthropology at Temple University.

Amínata Maraesa is a lecturer in the Department of Anthropology at Hunter College of the City University of New York and the Department of Latin American and Puerto Rican Studies at Lehman College of the City University of New York.

Rayna Rapp is a professor of anthropology in the Department of Anthropology at New York University. She is the author of *Testing Women, Testing the Fetus: The Social Impact of Amniocentesis in America* (Routledge, 1999), and coeditor with Faye Ginsburg of *Conceiving the New World Order: The Global Politics of Reproduction* (University of California Press, 1995).

Vania Smith-Oka is an assistant professor in the Department of Anthropology at the University of Notre Dame. Her books include the translation of *Report on the Fables and Rites of the Incas by Cristóbal de Molina*, with Brian S. Bauer and Gabriel Cantarutti (University of Texas Press, 2011), and *The History of the Incas by Pedro Sarmiento de Gamboa*, also with Brian S. Bauer and Gabriel Cantarutti (University of Texas Press, 2007).

Alyson G. Young is an assistant professor in the Department of Anthropology at the University of Florida.

Index

Amatlán (Mexico), midwives in, 107
amniocentesis, 200–201
autocuidado (self-care), 6, 130

bad-mother label in Mexico, 117
bañeras (herbal bath specialists), 49
Beck, Ulrich, 4
Belize
    anemic women in, 218–20
    cesarean section in, 224
    eclampsia in, 223
    late onset of prenatal care in, 215–16
    maternal mortality rate in, 223
    nurse-midwives authority in, 225–26
    prenatal risk assessment in, 211–26
Belizean Ministry of Health, 215, 216, 218, 220, 225
biomedical care
    among Datoga, 162, 164–66
    in Ghana, 176–78, 183–86
    in Guatemala, 19–22, 88–89
    in Mexico, 103
biomedical models of blame, 183–86
birth weight paradox, 37, 39–40
blame, assessment and assignment of, 178, 181–86
brujos (witch doctors), 49

Cantel (Guatemala), reproduction risk in.
    See Guatemala: risk and reproduction in
cesarean section
    Belizean beliefs on, 224
    as general risk factor, 88
    Guatemalan beliefs on, 93, 94–95
    Mexican immigrant women and, 50–51
    as ultimatum in Mexico, 111, 114, 116
Child Protective Services, 63
China. *See* Larger Shangri-la Project (China)

clinical setting, authority in, 111–12
Colom, Alváro, 81–82
comadrona (midwife), 2, 17
    defined, 83, 84
    interviews of, 26–27
    oxytocin injections by, 28–29
    supernatural pacts and, 24–25
    training, 23
Cosminsky, Sheila, 6, 81–97
County Population and Family Planning Commission (China), 149
curanderos (ritual specialists), 107, 108

Datoga mothers and children
    biomedical care practices of, 162
    biomedical risk indicators and, 164–66
    clinical staff view of, 167
    communication and child health responsibility in, 167–68
    culture and newborn children, 161–62
    ethnographic data for, 158–59
    ethnomedical knowledge in, 162–64
    health among, 157–68
    health disparities in, 159
    infant breastfeeding and, 163–64
    infant care constraints in, 164–66
    infant vulnerability to illness and, 160–62
    vulnerable children, identifying, 160–62
    Western biomedicine and, 168
    See also diarrheal illness, in Datoga infants and children
Deng Xiaoping, 145
Denham, Aaron R., 8, 173–87
destiny, 29–31
diarrheal illness, in Datoga infants and children
    causes of, 162–63

www.ingramcontent.com/pod-product-compliance
Lightning Source LLC
Chambersburg PA
CBHW080416270326
41929CB00018B/3052